Progress in Pain Research and Management
Volume 31

The Pain System in Normal and Pathological States: A Primer for Clinicians

Mission Statement of IASP Press®

The International Association for the Study of Pain (IASP) is a nonprofit, interdisciplinary organization devoted to understanding the mechanisms of pain and improving the care of patients with pain through research, education, and communication. The organization includes scientists and health care professionals dedicated to these goals. The IASP sponsors scientific meetings and publishes newsletters, technical bulletins, the journal *Pain*, and books.

The goal of IASP Press is to provide the IASP membership with timely, high-quality, attractive, low-cost publications relevant to the problem of pain. These publications are also intended to appeal to a wider audience of scientists and clinicians interested in the problem of pain.

Progress in Pain Research and Management
Volume 31

The Pain System in Normal and Pathological States: A Primer for Clinicians

Editors

Luis Villanueva, DDS, PhD

Faculty of Dental Surgery, INSERM E-216,
Clermont-Ferrand, France

Anthony H. Dickenson, PhD

Department of Pharmacology, University College London,
United Kingdom

Hélène Ollat, MD

Association for Neuro-Psychiatry; Neurology Department,
Hospital Lariboisière, Paris, France

IASP PRESS® • **SEATTLE**

Library of Congress Cataloging-in-Publication Data

The pain system in normal and pathological states : a primer for clinicians / editors, Luis
  Villanueva, Anthony H. Dickenson, Hélène Ollat.
     p. ; cm. -- (Progress in pain research and management ; v. 31)
   Includes bibliographical references and index.
   ISBN 0-931092-53-1 (alk. paper)
   1. Pain--Congresses. I. Villanueva, Luis, 1957- II. Dickenson, A. H. III. Ollat, H. IV.
  Series.
   [DNLM: 1. Pain--physiopathology--Congresses. WL 704 P14775 2004]
   RB127.P353 2004
   616'.0472--dc22

                                                                              2004042172

Published by:

IASP Press
International Association for the Study of Pain
909 NE 43rd Street, Suite 306
Seattle, WA 98105-6020 USA
Fax: 206-547-1703
www.iasp-pain.org
www.painbooks.org

Printed in the United States of America

This volume is dedicated to Jean-Marie Besson

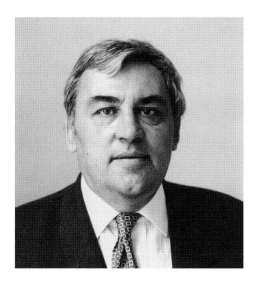

Born in Belfort, France, in 1938, Jean-Marie Besson obtained his doctorate in pharmacy in 1962. His interest in the neurophysiology of pain then started at the Marey Institute in Paris, where after completing his PhD in neurophysiology he joined the CNRS and became the leader of a group devoted to the study of central mechanisms of pain. Jean-Marie's seminal contributions to our understanding of pain mechanisms include the first demonstration of a selective antinociceptive action of opiates on spinal dorsal horn neurons and of the participation of descending serotoninergic systems in the modulation of pain.

He then founded in Paris the first INSERM (French National Institute of Health and Medical Research) unit devoted to preclinical studies of pain mechanisms and analgesia. Over 25 years his laboratory trained both scientists and clinicians from many countries, making major contributions to our knowledge of the mechanisms of pain and analgesia. Jean-Marie participated actively in the creation and development of the International Association for the Study of Pain (IASP), as a founding member and then as president. His brilliant scientific career is illustrated by a remarkable number of peer-reviewed articles, several major reviews and books, and a series of major awards in the field of pain research. These include the Bristol-Myers-Squibb Award for Distinguished Achievement in Pain Research, the IASP John J. Bonica Distinguished Lecture Award, and the F.W.L. Kerr Award of the American Pain Society. This book honors one of the leaders in our field who has dedicated his life to building bridges between scientists and clinicians with the aim of winning the race against pain.

Contents

Part IV Endogenous Modulatory Systems: Their Role in Analgesia and Pain

Part V Novel Therapeutic Strategies: Preclinical and Clinical Approaches

Contributing Authors

Nadine Attal, MD, PhD *Center for the Evaluation and Treatment of Pain, INSERM E-332, Ambroise Paré Hospital, Boulogne-Billancourt, France; and University of Versailles-Saint-Quentin, France*

Ralf Baron, Dr med *Neurological Clinic, Christian Albrechts University, Kiel, Germany*

Allan I. Basbaum, PhD *Departments of Anatomy and Physiology and W.M. Keck Foundation Center for Integrative Neuroscience, University of California San Francisco, San Francisco, California, USA*

Jean-François Bernard, MD, PhD *Faculty of Medicine Pitié-Salpêtrière, INSERM U-288, Paris, France*

Didier Bouhassira, MD, PhD *Center for the Evaluation and Treatment of Pain, INSERM E-332, Ambroise Paré Hospital, Boulogne-Billancourt, France; University of Versailles-Saint-Quentin, France*

Rami Burstein, PhD *Departments of Anesthesia and Critical Care, Beth Israel Deaconess Medical Center, Boston, Massachusetts, USA; Department of Neurobiology and Program in Neuroscience, Harvard Medical School, Boston, Massachusetts, USA*

Kenneth L. Casey, MD *Departments of Neurology and Molecular and Integrative Physiology, University of Michigan, Ann Arbor, Michigan, USA; Neurology Service, Veterans Affairs Medical Center, Ann Arbor, Michigan, USA*

Pierre Cesaro, MD, PhD *Department of Neurology, INSERM U-421, Henri Mondor Hospital, Créteil, France*

Anthony H. Dickenson, PhD *Department of Pharmacology, University College London, London, United Kingdom*

Liam J. Drew, PhD *Molecular Nociception Group, Biology Department, University College, London, United Kingdom*

Ronald Dubner, DDS, PhD *Department of Biomedical Sciences, University of Maryland Dental School, Baltimore, Maryland, USA*

Howard L. Fields, MD, PhD *Department of Neurology, University of California, San Francisco, California, USA*

Nanna B. Finnerup, MD *Department of Neurology and Danish Pain Research Center, Aarhus University, Aarhus, Denmark*

Caroline Gauriau, PhD *Faculty of Medicine Pitié-Salpêtrière, INSERM U-288, Paris, France*

Itay Goor-Aryeh, MD *Departments of Anesthesia and Critical Care, Beth Israel Deaconess Medical Center, Boston, Massachusetts, USA*

Hermann O. Handwerker, MD *Department of Physiology and Experimental Pathophysiology, University of Erlangen/Nürnberg, Erlangen, Germany*

Raymond G. Hill, PhD *The Neuroscience Research Centre, Merck, Sharp and Dohme Research Laboratories, Terlings Park, Harlow, Essex, United Kingdom; currently Licensing and External Research, Europe, Merck, Sharp and Dohme Research Laboratories, Terlings Park, Harlow, Essex, United Kingdom*

Stephen P. Hunt, PhD *Department of Anatomy and Developmental Biology, University College London, Gower Street, London, United Kingdom*

Moshe Jakubowski, PhD *Departments of Anesthesia and Critical Care, Beth Israel Deaconess Medical Center, Boston, Massachusetts, USA*

Wilfrid Jänig, Dr med *Department of Physiology, Christian Albrechts University, Kiel, Germany*

Troels S. Jensen, MD, PhD *Department of Neurology and Danish Pain Research Center, Aarhus University, Aarhus, Denmark*

Yves Keravel, MD *Department of Neurosurgery, Henri Mondor Hospital, Créteil, France*

Martin Koltzenburg, Dr med, FRCP *Neural Plasticity Unit, Institute of Child Health, University College London, London, United Kingdom*

Jean Pascal Lefaucheur, MD *Department of Neurophysiology, Henri Mondor Hospital, Créteil, France*

Jürgen Lorenz, Dr med *Center for Experimental Medicine, Institute of Neurophysiology and Pathophysiology, University Clinic Hamburg-Eppendorf, Hamburg, Germany; currently Department of Applied Natural Sciences, Hamburg University of Applied Sciences, Hamburg, Germany*

Patrick W. Mantyh, PhD *Neurosystems Center and Departments of Preventive Sciences, Psychiatry, Neuroscience, and Cancer Center, University of Minnesota, and Veterans Affairs Medical Center, Minneapolis, Minnesota, USA*

Elizabeth A. Matthews, PhD *Department of Pharmacology, University College London, London, United Kingdom*

Henry J. McQuay, DM *Pain Relief Unit, Churchill Hospital, University of Oxford, Oxford, United Kingdom*

Thomas J. Morrow, MD, PhD *Departments of Neurology and Molecular and Integrative Physiology, University of Michigan, Ann Arbor, Michigan, USA; Neurology Service, Veterans Affairs Medical Center, Ann Arbor, Michigan, USA*

Karim Moubarak, MD *Department of Neurosurgery, Henri Mondor Hospital, Créteil, France*

Jean Paul Nguyen, MD *Department of Neurosurgery, Henri Mondor Hospital, Créteil, France*

Stéphane Palfi, MD, PhD *Department of Neurosurgery, INSERM U-421, Henri Mondor Hospital, Créteil, France*

Wahida Rahman, PhD *Department of Pharmacology, University College London, London, United Kingdom*

Ke Ren, MD, PhD *Department of Biomedical Sciences, University of Maryland Dental School, Baltimore, Maryland, USA*

Lars Rygh, MD, PhD *Department of Pharmacology, University College London, London, United Kingdom*

Martin Schmelz, MD *Department of Anesthesiology, Mannheim Clinic, University of Heidelberg, Mannheim, Germany*

Lucinda Seagrove, PhD *Department of Pharmacology, University College London, London, United Kingdom*

Rie Suzuki, PhD *Department of Pharmacology, University College London, London, United Kingdom*

Catherine Urch, MD, PhD *Department of Pharmacology, University College London, London, United Kingdom*

Luis Villanueva, DDS, PhD *Faculty of Dental Surgery, INSERM E-216, Clermont-Ferrand, France*

William D. Willis, Jr., MD, PhD *Department of Neuroscience and Cell Biology, University of Texas Medical Branch, Galveston, Texas, USA*

John N. Wood, PhD, DSc *Molecular Nociception Group, Biology Department, University College, London, United Kingdom*

Preface

The idea of producing this primer for clinicians emerged when we decided to organize a symposium in honor of Jean-Marie Besson's work over many years on the subject of pain mechanisms and modulation. According to Jean-Marie's aims, this book is primarily devoted to providing a comprehensive view of pain mechanisms to both teachers and clinicians. Jean-Marie's interest in building bridges between clinicians and scientists started early at the Institut Marey following his pioneering work that demonstrated a selective depression by opiates of spinal dorsal horn nociceptive activities and revealed the participation of descending serotoninergic systems in the modulation of pain. His work on opiates was of paramount importance because it was the starting point for subsequent preclinical and clinical studies of the direct, spinal analgesic effects of morphine. This basic finding has had many clinical applications.

Jean-Marie founded in Paris the first INSERM (French national institute of health and medical research) unit devoted to preclinical studies of pain mechanisms and analgesia. This laboratory trained both scientists and clinicians in a wide range of studies using many different techniques. These studies contributed to a better knowledge of the mechanisms of opioid and non-opioid analgesia, endogenous control mechanisms of pain, the anatomical and functional organization of pain networks, and the development of preclinical pain models. Rue d'Alésia became quickly one of the leading laboratories, attracting a number of young and senior scientists from many countries, many of whom now have leadership positions at several INSERM laboratories and at many other institutes around the world.

Jean-Marie participated actively in the creation of IASP as a founding member. As IASP president he continued to contribute to its development, with a special interest in broadening IASP activities to include developing countries. As an example of how this goal concerned Jean-Marie, soon after Algeria gained independence, he began participating in training programs there.

In addition to the intellectual qualities that brought Jean-Marie to a leadership position, his captivating personality allowed many of us to establish a deep and lasting friendship with him. The warm, interactive, and friendly atmosphere in which the symposium in his honor took place was perhaps a major impetus for our colleagues to devote such care to writing the chapters of this book.

The first part of this volume is devoted to the analysis of peripheral nociceptive inputs to the dorsal horn. By employing molecular approaches, Liam J. Drew and John N. Wood describe the role of ion channels and receptors in primary transduction mechanisms, the regulation of sensory neuron excitability, and how these channels participate in the induction of pain. Martin Koltzenburg describes the expression and the cellular and molecular features of ion channels that have a widespread distribution on sensory neurons and are activated by temperature changes and inflammatory mediators. On the basis of microneurography and psychophysical experiments, Hermann Handwerker and Martin Schmelz analyze the mechanisms of allodynia and hyperalgesia caused by inflammation. Different forms of hyperalgesia are mediated by quite different peripheral, and probably also central, mechanisms. These chapters show that cellular, molecular, and human experimental models are essential for better understanding of peripheral transduction mechanisms of pain. Such multiple approaches are thus essential for the development of new therapeutic strategies to control inflammatory and neuropathic pains.

The second part of the book analyzes the consequences of injury at the dorsal horn level. Stephen P. Hunt underlines the impact of molecular biology tools that allow the study of the role of peptides and early genes together with the use of gene knockout mice in spinal nociception. Such techniques also build bridges with more classical approaches for a further elucidation of long-term alterations in spinal processing following injury. These plasticity mechanisms, namely the ability of neuronal function to change after activity or injury-evoked dysfunction that leads to changes throughout the pain pathways, are also examined by Anthony Dickenson and colleagues. They illustrate that the central nervous system (CNS) has numerous systems that can act at many levels to increase or decrease incoming messages. Such central inhibitory and excitatory interactions between spinal and brainstem systems probably determine the level and the duration of pain, but just as importantly, affect the analgesic efficacy of drugs in particular contexts. In this respect, Ronald Dubner and Ke Ren provide evidence that descending modulation of spinal nociceptive transmission from the rostral ventromedial medulla (RVM) undergoes early facilitation and dominant, late inhibition following persistent inflammation, as shown by the activation and expression of genes for excitatory amino acid receptors within the RVM. They propose that an imbalance between these time-dependent changes may be one mechanism underlying variability in persistent or chronic pain conditions.

In the third part of the book, devoted to the anatomical and functional organization of ascending pain pathways, Allan I. Basbaum proposes a novel strategy to identify "pain" networks in the CNS. He developed transgenic mice in which transneuronal labeling of circuits originating from any region of the brain or spinal cord can be induced. Since the transneuronal tracer can be triggered before or after tissue or nerve injury, this approach to circuit analysis can be used to study normal and altered pain circuits in the CNS, both during development and in the adult. Based on the use of high-resolution anatomical tracing and electrophysiological studies in rats, Jean-François Bernard and Caroline Gauriau show the existence of two main ascending nociceptive systems relaying in the brainstem. The first is a main target of lamina I (spino-parabrachial) neurons that distributes inputs to the amygdala and hypothalamus. The second, which originates from the deep dorsal horn, innervates the medullary subnucleus reticularis dorsalis and parabrachial areas that project in turn to the medial thalamus. These studies clearly show that brainstem areas have a complementary role with regard to the direct spinothalamic tract in conveying noxious inputs to the cortex. William D. Willis describes the detailed organization of multiple spinothalamocortical nociceptive systems in the monkey. These circuits originate from both the superficial and deep dorsal horn and ascend through the anterolateral columns. He suggests that the return of pain or the development of central neuropathic pain following an initially successful cordotomy may be due to enhanced effectiveness of other nociceptive pathways, such as those traveling within the dorsal columns. Kenneth L. Casey and colleagues describe a number of animal and human functional imaging studies that show that pain evoked in normal subjects in controlled experiments elicits forebrain activities in specific neuronal subsets that are now reasonably predictable. They also present ongoing studies of clinically relevant pain states that modify central processing in a way that alters both the forebrain responses to ascending nociceptive information and the initiation of central control mechanisms that modulate the perception of pain. They suggest that pathologically induced forebrain changes will alter the clinical response to drugs or any other form of treatment. Thus, a major challenge for better analgesic treatment for chronic pain will be to determine which of these forebrain changes assist or impede therapeutic efforts.

The fourth part of the book deals with the role that other endogenous neuronal mechanisms may play in pain processing. Ralf Baron and Wilfrid Jänig review both basic and clinical observations that address the role of the sympathetic nervous system in neuropathic pain. Their studies strongly suggest that the sympathetic nervous system is involved in the generation of pain. Primary afferent nociceptors are excited and possibly sensitized by norepinephrine released by the sympathetic fibers. The vascular bed or the inflammatory cells in the environment of the nociceptive neurons may have a permissive effect on sympathetic to nociceptor coupling or may be modulated directly by molecules released from sympathetic postganglionic neurons. Sympathetically maintained spontaneous and evoked activity in nociceptive neurons may generate a state of central sensitization/hyperexcitability that leads to spontaneous pain and pain evoked by stimulation of mechanoreceptors, thermoreceptors, or nociceptors. The authors believe that the exact mechanisms of afferent adrenergic sensitivity in human neuropathies of different etiologies and in particular the time course during the disease process and the genetic predisposition for the development of adrenergic sensitivity are major challenges to be addressed in future research. On the basis of clinical observations showing that migraine is associated with a high incidence of cutaneous allodynia, Rami Burstein and colleagues propose that there is a peripheral mechanism that drives throbbing, which begins a few minutes after the onset of the headache, followed by central sensitization expressed as cutaneous allodynia. Such sensitization starts shortly after the onset of the pain, becomes detectable within the first hour, and reaches maximal severity within 2–4 hours. With regard to commonly prescribed migraine drugs such as triptans, rather than rely on individual trial-and-error experience, he suggests a rational treatment strategy based on the timing of administration of sumatriptan that can block the development of peripheral or central sensitization, and discusses the site of action critical for terminating migraine headache with triptans. Luis Villanueva and Howard L. Fields consider the endogenous central mechanisms of pain modulation. They suggest that perhaps the main difficulty in attempting to correlate the activity of bulbospinal modulatory systems with behavioral analgesia is that several pain modulation systems operate in parallel, and so the net effect cannot be attributed exclusively to activity in any single network. In this respect, the most important, widespread source of top-down modulation arises from the cortex, given that almost all nociceptive relays within the CNS are under corticofugal modulation, including the networks involved in segmental and heterosegmental modulation at the dorsal horn level. In contrast to bulbospinal descending controls, corticofugal modulation often occurs in the absence of a painful stimulus. The authors underline the relevance of corticofugal controls in pathological pain by their role in phantom limb perception and in the pain that occurs in the absence of detectable organic lesions.

The last part of the book relates to preclinical and clinical approaches to novel therapeutic strategies. Raymond G. Hill recalls that in the recent past, classical animal models were able to predict the analgesic properties of the cyclooxygenase-2 inhibitors in humans, whereas they have been unsuccessful in predicting the potential efficacy of other putative analgesics such as neuropeptide receptor antagonists. He raises the key question as to whether animal tests can be assumed to be reliably predictive as we go forward and try to exploit potential pain targets emerging from the elucidation of the human genome. He suggests that recent advances including genetic approaches, imaging techniques, and the development of more disease-relevant models are useful tools that could be employed in both small animals and human subjects. Interestingly, in this respect, despite its prevalence as a pain condition, models of cancer pain have only recently been described. Patrick W. Mantyh presents a mouse model using intramedullary injection and containment of osteolytic sarcoma cells into the mouse femur. These tumor cells induced bone destruction as well as ongoing and movement-evoked pain behavior similar to that found in patients with bone cancer pain. This reorganization generated a neurochemical signature of bone cancer pain that was different from that observed in mouse models of chronic neuropathic or inflammatory pain. He suggests that defining when and how these different components drive bone cancer pain may allow the development of more selective analgesic agents to treat this chronic pain state. Troels S. Jensen and Nanna Finnerup analyze the clinical manifestations of neuropathic pain after peripheral nerve injury and after damage to the CNS, with particular emphasis on sensory abnormalities. They explain that the relationship between symptoms and signs versus mechanisms on the other is unclear because one mechanism may give rise to several symptoms, and one specific symptom can be caused by different mechanisms. They emphasize the importance of a possible translation of neuronal hyperexcitability into clinical symptoms because this area represents a window to understanding potential mechanisms underlying various neuropathic pain conditions and thereby a rational approach by which these conditions can be targeted pharmacologically. Didier Bouhassira and Nadine Attal explain that new approaches to neuropathic and other types of pain based on the current understanding of their mechanisms and aiming to target treatments specifically at those mechanisms are attractive, but do not yet seem to be attainable, mainly because of the difficulties of translating to the clinic the pathophysiological mechanisms identified in animal studies. They present recent data tending to support more clinically oriented approaches, based on the evidence that neuropathic pains constitute a multidimensional category. Thus, the development of novel treatment strategies might well depend on the identification of relevant criteria allowing diagnosis and classification of patients in several subgroups that might respond differentially to treatments. They conclude that numerous data tend to favor an approach based on symptoms or combinations of symptoms of neuropathic pain, but that this hypothesis should be confirmed in further studies. Jean-Paul Nguyen and colleagues describe chronic motor cortex stimulation, describing steps aimed at improving surgical procedures, the current main indications, and some hypotheses concerning the mechanism of analgesic action. This rapidly growing technique is essentially indicated for the treatment of certain pains that cannot be controlled by spinal cord stimulation—central pain and neuropathic facial pain. The authors explain that optimal selection of the best indications must be based on a technique that precisely identifies the cortical zone to be stimulated. A relatively large craniotomy and the use of a neuronavigation system appear to be essential. Other indications need to be confirmed, especially paraplegic pain, phantom limb pain, and plexus injury pain. The authors conclude that the identification of the neuronal substrates and the mechanisms underlying analgesia elicited by motor cortex stimulation is essential to improve the stimulation parameters that remain empirical. In his clinical viewpoint, Henry McQuay states that over the past decade clinicians have been dismayed by the failure of a number of promising ideas from basic research to produce clinical benefit. He explains that this is not an argument against basic research, but a signal perhaps that divorcing clinical and basic research can lead us down blind alleys. This awareness is necessary in the current debate about the mechanistic approach, where pragmatic clinicians know that the same drugs work, for instance antidepressants and anticonvulsants in neuropathic pain, independent of the underlying mechanism. The author believes that clinical trials showing differential efficacy in different underlying mechanisms could illuminate this area. Clinical pain research needs to be able to study packages of care, as well as to be able to study single intervention efficacy. Just as basic researchers need fresh ideas about how to study neuropathic pain, clinicians need a methodology that allows them to compare different packages of care, each with a selection of different interventions. In other words, as Jean-Marie has often said: "tout un programme!"

In conclusion, this book promotes the development of open approaches with the aim of integrating nociception and pain, thus building bridges between scientists and clinicians. With this holistic framework, we will continue to follow pain research into the future based on Jean-Marie's aims.

Luis Villanueva, DDS, PhD
Anthony H. Dickenson, PhD
Hélène Ollat, MD

Part I

Nociceptive Inputs to the Dorsal Horn

*The Pain System in Normal and Pathological States:
A Primer for Clinicians,* Progress in Pain Research
and Management, Vol. 31, edited by Luis Villanueva,
Anthony Dickenson, and Hélène Ollat, IASP Press,
Seattle, © 2004.

1

Molecular Mechanisms of Noxious Mechanosensation

Liam J. Drew and John N. Wood

*Molecular Nociception Group, Biology Department, University College,
London, United Kingdom*

Molecular cloning and functional expression studies have provided us with a catalogue of chemically and thermally activated ion channels and seven-transmembrane receptors present on nociceptive sensory neurons. In addition, the properties of voltage-gated potassium, sodium, and calcium channels, some of them unique to sensory neurons, have been extensively explored. In contrast, we know almost nothing about the receptors that transduce noxious mechanosensation. Given the clinical importance of mechanosensation in chronic pain, identifying the receptors and channels involved in mechanotransduction could provide new routes to analgesic drug development. This chapter describes candidate mechanotransducing mechanisms, the properties of mechanically activated ion channels in sensory neurons in vitro, and the use of null mutant mice to identify components of mammalian noxious mechanosensors.

UNDERSTANDING MECHANOSENSORY MECHANISMS

Altered mechanical pain thresholds are arguably the most troublesome problems in pain pathology. Mechanical allodynia is associated with a variety of neuropathic insults, and with many conditions where the site of the malfunction is unknown. For example, the lifetime incidence of low back pain (LBP) ranges from 60% to 90% with a 5% annual incidence. No consensus exists concerning the mechanism or most appropriate treatment and management of mechanical LBP. It is a reasonable assumption that every reader of this chapter will suffer from lowered mechanical pain thresholds at some time, and will attempt to treat the condition with drugs that act at sites other than the primary mechanotransducing channels.

Most research on mammalian mechanosensation supports the notion that the mechanosensitive channels are present on the peripheral terminals of the dorsal root ganglion (DRG) nerve fiber (Lewin and Stucky 2000). This view is supported by a number of observations; first, the rapidity of sensory transduction precludes the contribution of a slow process such as communication between the nerve ending and an auxiliary mechanotransducing cell. Second, the peripheral termination of mechanosensitive nociceptive neurons as bare, unspecialized sensory endings indicates that transduction occurs in cells in the absence of complex end organs. Third, despite the association of low-threshold mechanoreceptors with specialized end organs (e.g., Pacinian corpuscles, Merkel cells), in the absence of such specializations transduction still proceeds (Mills and Diamond 1995; Kinkelin et al. 1999). Fourth, when afferent nerves are ligated or cut, the resultant neuroma acquires mechanosensitivity, indicative of the insertion of the mechanotransduction apparatus into the cell membrane at this point (Welk et al. 1990). Finally, a number of studies have demonstrated that mechanical stimuli depolarize cultured sensory neurons (McCarter et al. 1999; Drew et al. 2002, 2004).

It is widely believed that mechanotransduction proceeds via the direct activation of mechanosensitive ion channels that are located on the peripheral, sensory terminals of DRG neurons, However, our understanding of mechanosensation at the molecular level lags behind that of all other sensory modalities (Gillespie and Walker 2001). To date, no eukaryotic ion channel has been shown to be both unequivocally mechanically gated and central to the sensation of mechanical events. Moreover, the degree of conservation of mechanosensory mechanisms is currently poorly defined. Bacterial ion channels gated by membrane stretch have been identified that have no clear eukaryotic homologues (see Blount and Moe 1999; Hamill and Martinac 2001; Sukharev and Corey 2004 for reviews), and it is uncertain if similar basic mechanisms of mechanotransduction function in the diverse array of mechanosensory cell types that have evolved across and within different animal classes. Likewise, the relatedness of ion channels that mediate mechanotransduction in distinct systems remains to be determined (Kernan and Zuker 1995). These uncertainties extend to mammalian somatic sensation, where it is unclear whether low-threshold mechanoreceptors and mechanosensitive nociceptors utilize the same transduction mechanisms.

Mechanically activated currents have been observed in numerous systems both at the single-channel and whole-cell levels (Sackin 1995; Hamill and Martinac 2001). However, approaches to uncovering the molecular identities of mechanically activated ion channels are compromised by a number of factors. First, the expression pattern of such channels precludes the harvesting of large amounts of protein enriched for transduction molecules. For example, in the cochlea a few thousand hair cells each express only around 100 channels, and somatosensory nerve terminals are diffusely distributed in peripheral tissues. Second, although antagonists of stretch-activated currents have been identified from three chemical classes (represented by amiloride, gentamicin, and gadolinium), none of these compounds act with high affinity or specificity (Hamill and McBride 1996). Consequently, although they have allowed for pharmacological characterization of mechanosensitive channels, no antagonist so far identified is able to act as a biochemical "tag." Finally, research on mechanotransduction by hair cells and by body touch receptors in *C. elegans* indicate that gating of mechanosensory ion channels is almost certainly dependent on their interactions with auxiliary proteins. Such complexity of mechanisms is likely to hamper the functional reconstitution of mechanosensitive ion channels in heterologous systems.

The field is further complicated by observations that numerous ion channels are mechanosensitive where there is no clear connection between this property and the established physiological function of the channel. For instance, the potassium channels TREK-1 (Patel et al. 1998), TRAAK (Maingret et al. 1999), and *Shaker* (Gu et al. 2001) are mechanically gated, and NMDA-receptor activity is modulated by membrane stretch (Paoletti and Ascher 1994). In such cases it is unclear if mechanical force represents a relevant physiological stimulus or if it is an artefact of multi-conformational gating; i.e., as membrane tension is altered, different channel conformations may be favored. Therefore, mechanosensitivity is insufficient evidence to ascribe a sensory function to an ion channel (Gu et al. 2001; Hamill and Martinac 2001; Goodman and Schwarz 2003). Moreover, mechanical gating of ion channels has been recorded at the single-channel level, when equivalent whole-cell currents have been absent (Morris and Horn 1991; Zhang and Hamill 2000). These findings have led some investigators to suggest that mechanical gating may not always be of physiological relevance (Morris and Horn 1991). Such discrepancies may be due (at least in part) to pathological effects on membrane morphology caused during or after seal formation, in particular the flattening of the membrane across the pipette tip and the decoupling of the membrane from the underlying cytoskeleton (Hamill and McBride 1997; Zhang and Hamill 2000).

Genetic screening of mechanosensory mutants in *Caenorhabditis elegans* (Chalfie and Sulston 1981) and *Drosophila* (Kernan et al. 1994) has proved the most fruitful approach to isolating genes implicated in mechanosensation. This research has focused attention on two classes of ion channel as potential mechanotransducers, namely the degenerin/epithelial sodium channel (DEG/

ENaC) and transient receptor potential (TRP) classes. In invertebrates, evidence is strong that members of these channel families form mechanosensory ion channels, whereas work investigating the function of their mammalian homologues has yet to conclusively implicate any ion channel in primary mechanotransduction.

ASIC FAMILY MEMBERS

In the nematode worm *C. elegans*, two MEC (mechanosensory abnormal) ion channel subunits, MEC-4 and MEC-10, are required for sensing light touch. In body touch neurons, these subunits putatively form a mechanosensitive ion channel within a transduction complex that includes intra- and extracellular binding proteins (see Tavernarakis and Driscoll 1997; Ernstrom and Chalfie 2002). MEC-4 and MEC-10 form a sodium channel when expressed in *Xenopus* oocytes that is regulated by the auxiliary proteins MEC-2 (Goodman et al. 2002) and MEC-6 (Chelur et al. 2002). Nematodes with loss-of-function mutations in MEC-4 and MEC-2 fail to show increases in intracellular calcium in response to mechanical stimulation (Suzuki et al. 2003a).

The mammalian acid-sensing ion channels (ASICs) are members of the same DEG/ENaC ion channel superfamily as MEC-4 and MEC-10, although the ASICs form a distinct branch of the DEG/ENaC phylogenetic tree that is relatively distant to the branch that contains the MEC channels (Goodman and Schwarz 2003). There are four identified genes encoding ASIC subunits, ASIC1–4, with two alternative splice variants of ASIC1 and 2 taking the number of known subunits to six. Most of these subunits are highly expressed in sensory neurons (Waldmann and Lazdunski 1998), and ASIC1b (Chen et al. 1998) and ASIC3 (Waldmann et al. 1997a) are selectively expressed in sensory ganglia. Although protons are the only confirmed activator of ASICs, the homology between ASICs and MEC channels, coupled to the expression pattern of ASICs, has led to the hypothesis that these channels function in mechanotransduction (Lewin and Stucky 2000; Welsh et al. 2001). However, the distribution of ASICs throughout the nervous system suggests that they have physiological functions in multiple systems. Consistent with this observation are multiple studies showing that numerous types of central and peripheral neurons exhibit proton-activated currents that are likely to be mediated by these channels (Waldmann and Lazdunski 1998). In contrast, evidence of ASIC gating by physiological processes such as synaptic activation or mechanical stimulation is currently absent (for example, see Alvarez de la Rosa et al. 2003).

A number of groups have investigated the distribution of ASIC channels across the cell types of the dorsal root ganglia (DRG). When Waldmann et al. (1997b) cloned ASIC1a, their in situ hybridization data suggested that this subunit was most highly expressed in small DRG neurons. Olson et al. (1998) reported that an antibody directed against a 15-amino-acid sequence in the C-terminus of ASIC1 stained predominantly small neurons that also displayed immunoreactivity to substance P and calcitonin gene-related peptide, although several nonpeptidergic, larger cells appeared to also display ASIC staining. Alvarez de la Rosa et al. (2002), also using a polyclonal antibody against a region of the C-terminus of ASIC1 (i.e., a region common to 1a and 1b), found expression of this protein in subsets of DRG neurons, both small (immunoreactive for peripherin) and large (immunoreactive for neurofilament 200). The results from Chen et al. (1998) suggest that immunoreactivity in larger neurons may represent the expression of ASIC1b; using in situ hybridization the investigators found ASIC1b transcripts predominantly in peripherin-negative neurons, whereas they found transcripts for ASIC1a, in agreement with Waldmann et al. (1997b), in peripherin-positive, small neurons.

Current data suggest that ASIC2a is expressed predominantly in medium to large DRG neurons; both García-Añoveros et al. (2001), using a splice-variant specific N-terminus directed antibody, and Alvarez de la Rosa et al. (2002), using an antibody against the shared ASIC2 C-terminus, detected immunoreactivity in neurofilament-200-positive, peripherin-negative neurons. Price et al. (2000), using in situ hybridization and immunocytochemistry (pan-ASIC2 C-terminus antibody), found the most intense staining for ASIC2 in large neurons, although staining was also present in small cells. The in situ hybridization data of Lingueglia et al. (1997) showed ASIC2b staining to be most intense in small neurons.

With regard to ASIC3, Lazdunski's group again reported that transcripts are found most abundantly in small neurons of the DRG (Waldmann et al. 1997a). Alvarez de la Rosa et al. (2002), in contrast, found immunoreactivity most abundantly in large neurons, for the most part colocalized with ASIC2, whereas Price et al. (2001) reported ASIC3 staining in most small and large DRG neurons and concluded that almost all substance-P-positive cells are immunoreactive for ASIC3.

Other groups have attempted to correlate channel activity observed in sensory neurons with that of heterologously expressed ASICs. Alvarez de la Rosa et al. (2002) made outside-out patch recordings from rat DRG neurons and compared the currents they recorded to currents generated by expression of either ASIC1a alone or ASIC2a and 3 together in *Xenopus* oocytes. Their results suggested that ASIC2a and 3 formed heteromeric channels whereas

ASIC1a formed homomeric channels in DRG neurons; the latter population was the predominant response of small DRG neurons. Conversely, Benson et al. (2002) analyzed transient low-pH-evoked currents in sensory neurons derived from wild-type and ASIC1, 2, and 3 knockout mice and in cell lines transiently expressing different combinations of ASIC subunits. Their conclusions were that the properties of whole-cell currents in wild-type DRG neurons were consistent with heteromerization of all three subunits. Proton-gated currents in wild-type DRG neurons desensitized more rapidly than did currents mediated by any single ASIC subunit, negating the possibility that low pH concurrently activated a combination of homomeric ASIC channels. Likewise, Drew et al. (2004) found that transient low-pH currents were exhibited by similar proportions of wild-type and ASIC2/3 double knockout neurons; in the former population, current kinetics were again consistent with coexpression of ASIC1, 2, and 3 subunits and in the latter population they were consistent with expression of ASIC1.

If ASICs partake in mechanotransduction, they must be expressed appropriately in the peripheral terminals of sensory neurons. García-Añoveros et al. (2001) undertook a study of ASIC2a distribution in DRG neurons. At the level of the cell body they found ASIC2a immunoreactivity in the cytoplasm, predominantly near the axon hillock, and showed that this channel subunit is selectively transported to the periphery by sensory neurons, precluding a role for it in spinal synaptic physiology. When nerve endings were stained for ASIC2a, immunoreactivity was largely colocalized with neurofilament 200 staining and was seen in nerve endings associated with Meissner corpuscles, Merkel disks, hair follicle afferents (circumferential and lanceolate), vibrissal afferents, and a subpopulation of intraepidermal terminals that expressed neurofilament 200. In agreement, Price et al. (2000), using a different ASIC2 antibody, reported staining of lanceolate nerve endings surrounding hair follicles, although they did not report the presence or absence of staining in other peripheral structures. Price et al. (2001) also detected ASIC3 immunoreactivity in the sensory terminals of DRG neurons. They reported staining in nerve fibers associated with Meissner's corpuscles, guard hair follicles, and Merkel cell complexes and also in fine epidermal nerve endings. With regards to ASIC1, Olson et al. (1998) presented data suggesting that this subunit is also located in nerve endings of the skin and claimed that it is often colocalized with substance P staining.

Together, the above studies show that ASIC subunits are found at appropriate sites to contribute to mechanosensation. However, studies (Olson et al. 1998; Price et al. 2000; 2001; García-Añoveros et al. 2001; Alvarez de la Rosa et al. 2002) show staining for ASIC subunits along the length of the fiber, not specifically enriched at the terminal. Although the resolution is often insufficient to determine if these channels are membrane associated or are being transported in the axoplasm, Alvarez de la Rosa et al. (2002) do suggest that ASIC1 staining is in the plasmalemma of axons. Such a distribution may implicate ASICs in a regulatory function not specific to the site of transduction.

Expression in sensory terminals is necessary for a role in the transduction of either acidic or mechanical stimuli. However, the finding that most sensory terminals of Aβ fibers are immunoreactive for ASICs is at odds with the long-known observation that low-threshold mechanoreceptors are not activated by low pH (see Lewin and Stucky 2000). Thus, Welsh et al. (2001) have proposed that ASICs may exist, like MEC-4 and MEC-10, in a multiprotein mechanotransduction complex that through an unknown mechanism masks the proton sensitivity of these channels.

ASIC NULL MUTANTS AND MECHANOSENSATION

To investigate the role of ASIC2 (Price et al. 2000) and ASIC3 (Price et al. 2001; Chen et al. 2002) in somatosensory physiology, null mutants for each of these genes were assayed electrophysiologically and behaviorally for sensory responses to a range of stimuli. In both mutants Gary Lewin's group (Price et al. 2001, 2002) used the skin-nerve preparation to study the response properties of DRG fibers to mechanical, thermal, and chemical stimulation. In ASIC2 knockouts, the primary finding was that Aβ-fiber mechanoreceptors of null mutants had a decreased firing rate in response to suprathreshold mechanical stimulation, whereas all other fiber types had normal responses in this modality. Rapidly adapting mechanoreceptors displayed firing rates that were approximately 50% of those seen in wild-types, whereas slowly adapting fibers had a slight reduction in firing (approximately 20% below control values at the highest stimulus intensity). The mechanosensitivity of all other fiber types was unchanged, and the responses of C fibers in ASIC2 nulls to acid injection into the paw were indistinguishable from those of wild-types. These data suggest that ASIC2 selectively plays a role in modulating the sensitivity of low-threshold mechanoreceptors, although it is notable that the threshold of activation of these fibers was unchanged in the knockouts. The authors showed with whole-cell patch-clamp recordings that there is no difference in action potential thresholds between nulls and controls, suggesting that electrical excitability per se is not disrupted. However, given that mechanical thresholds are normal but sustained firing is diminished, it would of interest to determine if the firing rates of all fiber types in response to electrical stimulation were similar in mutant and wild-type animals.

In mice lacking the gene for ASIC3, Price et al. (2001) found deficits in the responses of nerve fibers to activation by heat, protons, and mechanical stimulation. With regard to mechanical stimulation, rapidly adapting mechanoreceptors showed enhanced firing to suprathreshold stimuli, the maximal difference being an approximate doubling of the firing rate. Conversely, at high stimulus intensities, Aδ-fiber mechanonociceptors showed reduced responses and also a minor increase in mechanical thresholds. No other fiber type was different from wild-type fibers. To determine if ASIC3 contributes to acid-induced firing in C-fiber mechanoheat (CMH) receptors, two strengths of acidic solutions were injected into the receptive field. Following the application of a pH 5 solution, CMH fibers in null mutants fired at a lower rate than in wild-types, although no difference was detectable at pH 4 owing to an increase in firing in the nulls and little change in evoked activity in wild-types. This finding may well represent differential contributions of TRPV1 at the two pHs, suggesting ASIC3 functions in the detection of smaller drops in pH. Finally, quite unexpectedly, a shortening of the response to noxious (52°C) heating was observed in ASIC3 knockouts.

At the behavioral level, both Price et al. (2001) and Chen et al. (2002) have assayed ASIC3 responses to painful stimuli. Saliently, neither group found changes in acute behavioral responses to mechanical stimuli (von Frey withdrawal thresholds). Price et al. (2001) also found no effect of ASIC3 gene ablation on paw-withdrawal latencies to radiant heat in carrageenan-inflamed or non-inflamed mice or on responses to injection of 0.6% acetic acid. However, interesting differences were found in two tests of hyperalgesia; mechanical withdrawal thresholds following carrageenan administration were lower in ASIC3 nulls than in controls and conversely, following hyperalgesia induced by intramuscular acid (pH 4) injection, ASIC3 nulls were much less responsive than wild-types. The overall conclusion of Chen et al.'s (2002) analysis was that ASIC3 has a modulatory role in responses to high-intensity pain. This group, in slight disagreement with Price et al. (2001), found no difference in responses to acute thermal or mechanical stimuli between groups following carrageenan-induced hyperalgesia. However, differences emerged between nulls and controls when high-intensity noxious stimuli were applied to non-inflamed animals. For instance, although there was no significant difference in the tail-flick test at 50°C, when the temperature was increased to 52.5°C or 55°C nulls had shorter withdrawal latencies. Likewise, when 0.1–0.5% acetic acid was injected intraperitoneally, no significant strain differences were apparent, but (in contrast to Price et al. 2001) at 0.6% writhing behavior was more frequent and onset latency was shorter in nulls. Finally, in the tail pressure assay, the pain threshold was reduced by approximately 40% in the absence of ASIC3.

In contrast to the ASIC2 knockouts, where abnormalities were limited to one modality, the picture that emerges from studying ASIC3 nulls is that this channel contributes to sensation in multiple modalities. The skin-nerve preparation data show that certain fibers have altered sensitivity to heat, protons, and pressure. Although the behavioral data are relatively confusing, with a mixture of hypo- and hyperalgesic changes, they are consistent with ASIC3 functioning in various modalities. It remains to be determined if the type of acid injection given in these studies is functionally relevant, in terms of the rate and magnitude of pH change, to the acidosis that occurs during inflammation.

Studies of the knockout animals are the most significant indication that ASICs play a role in mammalian mechanosensation. However, no studies have reported mechanically activated currents, either at the whole-cell or single-channel level, that are attributable to ASICs. Moreover, the observation that amiloride and its analogues block a number of mechanosensitive ion channels is not strong evidence implicating ASICs, as this compound does not have specific affinity for a single class of channels. The skin-nerve preparation is a powerful approach for studying the response properties of DRG fibers, but in recording action potential discharge it gathers data a number of steps downstream of transduction. Hence, ablation of ASICs could affect firing by decreasing the efficiency of transduction or dysregulation of action potential generation, possibly specifically, during high-frequency firing. If the latter scenario were true, the modality-specific changes in ASIC2 knockouts could be due to the predominant expression of ASIC2a in large neurons, likely to be low-threshold mechanoreceptors, whereas, consistent with the broader consequences of its ablation, ASIC3 appears to be more widely distributed across different cell types.

TRANSIENT RECEPTOR POTENTIAL CHANNELS

The TRP ion channel superfamily contains a remarkably diverse array of channels that display a multitude of functions (Clapham et al. 2001), although Clapham (2003) has recently emphasized that most of these channels have sensory roles. In mammals there are three main classes of TRP channels: TRPC (classical/short), TRPV (vanilloid receptors), and TRPM (melastatin/long), and in addition there are the related polcystins, mucolipins, and ANKTM1. TRP channels are characterized by six transmembrane domains, cationic conductances (usually including permeability to Ca^{2+}), and intracellular C- and N-termini, the latter often containing ankyrin domains. A number of TRP-related channels are believed to function in thermal transduction by sensory neurons (Jordt et al. 2003; Patapoutian et al. 2003). However, following recent work performed in *C. elegans* and *Drosophila*, attention has focused on the idea that certain TRP channels may act as mechanosensors.

TRP CHANNELS IN NON-MAMMALIAN MECHANOSENSATION

The first TRP-related channel to be implicated in mechanosensation was the osmosensory abnormal channel OSM-9, cloned by Colbert et al. (1997). Nematodes with mutant forms of this channel have severe defects in olfaction and in avoidance behaviors evoked by nose touch and hyperosmolarity. Nose touch avoidance is mediated by three ciliated sensory neurons. In transgenic nematodes, each of these neurons expressed OSM-9::GFP fusion protein, and consistent with OSM-9 playing a role in sensory transduction, this protein localized to the sensory cilia. It remains to be determined whether OSM-9 is directly activated by sensory stimuli or acts downstream of the transduction process. In response to osmotic stimuli, ASH-directed behaviors also require the functional expression of genes for OCR-2 (another TRP-related ion channel, Tobin et al. 2002), ODR-3 (a Gα-protein, Roayaie et al. 1998), and OSM-10 (a cytoplasmic protein, Hart et al. 1999), but requires only the former two to respond to nose touch. The dependence of osmotic but not mechanical responses on functional OSM-10 expression suggests that distinct transduction mechanisms operate in each modality, potentially converging on OSM-9 activation, although such data do not preclude direct mechanical activation of OSM-9.

Also identified via genetic screening was the *Drosophila* TRP-like channel NOMPC (Walker et al. 2000). The basis for NOMPC's discovery was a screen for mutants insensitive to touch as larvae or that displayed uncoordinated movement as adults (Kernan et al. 1994). Recordings made from type I sensory bristle neurons revealed that a number of these mutants had no mechanoreceptor potential (NOMP), suggestive of deficits in transduction events. Of these mutants two have been characterized molecularly; one is NOMPA, an extracellular protein that is proposed to tether the neuronal transduction machinery to the moving bristle (Chung et al. 2001), and the other is NOMPC (Walker et al. 2000). Mutants with truncated forms of *nompC* are morphologically normal but lose the rapidly adapting component of mechanically evoked receptor currents. In addition, substitution of a cysteine by a tyrosine at position 1400 (between the third and fourth transmembrane domains) produces a mutant (*nompC4*) that displays transduction currents that adapt much more rapidly than wild-type responses. NOMPC displays a predicted membrane topology similar to known TRP channels and shows homology in the conserved pore-forming domain. It also has 29 ankyrin repeats in its N-terminal, the most of any known protein, which may be involved in the anchoring and gating of the channel. The subcellular distribution of NOMPC remains to be characterized, and again it is conceivable that it acts downstream of transduction events, although the rapidity of transduction in these cell types argues against this possibility. However, a small non-adapting receptor potential remains in *nompC* mutants, perhaps indicating that another transduction channel operates independently in these cells or that in a heteromultimeric complex NOMPC regulates the gating of this channel.

Fruit flies with *nompC* mutations were reported to have only moderate deficits in auditory responses, mediated by the chordotonal neurons of Johnston's organ (Eberl et al. 2000). This phenomenon appears to be due to the expression of an alternative transduction channel in these neurons; Kim et al. (2003) recently identified Nanchung (Nan) as a TRP-like channel required for responses of chordotonal neurons to sound waves. Nan is related to OSM-9 and the mammalian TRPV channels and is selectively expressed in chordotonal neurons. In animals lacking functional Nan channels, extracellular recordings revealed an absence of sound-evoked activity in antennal afferent nerves, suggestive of a key role in transduction. When Nan was expressed in Chinese hamster ovary cells it generated Ca^{2+} permeant, cationic currents in response to hypotonic solutions, although these currents developed slowly, and it is uncertain if such gating occurs via the same mechanism that operates during hearing.

Despite the apparently minor role played by NOMPC in *Drosophila* audition, Sidi et al. (2003) found that the zebrafish homologue of this channel is fundamental to hair cell physiology in larvae of this species. They selectively detected *nompC* mRNA in the larval and embryonic hair cells of the inner ear of zebrafish. Knockdown of *nompC* expression using morpholino antisense oligonucleotides produced larvae that, although morphologically normal and touch responsive, failed to respond to acoustic stimuli and showed vestibular defects. In treated larvae, extracellular recordings from hair cell afferents revealed an ablation of movement-evoked activity. This study suggests a conservation of NOMPC function across phyla, and cluster analysis performed by this group suggests that *nompC* exists in its own class of TRP-related channels, distantly but most closely related to TRPV/OSM-9 channels. Walker et al. (2000) had also identified a *C. elegans* homologue of *nompC* and showed that NOMPC::GFP fusion proteins are expressed in the sensory cilia of nematode mechanosensory neurons (and some interneurons), but functional studies of this channel in worms have yet to be reported.

Finally, in *Drosophila* a third TRP-related ion channel, known as "pain-less," has been implicated in noxious mechanosensation by Tracey et al. (2003). This group developed a genetic screen for studying nocifensive be-havior in *Drosophila* larvae and showed that animals lacking functional expression of the *painless* gene showed defective behavioral responses to noxious temperatures and noxious pressure. Painless is expressed in a dis-crete punctate fashion on the dendrites of putative nociceptors, and the sensory deficits of mutants led to the idea that the painless channel func-tions, analogously to TRPV1, as a transducer of noxious stimuli in multiple modalities. Again, although the data are consistent with such a hypothesis, direct channel activation by physical stimuli was not demonstrated, thus it is possible that the protein acts up- or downstream of transduction.

ARE THERE MECHANICALLY GATED TRP CHANNELS IN DRG NEURONS?

The studies outlined above have naturally led to much speculation on the role of TRP channels in mammalian mechanosensation. To date no chan-nels with close homology to either NOMPC or Nan have been reported in mammals, but TRPV4 (Liedtke et al. 2000; Strotmann et al. 2000) shows moderate homology to OSM-9 (26% amino acid identity, 44% identity or conservative change; Liedtke et al. 2003). TRPV4 is widely expressed in rodents, with the highest expression levels in the kidney and significant expression in the liver, heart, testes, and brain. Interestingly, expression is also seen in cochlea, trigeminal ganglia, and Merkel cells, all of which are associated with mechanosensation (Liedtke et al. 2000; Strotmann et al. 2000). When heterologously expressed, TRPV4 is gated by hypotonicity (Liedtke et al. 2000; Strotmann et al. 2000) and also by phorbol esters, lipids, and moderate temperatures. The channel gives rise to a nonselective cationic conductance that can be blocked by La^{3+}, Gd^{3+}, and ruthenium red (Liedtke et al. 2000; Strotmann et al. 2000). Gating by multiple stimuli has also been demonstrated for the related TRPV1 channel and has led to the suggestion that this channel acts as an integrator of multiple sensory stimuli. This may be the case for TRPV4, but it is necessary to demonstrate that stimuli that activate this channel in vitro are physiologically relevant in the whole animal. Gating by hypotonicity has fueled conjecture that TRPV4 is mechanically gated. However, when recording from cell-attached patches, Strotmann et al. (2000) found that although reducing external osmolarity increased channel activity, application of negative or positive pressure through the pipette did not alter gating. Moreover, gating of TRPV4 by hypotonicity occurs slowly, after a lag of "a few seconds to 2 minutes" (Liedtke et al.

2000; Strotmann et al. 2000). Hence, it is unclear if activation induced by osmotic stimuli occurs via membrane effects or if this stimulus induces biochemical changes that activate the channel via intracellular signaling. The latter hypothesis is strongly supported by recent data of Xu et al. (2003). This study showed that hypotonicity rapidly induced tyrosine phosphorylation of TRPV4 that increased with stimulus duration. Inhibitors of kinases of the Src family blocked phosphorylation of TRPV4; the study demonstrated that one such kinase, Lyn, coimmunoprecipitates with TRPV4, is activated by hypotonicity, and can phosphorylate TRPV4 at tyrosine-253. Consistent with indirect gating by osmolarity, mutation of tyrosine-253 to a phenylalanine abolished hypotonic gating of TRPV4.

In a study of TRPV4 null mutant mice, Suzuki et al. (2003b) reported impaired pressure sensation in these animals. In the tail-pressure behavioral assay, TRPV4 nulls had thresholds around twice those of controls, whereas von Frey withdrawal thresholds were unchanged. In an electrophysiological analysis of these mice, the authors found that activation thresholds of "rapid-response" and "slow-response" A fibers were approximately trebled and doubled, respectively. The authors report that mechanically sensitive C fibers were absent in mutants, but only report six such fibers out of 300 recordings in wild-type mice. It would be of interest to analyze the response properties of DRG fiber types in these animals using the skin-nerve preparation (Koltzenburg et al. 1997), as used in the analysis of ASIC2/3 knockouts.

Alessandri-Haber et al. (2003) reported that the expression of TRPV4, assayed by single-cell reverse transcription polymerase chain reaction, correlated entirely with the expression of hypotonicity-induced changes in the excitability of cultured DRG neurons. The frequency of such neurons was approximately one in three, and around 90% of responsive cells had wide action potentials indicative of nociceptors. Despite the authors' inability to detect TRPV4 immunoreactivity in the somata of DRG neurons, Western blots from saphenous nerve suggested that this protein was transported to the periphery by sensory neurons. These investigators recorded primary afferent activity evoked by water injection that was potentiated by prostaglandin E_2 (PGE$_2$). This stimulus evoked pain behaviors, but only after PGE$_2$ sensitization. In support of a role of TRPV4 in this modality, when rats were treated with antisense oligonucleotides against this channel, water-evoked pain responses were significantly reduced. Unfortunately, no nerve fiber recordings are reported from antisense-treated animals, but behavioral data show that downregulation of TRPV4 did not alter mechanical hyperalgesia or acute mechanical withdrawal thresholds.

A novel approach to the study of ion channel function was employed by Liedtke et al. (2003) to study TRPV4. Given the homology of TRPV4 to OSM-9, this group expressed TRPV4 in *C. elegans* on an *osm-9* mutant background to assess whether this channel could phenotypically rescue these animals. Interestingly, expression of TRPV4 restored responses of mutants to mechanical stimulation of the nose and to hypertonic stimuli but not to repellent odorants. TRPV4::GFP was expressed in the sensory cilia of receptor neurons, and phenotypic rescue was absent when these cells were ablated. However, just as it is unclear if OSM-9 acts as a primary transducer of sensory stimuli, it remains ambiguous if TRPV4 is being activated directly or is acting downstream of other transduction events; TRPV4 does not rescue the phenotype of OSM-9 mutants that also lack functional OCR-2, ODR-3, or OSM-10. Finally, TRPV4 is gated by *hypo*tonicity in mammalian cells and here it is mediating responses to *hyper*tonicity, which suggests that different mechanisms are in operation. One possible route to resolving these issues would be to express the T253F mutant form of TRPV4 in *osm-9* mutants to determine whether this channel rescued either osmotic or touch sensitivity, and to ascertain whether both of these stimuli converge upon tyrosine-253 phosphorylation or rather gate the channel via independent mechanisms.

Overall, it is unclear if TRPV4 can be directly mechanically activated or if it participates in the detection of mechanical stimuli in situ; the striking phenotype reported by Suzuki et al. (2003b) using electrophysiology is at odds with the relatively sparse expression of TRPV4 in DRG neurons and the limited behavioral changes observed by Alessandri-Haber et al. (2003) and Suzuki et al. (2003b). It also remains to be determined if hypotonicity is a relevant stimuli, and thus a physiological activator of TRPV4, in pain pathways. It may be the case that osmosensitivity is important for this channel's function in other systems such as hypothalamic osmosensation (see Liedtke and Friedman 2003). Additionally, the contributions made to sensory function by thermal and lipid gating of TRPV4 are currently unknown.

In addition to TRPV4, a role for TRPV1 has been postulated in bladder mechanosensation. Birder et al. (2002) demonstrated that, despite having apparently morphologically normal bladders, TRPV1 knockout mice had deficits in voiding reflexes and spinal signaling of bladder volume. Distension of the bladder is known to evoke release of adenosine triphosphate (ATP); however, the absence of TRPV1 caused a reduction in the amount of ATP released both from stretched whole bladders and from hypotonically swollen urothelial cells. Moreover, stimulation of cultured urothelial cells with capsaicin evoked ATP release, suggesting that TRPV1 activation is both necessary and sufficient to evoke ATP release. No group has reported gating of TRPV1 by mechanical stimuli, and despite high levels of expression of TRPV1 in nociceptive neurons, cutaneous mechanosensation is seemingly normal in mice lacking this receptor (Caterina et al. 2000).

CHEMICALLY MEDIATED MECHANOSENSATION

In addition to direct activation of mechanosensitive ion channels, organisms can also sense changes in mechanical forces via the release of chemical mediators. This hypothesis purports that mechanical force induces chemical release from cells in close proximity to sensory endings and that these mediators act in a paracrine fashion to activate sensory neurons via ligand-gated ion channels or G-protein-coupled receptors (GPCRs).

It has long been known that endothelial cells release a number of factors, including nitric oxide, ATP, and substance P, in response to changes in blood flow (see Burnstock 1999). Burnstock (1999) also suggested that purinergic signaling might be important in nociception due to activation of damage-sensing neurons by endothelial cells in the microcirculation and that the sensing of mechanical distension of tubes (e.g., the gut, vagina, and urethra) or sacs (e.g., the bladder or lung) may be mediated by mechanically induced ATP release from epithelial cells. Empirical support for this idea came from studies of $P2X_3$ null mutants. Cockayne et al. (2000) showed that mice lacking this receptor displayed a marked bladder hyporeflexia, demonstrating reduced micturition frequency and increased bladder volume. They also showed that normally $P2X_3$ receptors are present on sensory nerves innervating the bladder. Subsequent work by the same group showed that bladder distension evoked a graded release of ATP and that the response of sensory fibers to bladder distension was attenuated in $P2X_3$ knockouts. In wild-type mice, ATP activated sensory fibers, and purinergic antagonists inhibited distension-evoked activity (Vlaskovska et al. 2001).

It is unclear how general this mechanism is; $P2X_3$ null mutants, for example, had no apparent deficits in cutaneous mechanosensation (Souslova et al. 2000). However, Cook et al. (2002) showed that when keratinocytes or fibroblasts were mechanically lysed in the vicinity of sensory neurons, neurons were depolarized by ATP acting at P2X receptors. This finding raises the possibility that some noxious mechanical stimuli may activate nociceptors via damage to nearby cells and consequent ATP release; the viability of this mechanism in vivo would be dependent on the actions of diffusion barriers to ATP and on the presence of ectonucleotidases. Nakamura and Strittmatter (1996) had previously proposed that $P2Y_1$ purinergic receptors might contribute to touch-induced impulse generation. They identified this GPCR from an expression-cloning screen of *Xenopus* oocytes expressing DRG cRNAs and found that eggs expressing $P2Y_1$ responded, via mechanically evoked ATP release, to a puff of external buffer with an inward current. Transcripts for $P2Y_1$ receptors were shown to be expressed in large-diameter rat DRG neurons. In a frog teased nerve-fiber preparation, ATP excited and sensitized mechanically sensitive fibers; touch-induced activity was attenuated by the purinergic receptor antagonist suramin and by the nucleotidase apyrase. It does seem unlikely, however, that increases in membrane excitability via activation of a GPCR would be rapid enough to act as a primary transduction mechanism. Similar findings have not been reported for mammalian mechanoreceptors, although nociceptors are activated by ATP (Hamilton et al. 2001; Molliver et al. 2002), and the expression of $P2Y_1$ in large nerve fibers suggests that it may modulate the excitability of these cells.

EXPERIMENTAL CHARACTERIZATION OF SENSORY NEURON MECHANOSENSORS

One approach to characterizing the components of mammalian mechanosensors is to study the properties of mechanosensitive ion channels in sensory neurons in vitro. A system for examining the properties of mechanically activated ion channels in sensory neurons was first described by Jon Levine's group (McCarter et al. 1999). This group showed that mechanical stimulation of the somatic membrane of cultured neurons evoked a nonselective cation current that was sensitive to gadolinium and high concentrations of the amiloride analogue benzamil. We have further characterized such ion channels (Drew et al. 2002, 2004), using the approach schematized in Fig. 1.

Using this approach, we have accumulated evidence that distinct mechanosensitive phenotypes are seen in cultured sensory neurons that are consistent with the predicted in vivo phenotypes of these neurons. When recording from neonatal rat neurons, we used capsaicin sensitivity to distinguish nociceptive neurons from putative low-threshold mechanoreceptors. Most of these sensory neurons responded to mechanical stimulation with rapidly adapting cationic currents (Drew et al. 2002). However, in capsaicin-insensitive neurons (the majority of which would be the cell bodies of low-threshold mechanoreceptors), currents were larger than and were activated at lower thresholds than mechanically activated currents in capsaicin-sensitive (i.e., nociceptive) neurons. A further population of capsaicin-insensitive neurons

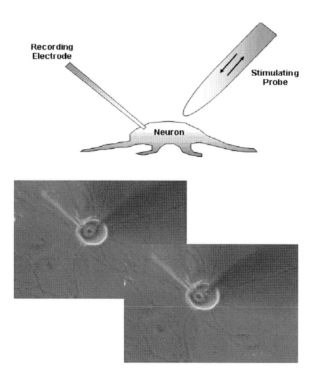

Fig. 1. Perforated-patch recordings were made from sensory neurons cultured for one day. Mechanical stimulation was applied using a heat-polished glass pipette controlled by a piezo crystal device. Incrementing stimuli allowed characterization of the mechanosensitivity of neurons classified as putative low-threshold mechanoreceptors or nociceptors.

displayed slowly adapting currents, which activated at similar thresholds to those in capsaicin-sensitive neurons.

In adult mouse neurons, given the maturation of action potential properties (Fitzgerald and Fulton 1992), action potential duration was used to classify neurons as low- and high-threshold mechanoreceptors (Rose et al. 1986; Koerber et al. 1988; Ritter and Mendell 1992). Thus, large neurons with narrow action potentials, indicative of low-threshold mechanoreceptors, had larger mechanically activated currents than those of comparably sized neurons with wide, inflected action potentials (i.e., nociceptors) (Drew et al. 2004). Mechanically activated (MA) currents were also kinetically distinct; in neurons with narrow action potentials, currents were rapidly adapting, and those of nociceptive neurons showed adaptation kinetics intermediate between rapidly and slowly adapting currents (Fig. 2). Mechanically evoked responses in small to medium neurons were of three types: rapidly, intermediately, and slowly adapting. The predominant current type

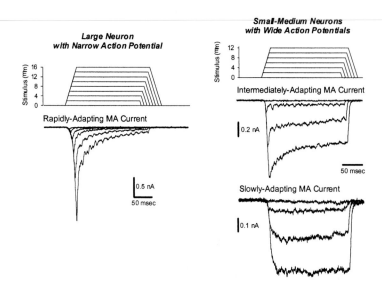

Fig. 2. Examples of mechanically activated (MA) currents generated by adult mouse sensory neurons. Low-threshold mechanoreceptor neurons (left) displayed distinctive rapidly adapting MA currents, whereas nociceptive neurons (right) that responded to mechanical stimulation displayed slowly or intermediately adapting MA currents.

had intermediately adapting kinetics and was characteristic of all responding neurons that bound isolectin B4 (IB4) and a subpopulation of IB4-negative neurons. Another IB4-negative subpopulation exhibited MA currents with rapidly adapting kinetics similar to those of large neurons with narrow action potentials. The majority of these neurons also displayed narrow action potentials and may also be low-threshold mechanoreceptors (Djouhri et al. 1998; Lawson 2002). The remaining neurons that responded displayed slowly adapting currents. Hence, intermediately adapting currents appear to be the response of most nociceptive neurons to membrane displacement. The identity of neurons that display slowly adapting responses is unclear, but this distribution and frequency and their physiological properties are consistent with them being Aδ-fiber mechanonociceptors (see Koltzenburg et al. 1997).

In an attempt to elucidate the molecular basis of MA currents in DRG neurons, we investigated if putative low-threshold mechanoreceptor neurons derived from ASIC2 and ASIC3 null mutants showed alterations in their responses to focal mechanical stimulation. As described above, Price et al. (2000, 2001) observed that certain classes of fibers in these mutants showed abnormal mechanically evoked firing. However, in our system the deletion

of the genes for ASIC2 and ASIC3, either alone or together, had no significant effect either on the sensitivity of large neurons to mechanical stimulation or on the kinetics of evoked responses. We therefore concluded that
neither of these ion channels contributes to the generation of MA currents in
isolated neurons. Mechanically evoked responses of small to medium-sized
neurons also showed no differences between wild-type neurons and those
lacking ASIC2 and ASIC3. The data of Price et al. (2001) suggest a reduced
sensitivity of Aδ-fiber nociceptors in ASIC3 knockouts, but no subpopulation showed any decrease in sensitivity in our assay.

Mechanosensitivity seems to be a property intrinsic to the sensory neuron (see Lewin and Stucky 2000 for discussion). Hence, the striking correlation between the phenotype of cultured neurons and the characteristics of
MA currents strongly suggests that the mechanosensitive ion channels found
at the soma are important in mechanosensation. We propose that in the in
vivo setting, these ion channels would be present at the sensory endings and
would contribute to the transduction of mechanical force into action potentials. Our studies show that mechanosensitive ion channels expressed by
DRG neurons can generate considerable whole-cell currents in an environment that is devoid of a complex extracellular matrix. However, it remains a
possibility that components of the external matrix can affect the behavior of
these channels, potentially regulating their sensitivity and their gating kinetics. It is also possible that in vivo, mechanosensitive ion channels are expressed in localized regions of membrane that are configured to respond to
mechanical displacement in a manner distinct from the somatic membrane
(Hamill and Martinac 2001).

The gating of the ion channels underlying mechanically activated currents is dependent on the actin cytoskeleton (Drew et al. 2002; P. Cesare,
unpublished observations). Although the identity of these ion channels is
unknown, mechanically activated currents are also inhibited by external calcium and gadolinium and, in a voltage-dependent manner, by ruthenium red
(Drew et al. 2002, 2004), all characteristics shared with members of the TRP
channel family (see Clapham et al. 2001; Gunthorpe et al. 2002).

Finally, the group of Uhtaek Oh (Cho et al. 2002) has published an
extensive study of DRG mechanosensitive ion channels at the single-channel level. Recording from cell-attached patches and applying negative pressure through the pipette, the investigators detected two classes of
mechanosensitive ion channels. First, they found low-threshold (LT) channels in 25.7% of patches that were activated at –10 to –20 mm Hg with a
$P_{1/2}$ (50% probability of opening) of 60.6 mm Hg and second, they saw
high-threshold (HT) channels in 23.6% of patches with a $P_{1/2}$ of 83.1 mm Hg
and a threshold of >60 mm Hg. Current voltage relationships and ionic

substitution experiments showed that both channel subtypes were nonspecific cation channels with significant permeability to Ca^{2+}. LT channels were outwardly rectifying, and HT channels had a more linear relationship. Both channels were blocked by Gd^{3+} and were inhibited by pretreatment of the patch with cytochalasin D (10 μM) or colchicine (500 μM) or by excision of a cell-attached patch to the inside-out configuration. In all three cases, the inhibitory effect was significantly more pronounced for LT channels than it was for HT channels. Another interesting finding of this study was that HT, but not LT, channels showed a marked sensitization following exposure to PGE_2. A major consideration regarding this study is the cell size distribution of both channel types. HT channels were found in a population of cells with diameters of 10–17.5 μm and LT channels in significantly larger cells with diameters of 10–30 μm. This distribution is significantly different from that found for neurons with mechanically activated whole-cell currents, strongly suggesting that the observed single channels do not underlie such currents. Moreover, it is conspicuous that the largest cells tested (30–40 μm), which would be expected to be low-threshold mechanoreceptors, showed no mechanically evoked activity. The molecular identities of these ion channels are unknown, yet it is notable that they had a number of properties that distinguished them from members of DEG/ENaC family.

CONCLUSION

The research discussed in this chapter highlights both the recent progress made in understanding the molecular basis of mechanosensation and also how far there is to go. Although numerous channels have been implicated in this sensory modality by genetic techniques, no metazoan ion channel has been shown to be both unequivocally mechanically gated and central to sensory mechanotransduction. Genetics and behavioral studies, and even electrophysiological investigations, are always open to the caveat that the identified channel is activated downstream of the primary transduction event. Heterologous expression of mechanically evoked channel activity is likely to prove technically demanding due to the elaborate sensory cell types in which such channels are expressed and their likely inclusion in multiprotein mechanosensory complexes. Strong evidence implicates MEC-4 and MEC-10 in *C. elegans* body touch sensation and implicates NOMPC and Nan in mechanosensation by type I receptors of *Drosophila*. Consequently, at present the primary candidates for the role of mammalian mechanotransducers are in the TRP and ENaC/DEG ion channel families, both of which are remarkably functionally diverse. However, in no case is the available evidence supporting a function for a mammalian channel in mechanotransduction as strong as it is in fruit flies or nematodes.

The findings in invertebrates suggest that there is not simply one family of mechanosensitive ion channels underlying metazoan mechanotransduction. The extensiveness of genetic screens in *C. elegans* and *Drosophila* suggest that other ion channels are unlikely to function in these species (although extensive studies of other submodalities, such as harsh body touch, have not been undertaken). However, if mechanosensitivity has evolved in two markedly distinct families of proteins, it is possible that it has also done so in further ion channel types. It is also of interest to note the diversity in DEG/ENaC channels in *C. elegans* and *Drosophila* (28 and 25 homologues, respectively) when compared to the number of related channels in vertebrates (8, for example, in mice) (Goodman and Schwarz 2003).

Related to the diversity of putative mechanosensing ion channels is the issue of diversity in cellular systems that mediate mechanosensation. Despite superficial similarities, which are often emphasized, the phylogenetic relationship between mammalian hair cells and primary somatosensory neurons and the analogous cell types in invertebrates is poorly established. It is certainly notable that in *C. elegans* body touch neurons, mechanosensation is critically dependent on microtubules, and that the cilia of *Drosophila* neurons innervating type I sensory organs contain typical microtubule arrangements. In contrast, at the site of transduction in mammalian hair cells and in somatosensory neurons, the cytoplasm is dominated by actin microfilaments. Finally, the extent to which various systems rely on chemically mediated mechanosensation remains to be determined. In some systems it may have a modulatory role in association with faster mechanisms, and in others, such as bladder stretch and perhaps nociception, it may have a primary role. Thus, much remains to be determined regarding the molecular basis of mechanotransduction in nociceptors. The molecular definition of noxious mechanotransducing receptors is an important challenge in terms of understanding mechanisms of activation of nociceptors and for defining new targets for analgesic drug development.

REFERENCES

Alessandri-Haber N, Yeh JJ, Boyd AE, et al. Hypotonicity induces TRPV4-mediated nociception in rat. *Neuron* 2003; 39:497–511.

Alvarez de la Rosa D, Zhang P, Shao D, White F, Canessa CM. Functional implications of the localization and activity of acid-sensitive channels in rat peripheral nervous system. *Proc Natl Acad Sci USA* 2002; 99:2326–2331.

Alvarez de la Rosa D, Krueger SR, Kolar A, et al. Distribution, subcellular localization and ontogeny of ASIC1 in the mammalian central nervous system. *J Physiol* 2003; 546:77–87.

Benson CJ, Xie J, Wemmie JA, et al. Heteromultimers of DEG/ENaC subunits form H⁺-gated channels in mouse sensory neurons. *Proc Natl Acad Sci USA* 2002; 99:2338–2343.

Birder LA, Nakamura Y, Kiss S, et al. Altered urinary bladder function in mice lacking the vanilloid receptor TRPV1. *Nat Neurosci* 2002; 5:856–860.

Blount P, Moe PC. Bacterial mechanosensitive channels: integrating physiology, structure and function. *Trends Microbiol* 1999; 7:420–424.

Burnstock G. Release of vasoactive substances from endothelial cells by shear stress and purinergic mechanosensory transduction. *J Anat* 1999; 194:335–342.

Caterina MJ, Leffler A, Malmberg AB, et al. Impaired nociception and pain sensation in mice lacking the capsaicin receptor. *Science* 2000; 288:306–313.

Chalfie M, Sulston J. Developmental genetics of the mechanosensory neurons of *Caenorhabditis elegans*. *Dev Biol* 1981; 82:358–370.

Chelur DS, Ernstrom GG, Goodman MB, et al. The mechano-sensory protein MEC-6 is a subunit of the *C. elegans* touch-cell degenerin channel. *Nature* 2002; 420:669–673.

Chen CC, England S, Akopian AN, Wood JN. A sensory neuron-specific, proton-gated ion channel. *Proc Natl Acad Sci USA* 1998; 95:10240–10245.

Chen CC, Zimmer A, Sun WH, et al. A role for ASIC3 in the modulation of high-intensity pain stimuli. *Proc Natl Acad Sci USA* 2002; 99:8992–8997.

Cho H, Shin J, Shin CY, Lee S-Y, Oh U. Mechanosensitive ion channels in cultured sensory neurons of neonatal rats. *J Neurosci* 2002; 22:1238–1247.

Chung YD, Zhu J, Han Y, Kernan MJ. *nompA* encodes a PNS-specific, ZP domain protein required to connect mechanosensory dendrites to sensory structures. *Neuron* 2001; 29:415–428.

Clapham DE. TRP channels as cellular sensors. *Nature* 2003; 426:517–524.

Clapham DE, Runnels LW, Strubing C. The TRP ion channel family. *Nat Rev Neurosci* 2001; 2:387–396.

Cockayne DA, Hamilton SG, Zhu QM, et al. Urinary bladder hyporeflexia and reduced pain-related behaviour in P2X₃-deficient mice. *Nature* 2000; 407:1011–1015.

Colbert HA, Smith TL, Bargmann CI. OSM-9, a novel protein with structural similarity to channels, is required for olfaction, mechanosensation, and olfactory adaptation in *Caenorhabditis elegans*. *J Neurosci* 1997; 17:8259–8269.

Cook SP, McCleskey EW. Cell damage excites nociceptors through release of cytosolic ATP. *Pain* 2002; 95:41–47.

Djouhri L, Bleazard L, Lawson SN. Association of somatic action potential shape with sensory receptive properties in guinea-pig dorsal root ganglion neurons. *J Physiol* 1998; 513:857–872.

Drew LJ, Wood JN, Cesare P. Distinct mechanosensitive properties of capsaicin-sensitive and -insensitive sensory neurons. *J Neurosci* 2002; 22:RC228.

Drew LJ, Rohrer DK, Price MP, et al. Acid-sensing ion channels ASIC2 and ASIC3 do not contribute to mechanically activated currents in mammalian sensory neurons. *J Physiol* 2004; 556(Pt 3):691–710 .

Eberl DF, Hardy RW, Kernan MJ. Genetically similar transduction mechanisms for touch and hearing in *Drosophila*. *J Neurosci* 2000; 20:5981–5988.

Ernstrom GG, Chalfie M. Genetics of sensory mechanotransduction. *Annu Rev Genet* 2002; 36:411–453.

Fitzgerald M, Fulton BP. The physiological properties of developing sensory neurons. In: Scott SA (Ed). *Sensory Neurons. Diversity, Development, and Plasticity*. New York: Oxford University Press, 1992, pp 287–306.

García-Añoveros J, Samad TA, Zuvela-Jelaska L, Woolf CJ, Corey DP. Transport and localization of the DEG/ENaC ion channel BNaC1-alpha to peripheral mechanosensory terminals of dorsal root ganglia neurons. *J Neurosci* 2001; 21:2678–2686.

Gillespie PG, Walker RG. Molecular basis of mechanosensory transduction. *Nature* 2001; 413:194–202.

Goodman MB, Schwarz EM. Transducing touch in *Caenorhabditis elegans*. *Annu Rev Physiol* 2003; 65:429–452.

Goodman MB, Ernstrom GG, Chelur DS, et al. MEC-2 regulates *C. elegans* DEG/ENaC channels needed for mechanosensation. *Nature* 2002; 415:1039–1042.

Gu CX, Juranka PF, Morris CE. Stretch-activation and stretch-inactivation of Shaker-IR, a voltage-gated K$^+$ channel. *Biophys J* 2001; 80:2678–2693.

Gunthorpe MJ, Benham CD, Randall A, Davis JB. The diversity in the vanilloid (TRPV) receptor family of ion channels. *Trends Pharmacol Sci* 2002; 23:183–191.

Hamill OP, Martinac B. Molecular basis of mechanotransduction in living cells. *Physiol Rev* 2001; 81:685–740.

Hamill OP, McBride DW Jr. The pharmacology of mechanogated membrane ion channels. *Pharmacol Rev* 1996; 48:231–252.

Hamill OP, McBride DW Jr. Induced membrane hypo/hyper-mechanosensitivity: a limitation of patch-clamp recording. *Annu Rev Physiol* 1997; 59:621–631.

Hamilton SG, McMahon SB, Lewin GR. Selective activation of nociceptors by P2X receptor agonists in normal and inflamed rat skin. *J Physiol* 2001; 534:437–445.

Hart AC, Kass J, Shapiro JE, Kaplan JM. Distinct signaling pathways mediate touch and osmosensory responses in a polymodal sensory neuron. *J Neurosci* 1999; 19:1952–1958.

Jordt SE, McKemy DD, Julius D. Lessons from peppers and peppermint: the molecular logic of thermosensation. *Curr Opin Neurobiol* 2003; 13:487–492.

Kernan M, Zuker C. Genetic approaches to mechanosensory transduction. *Curr Opin Neurobiol* 1995; 5:443–448.

Kernan M, Cowan D, Zuker C. Genetic dissection of mechanosensory transduction: mechanoreception-defective mutations of *Drosophila*. *Neuron* 1994; 12:1195–1206.

Kim J, Chung YD, Park DY, et al. A TRPV family ion channel required for hearing in *Drosophila*. *Nature* 2003; 424:81–84.

Kinkelin I, Stucky CL, Koltzenburg M. Postnatal loss of Merkel cells, but not of slowly adapting mechanoreceptors in mice lacking the neurotrophin receptor p75. *Eur J Neurosci* 1999; 11:3963–3969.

Koerber HR, Druzinsky RE, Mendell LM. Properties of somata of spinal dorsal root ganglion cells differ according to peripheral receptor innervated. *J Neurophysiol* 1988; 60:1584–1596.

Koltzenburg M, Stucky CL, Lewin GR. Receptive properties of mouse sensory neurons innervating hairy skin. *J Neurophysiol* 1997; 78:1841–1850.

Lawson SN. Phenotype and function of somatic primary afferent nociceptive neurons with C-, A-delta- or A-alpha/beta-fibres. *Exp Physiol* 2002; 87:239–244.

Lewin GR, Stucky CL. Sensory neuron mechanotransduction: regulation and underlying molecular mechanisms. In: Wood JN (Ed). *Molecular Basis of Pain Transduction*. Wiley-Liss, 2000, pp 129–148.

Liedtke W, Friedman JM. Abnormal osmotic regulation in trpv4-/- mice. *Proc Natl Acad Sci USA* 2003; 100:13698–13703.

Liedtke W, Choe Y, Martí-Renom MA, et al. Vanilloid receptor-related osmotically activated channel (VR-OAC), a candidate vertebrate osmoreceptor. *Cell* 2000; 103:525–535.

Liedtke W, Tobin DM, Bargmann CI, Friedman JM. Mammalian TRPV4 (VR-OAC) directs behavioral responses to osmotic and mechanical stimuli in *Caenorhabditis elegans*. *Proc Natl Acad Sci USA* 2003; 100(Suppl 2):14531–14536.

Lingueglia E, de Weille JR, Bassilana F, et al. A modulatory subunit of acid sensing ion channels in brain and dorsal root ganglion cells. *J Biol Chem* 1997; 272:29778–29783.

Maingret F, Fosset M, Lesage F, Lazdunski M, Honore E. TRAAK is a mammalian neuronal mechano-gated K$^+$ channel. *J Biol Chem* 1999; 274:1381–1387.

McCarter GC, Reichling DB, Levine JD. Mechanical transduction by rat dorsal root ganglion neurons *in vitro*. *Neurosci Lett* 1999; 273:179–182.

Mills LR, Diamond J. Merkel cells are not the mechanosensory transducers in the touch dome of the rat. *J Neurocytol* 1995; 24:117–134.

Molliver DC, Cook SP, Carlsten JA, Wright DE, McCleskey EW. ATP and UTP excite sensory neurons and induce CREB phosphorylation through the metabotropic receptor, P2Y$_2$. *Eur J Neurosci* 2002; 16:1850–1860.

Morris CE, Horn R. Failure to elicit neuronal macroscopic mechanosensitive currents anticipated by single-channel studies. *Science* 1991; 251:1246–1249.

Nakamura F, Strittmatter SM. P2Y$_1$ purinergic receptors in sensory neurons: contribution to touch-induced impulse generation. *Proc Natl Acad Sci USA* 1996; 93:10465–10470.

Olson TH, Riedl MS, Vulchanova L, Ortiz-Gonzalez XR, Elde R. An acid sensing ion channel (ASIC) localizes to small primary afferent neurons in rats. *Neuroreport* 1998; 9:1109–1113.

Paoletti P, Ascher P. Mechanosensitivity of NMDA receptors in cultured mouse central neurons. *Neuron* 1994; 13:645–655.

Patapoutian A, Peier AM, Story GM, Viswanath V. ThermoTRP channels and beyond: mechanisms of temperature sensation. *Nat Rev Neurosci* 2003; 4:529–539.

Patel AJ, Honore E, Maingret F, et al. A mammalian two pore domain mechano-gated S-like K$^+$ channel. *EMBO J* 1998; 17:4283–4290.

Price MP, Lewin GR, McIlwrath SL, et al. The mammalian sodium channel BNC1 is required for normal touch sensation. *Nature* 2000; 407:1007–1011.

Price MP, McIlwrath SL, Xie J, et al. The DRASIC cation channel contributes to the detection of cutaneous touch and acid stimuli in mice. *Neuron* 2001; 32:1071–1083.

Ritter AM, Mendell LM. Somal membrane properties of physiologically identified sensory neurons in the rat: effects of nerve growth factor. *J Neurophysiol* 1992; 68:2033–2041.

Roayaie K, Crump JG, Sagasti A, Bargmann CI. The G alpha protein ODR-3 mediates olfactory and nociceptive function and controls cilium morphogenesis in *C. elegans* olfactory neurons. *Neuron* 1998; 20:55–67.

Rose RD, Koerber HR, Sedivec MJ, Mendell LM. Somal action potential duration differs in identified primary afferents. *Neurosci Lett* 1986; 63:259–264.

Sackin H. Mechanosensitive channels. *Annu Rev Physiol* 1995; 57:333–353.

Sidi S, Friedrich RW, Nicolson T. NompC TRP channel required for vertebrate sensory hair cell mechanotransduction. *Science* 2003; 301:96–99.

Souslova V, Cesare P, Ding Y, et al. Warm-coding deficits and aberrant inflammatory pain in mice lacking P2X3 receptors. *Nature* 2000; 407:1015–1017.

Strotmann R, Harteneck C, Nunnenmacher K, Schultz G. Plant TD OTRPC4, a nonselective cation channel that confers sensitivity to extracellular osmolarity. *Nat Cell Biol* 2000; 2:695–702.

Sukharev S, Corey DP. Mechanosensitive channels: multiplicity of families and gating paradigms. *Sci STKE* 2004; 219:re4.

Suzuki H, Kerr R, Bianchi L, et al. *In vivo* imaging of *C. elegans* mechanosensory neurons demonstrates a specific role for the MEC-4 channel in the process of gentle touch sensation. *Neuron* 2003a; 39:1005–1017.

Suzuki M, Mizuno A, Kodaira K, Imai M. Impaired pressure sensation in mice lacking TRPV4. *J Biol Chem* 2003b; 278:22664–22668.

Tavernarakis N, Driscoll M. Molecular modeling of mechanotransduction in the nematode *Caenorhabditis elegans*. *Annu Rev Physiol* 1997; 59:659–689.

Tobin D, Madsen D, Kahn-Kirby A, et al. Combinatorial expression of TRPV channel proteins defines their sensory functions and subcellular localization in *C. elegans* neurons. *Neuron* 2002; 35:307–318.

Tracey WD Jr, Wilson RI, Laurent G, Benzer S. *painless*, a *Drosophila* gene essential for nociception. *Cell* 2003; 113:261–273.

Vlaskovska M, Kasakov L, Rong W, et al. P2X$_3$ knock-out mice reveal a major sensory role for urothelially released ATP. *J Neurosci* 2001; 21:5670–5677.

Waldmann R, Lazdunski M. H$^+$-gated cation channels: neuronal acid sensors in the NaC/DEG family of ion channels. *Curr Opin Neurobiol* 1998; 8:418–424.

Waldmann R, Bassilana F, de Weille J, et al. Molecular cloning of a non-inactivating proton-gated Na⁺ channel specific for sensory neurons. *J Biol Chem* 1997a; 272:20975–20978.

Waldmann R, Champigny G, Bassilana F, Heurteaux C, Lazdunski M. A proton-gated cation channel involved in acid-sensing. *Nature* 1997b; 386:173–177.

Walker RG, Willingham AT, Zuker CS. A *Drosophila* mechanosensory transduction channel. *Science* 2000; 287:2229–2234.

Welk E, Leah JD, Zimmermann M. Characteristics of A- and C-fibers ending in a sensory nerve neuroma in the rat. *J Neurophysiol* 1990; 63:759–766.

Welsh MJ, Price MP, Xie J. Biochemical basis of touch perception: mechanosensory function of DEG/ENaC channels. *J Biol Chem* 2001; 277:2369–2372.

Xu H, Zhao H, Tian W, et al. Regulation of a transient receptor potential (TRP) channel by tyrosine phosphorylation. SRC family kinase-dependent tyrosine phosphorylation of TRPV4 on TYR-253 mediates its response to hypotonic stress. *J Biol Chem* 2003; 278:11520–11527.

Zhang Y, Hamill OP. On the discrepancy between whole-cell and membrane patch mechano-sensitivity in *Xenopus* oocytes. *J Physiol* 2000; 523:101–115.

Correspondence to: John N. Wood, PhD, DSc, Molecular Nociception Group, Biology Department, University College, London WC1E 6BT, United Kingdom. Email: j.wood@ucl.ac.uk.

The Pain System in Normal and Pathological States: A Primer for Clinicians, Progress in Pain Research and Management, Vol. 31, edited by Luis Villanueva, Anthony Dickenson, and Hélène Ollat, IASP Press, Seattle, © 2004.

2

Thermal Sensitivity of Sensory Neurons

Martin Koltzenburg

Neural Plasticity Unit, Institute of Child Health, University College London, London, United Kingdom

Recent significant progress in the discovery of the molecular transduction mechanisms underlying thermosensation could provide a cellular explanation for the distinct receptive properties of sensory neurons. This chapter provides a short overview of how transient receptor potential (TRP) channels could contribute to acute and chronic pain states and how they contribute to the signaling of noxious and innocuous temperature changes. TRP channels of the vanilloid family (TRPV1, TRPV2, TRPV3, and TRPV4) are excited by cutaneous heat stimuli, whereas TRPM8 and TRPA1 (Clapham et al. 2003) are responsive to cold. TRPV1 and TRPA1 are also implicated in mediating the pungency of nociceptor-specific chemicals such as capsaicin or mustard oil. Sensitization of TRPV1 is an important mechanism for heat hyperalgesia and thus for the generation of chronic pain symptoms.

TRP CHANNELS EXPRESSED IN PRIMARY SENSORY NEURONS

TRP channels were first described in the photoreceptors of the fruit fly *Drosophila.* In mammals TRP channels fulfill diverse functions, and to date six subfamilies are recognized based on their structural homology (Minke and Cook 2002; Clapham 2003). The seminal discovery of the capsaicin receptor TRPV1 (previously known as VR1) (Caterina et al. 1997) was followed by identification of several other TRP channels expressed in dorsal root ganglia (DRG) or peripheral tissues innervated by sensory neurons. These include TRPV2 (Caterina et al. 1999), TRPV3 (Peier et al. 2002b; Smith et al. 2002; Xu et al. 2002), TRPV4 (Trost et al. 2001; Guler et al. 2002; Nilius et al. 2003; Vriens et al. 2004), TRPM8 (previously known as CMR1; McKemy et al. 2002; Peier et al. 2002a), and TRPA1 (previously known as ANKTM1; Story et al. 2003; Jordt et al. 2004). Some controversy centers on how the expression and properties of these receptors correlate with the functional properties of sensory neurons that signal thermal or noxious events.

SENSITIVITY OF NOCICEPTORS IN NORMAL TISSUES

A broad consensus holds that acute pains studied under laboratory conditions are evoked by excitation of nociceptors with thin myelinated or unmyelinated axons (Meyer et al. 1994; Handwerker 1996; Raja et al. 1999). Investigators simultaneously using microneurographic recordings of primary afferents and psychophysical magnitude estimation techniques in conscious humans have shown that cutaneous nociceptors can encode the intensity of painful heat (Gybels et al. 1979), mechanical (Koltzenburg and Handwerker 1994; Schmidt et al. 2000; Schmelz et al. 2003), or chemical stimuli (Schmelz et al. 2003). However, investigators also agree that firing of a single nociceptor cannot necessarily be equated with the perception of pain. In human microneurographic experiments, it is not uncommon to activate individual nociceptors with painless stimuli. Moreover, mechano-heat-sensitive C fibers (CMH units, also known as polymodal nociceptors) innervating the hairy skin have thresholds around 41°–43°C, but the psychophysical heat-pain threshold of individuals is often considerably higher (LaMotte et al. 1984). Correspondingly, increases of skin temperature that evoke a low discharge rate of less than 0.3 impulses per second over short periods are usually painless (Van Hees and Gybels 1981). Furthermore, brief mechanical impact stimuli can elicit bursts of activity with instantaneous frequencies exceeding 10 Hz without being called painful (Koltzenburg and Handwerker 1994). The time lag between the firing of nociceptors and the appearance of pain following application of algesic chemicals is often considerable (Adriaensen et al. 1980). In aggregate, these results lead to the conclusion that both temporal summation and spatial summation in a population of nociceptors are important for encoding the magnitude of pain (Raja et al. 1999).

THERMAL SENSITIVITY OF THIN MYELINATED
OR UNMYELINATED AFFERENTS

Humans can readily distinguish innocuous warm sensations from noxious heat sensations. It is generally thought that warm sensation is signaled by unmyelinated fibers, whereas heat pain is signaled by unmyelinated and large myelinated fibers (Konietzny 1984; Raja et al. 1999). The properties of warm receptors have primarily been studied in carnivores and nonhuman primates, and relatively little information exists about the properties of thermal receptors in rodents (Konietzny 1984). Thermoreceptors responding to innocuous warming have been described in studies on the scrotal skin of the rat (Hensel and Schafer 1974; Hellon et al. 1975; Pierau et al. 1975), but they are generally not mentioned in reports investigating the receptive properties of fine afferents in cutaneous limb nerves of rats and mice. The obvious sparseness of these fibers in peripheral nerves of rodents is not fully understood; possible explanations are (1) they are genuinely scarce; (2) they become desensitized and unresponsive after repeated application of strong thermal stimuli, a procedure used in many electrophysiological recordings; or (3) in contrast to the classical view that they are mechanically insensitive in primates, they may be mechanically sensitive in rodents, which might lead to their classification as a nociceptors. The reported percentage of heat-sensitive myelinated mechanosensitive nociceptors in rat hairy skin ranges from 0% to 21% (Lynn and Carpenter 1982; Lynn and Shakhanbeh 1988; Leem et al. 1993; Simone and Kajander 1996, 1997; Bennett et al. 1998). For unmyelinated fibers the percentage of CMH fibers is in the range of 34–73% (Lynn and Carpenter 1982; Fleischer et al. 1983; Kress et al. 1992; Leem et al. 1993; Bennett et al. 1998). Some of these studies investigated the cold sensitivity of CMH units, finding that as many as a third of these units also appear to be excited by strong cold stimuli. The thermosensitivity of myelinated nociceptors in the mouse was comparable to rats for identical nerves and recording conditions, whereas heat-sensitive unmyelinated nociceptors appeared to be less abundant in mice, in the range of 40% (Koltzenburg et al. 1997).

In humans, thin or unmyelinated sensory fibers signal the conscious sensation of innocuous or noxious cold. This conclusion is primarily based on reaction time measurements and differential nerve blocks (Hensel et al. 1974; Konietzny 1984; Wasner et al. 2004). Compression block experiments generally indicate that Aδ fibers signal sensitivity to innocuous cold (Torebjörk and Hallin 1973; Mackenzie et al. 1975). Intriguingly, however, none of the microneurographic recordings have convincingly shown this type of Aδ fiber in humans (Adriaensen et al. 1983; Schmidt et al. 1995; Schmelz et al. 2000), and more recent microneurographic recordings from distal peripheral nerves have found that fibers responding to innocuous cold are conducting in the C-fiber range (Campero et al. 2001).

The threshold for cold pain is less clearly defined than that for heat pain. Psychophysical studies have recognized at least three types of cold sensation. The first two types are: (1) cool detection threshold, usually 0.5°C below ambient skin temperature; and (2) cold pain threshold, usually below 15°C.

The threshold for cold pain depends on skin area, rate of cooling, the size of the probe, and how subjects are instructed (Davis 1998; Harrison and Davis 1999). Some people recognize the burning component of cold pain, others the deep aching aspects. The third type of cold sensation is pain of freezing, a stinging type of pain that is qualitatively distinct from cool sensation and painful cold (Simone and Kajander 1997). Cooling can also induce a "paradoxical heat" sensation (Hamalainen et al. 1982; Susser et al. 1999), which is distinct from the "paradoxical cold" at the onset of a strong noxious heat stimulus (Dodt and Zotterman 1952). Whereas the sensation of paradoxical heat is conducted by unmyelinated, probably nociceptive, afferent fibers, the sensation of paradoxical cold is probably signaled by the excitation of sensitive cold afferents (Dodt and Zotterman 1952; Long 1977). Psychophysical studies have also shown that activation of cool-specific receptors by nonpainful cold stimuli inhibits nociceptor input by a central mechanism (Bini et al. 1984; Wahren et al. 1989; Yarnitsky and Ochoa 1990; Craig et al. 1996). Thus, in comparing psychophysical studies with properties of primary afferent neurons or isolated native sensory neurons, we must consider that the excitation threshold of nociceptors probably occurs at warmer temperatures than the psychophysical threshold of cold pain.

Many mechanosensitive fibers with large myelinated fibers are influenced by cold temperature (Werner and Mountcastle 1965; Iggo 1969; Casey and Hahn 1970; Burton et al. 1972; Duclaux and Kenshalo 1972; Booth and Hahn 1974; Konietzny 1984). While type I slowly adapting (SAI) fibers usually have a lower response to mechanical stimuli at cold temperatures, rapid dynamic cooling stimuli can excite these receptors (Burton et al. 1972; Duclaux and Kenshalo 1972; Konietzny 1984). In contrast, type II slowly adapting (SAII) fibers, which often exhibit spontaneous activity, increase their regular discharge at colder temperatures and often exhibit very dynamic discharges to rapid cooling, sometimes resembling the firing pattern of true cold-specific afferents (Iggo 1969; Burton et al. 1972; Booth and Hahn 1974; Konietzny 1984). While it is generally thought that this excitation or increased sensitivity of mechanoreceptors does not signal cold sensations, it may account for Weber's illusion that objects of equal weight feel heavier when cold (Werner and Mountcastle 1965).

Three distinct responses to cold can be identified among the thin myelinated and unmyelinated fibers. First, cold-sensitive receptors signal the sensation of cooling. They are mechanically insensitive units (in rodents also referred to as CC, cold-sensitive C fibers) that respond vigorously to small temperature reductions in the innocuous range. These units display a characteristic bursting discharge, respond dynamically, and are often excited by menthol. They show a plateau or even a reduced response to cold temperatures in the noxious range. Few studies have investigated these receptors in rodents (Kress et al. 1992). Second, many mechanosensitive nociceptors respond to cold stimuli in the noxious range. Up to 10% of the nociceptive Aδ fibers and up to a third of the C fibers in rats or mice also respond to noxious cold (Lynn and Carpenter 1982; Fleischer et al. 1983; Kress et al. 1992; Leem et al. 1993; Koltzenburg et al. 1997; Bennett et al. 1998). Units would typically discharge vigorously at the onset of a cold stimulus and rapidly inactivate when the temperature stimulus has passed its nadir. Some nociceptive units only discharge during the rewarming of the receptive field, but not during the cold stimulus itself, and thus probably do not constitute a genuine cold response (Kress et al. 1992; Koltzenburg et al. 1997). Third, most nociceptive Aδ and C fibers respond to temperatures below freezing, a stimulus that typically evokes a stinging, sharp pain (Simone and Kajander 1996, 1997; Cain et al. 2001).

The percentage of cold-sensitive units in rodents varies widely between studies and depends on both the search stimulus for the units and the cold stimulus. For example, some studies employed cold stimuli only down to 12°C, which could have activated a lower percentage of cold-sensitive units (Leem et al. 1993), whereas others used stimuli as cold as –20°C, which excited a much larger proportion of nociceptors (Simone and Kajander 1996, 1997). The temporal and spatial configuration of a cold stimulus is probably more crucial for cold than for heat stimulation. For example, it takes a 30–60-second application of a piece of ice to bring down the subepidermal temperature of an anesthetized rat to freezing, and most studies will not apply the stimulus for that long. The question of what constitutes an adequate cold stimulus (i.e., freezing the tissue or not) is also somewhat reminiscent of previous discussions about an appropriate heat stimulus for nociceptors. For example, it had been argued that the heat response of many Aδ nociceptors in normal skin is beyond the heat–pain withdrawal threshold. This assumption is the rationale for describing them as thermo-insensitive high-threshold mechanoreceptors rather than A-fiber mechanoheat fibers. Another confounding problem of electrophysiological experiments is that the same skin area is typically retested and re-exposed to noxious thermal stimuli, which could lead to sensitization or desensitization, a problem that is also apparent in psychophysical studies (Beise et al. 1998).

The first studies of fine afferents in rats mentioned cold sensitivity only briefly. They used mechanical search stimuli and briefly applied pieces of ice as a cold stimulus (probably leading to an underestimate of the percentage of units responding to noxious cold) (Lynn and Carpenter 1982; Fleischer et al. 1983). Lynn and Carpenter (1982) reported 6% of C fibers to be cold-sensitive units, which were all mechanosensitive. Fleischer reported 14% of mechanically insensitive cold fibers for the saphenous nerve and 25% for the coccygeal nerve, which were primarily identified by their characteristic bursting spontaneous activity rather than by a systematic search. This finding could point to differences in the percentage of cold-specific fibers in different body regions, which might, however, be partly explained by a bias introduced by the different temperatures at these sites. A study using unbiased electrical search stimuli in vitro and in vivo found that 5% and 8% of the C fibers in the saphenous nerve of the rat were typical cold-sensitive receptors (Kress et al. 1992; Lewin and Mendell 1994). In vitro, 15% of C fibers were mechano-cold-sensitive (CMC) and 4% were mechano-heat and cold-sensitive (CMHC). In the rat, heat-insensitive CMC fibers were absent during in vivo recordings, even though these units were specifically sought and even though cold stimuli were applied for a time sufficient to result in temperatures close to freezing (Kress et al. 1992). The percentage of CMHC fibers among the unmyelinated afferents was 14% in vivo. Thus, approximately a third of the CMH fibers in the rat also respond to cold.

Cold sensitivity of primary afferents has not been extensively studied in mice, partially due to the difficulty of applying focal cold stimuli. One in vitro study using a mechanical search stimulus found that approximately 10–20% of C fibers were CMC and another 10–20% were CMHC. Approximately 10% of the myelinated nociceptors responded to cold. In mice, cold-specific fibers with ongoing activity are virtually absent at the organ bath temperature of 32°C, but they can be recruited by using a cold search stimulus. Studies in vivo have found that more than two-thirds of C fibers innervating the glabrous skin respond to cold below freezing temperatures (Cain et al. 2001) and that approximately 20% of C fibers are excited by stimuli in the range of 0°–20°C (D.A. Simone, personal communication).

Rodents and humans have a similar percentage of cold-sensitive afferent nociceptors. In humans, 40% of CMH fibers were also excited by non-freezing, noxious cold stimuli (Campero et al. 1996), whereas the percentage of C fibers responding to innocuous cold appeared to be slightly higher at approximately 15% (Serra et al. 1999; Campero et al. 2001).

If we assume that the functional properties of sensory neurons are represented in vitro, we can make the following estimates. Approximately 70–80% of the neurons in culture are C fibers, and most innervate skin. Some 5% represent visceral afferents, and 10–20% innervate muscle or other deep somatic tissues. This means that approximately 5% of cells in culture are cold-specific receptors and a third are either CMHC or CMC units. The prevalence of A fibers in each category would be 0.5% and 3%, respectively. No studies published to date have systematically investigated in rats or mice the percentage of CC, CMHC, or CMC fibers that respond to menthol or capsaicin.

Apart from anatomical studies that have localized many TRP channels to sensory neurons, significant evidence now indicates that TRP channels are the molecular correlate for many of the receptive properties of nociceptors. Heterologous expression studies have shown that TRPV1 (Caterina et al. 1997), TRPV2 (Caterina et al. 1999), TRPV3 (Peier et al. 2002b; Smith et al. 2002; Xu et al. 2002), and TRPV4 (Guler et al. 2002) respond to heat. Mutant mice lacking TRP channels have been very informative in revealing the contribution these channels make to the functional properties of sensory neurons. Capsaicin has long been known to specifically excite nociceptors, and mice lacking TRPV1 are completely insensitive to this and related irritants. They display a strongly reduced response to protons, which indicates that TRPV1 is a main transducer in the peripheral pain pathway (Caterina et al. 2000; Davis et al. 2000). TRPV1 knockout mice also show a reduced sensitivity to strong noxious heat stimuli. However, while the heat-induced currents of DRG in culture are completely abolished, sensory neurons recorded in situ retain a significant heat sensitivity (Caterina et al. 2000). This discrepancy is not fully understood. However, one possible explanation that would be compatible with these findings is that other heat-transducing receptors in the target tissue could release mediators and thereby indirectly excite heat-sensitive nociceptors by a TRPV1-independent mechanism. Indeed, other heat-sensitive TRP channels such as TRPV3 and TRPV4 are found in keratinocytes or other epithelial cells; although well positioned for such a task, their relatively low heat thresholds are not compatible with a role in nociception (Caterina 2003; Chung et al. 2003).

TRPV2 is a very strong candidate to mediate the heat sensitivity of thin myelinated nociceptors. TRPV2 is found in neurons that do not express TRPV1; their cells are larger than those of TRPV1-containing neurons and they are co-expressed with markers for myelinated fibers (Caterina et al. 1999). Importantly, the properties in the heterologous system resemble the heat currents in some capsaicin-insensitive sensory neurons recorded in culture (Nagy and Rang 1999). This finding has led to the suggestion that TRPV2 is the key heat-transducing molecule on myelinated capsaicin-insensitive nociceptors, whereas TRPV1 is the important heat sensor on thin myelinated and unmyelinated capsaicin-sensitive nociceptors (Caterina and Julius 2001).

Because both TRPV3 and TRPV4 are readily activated by innocuous temperatures, they are unlikely to play a significant role in nociception in isolation. However, because TRPV3 is found in many capsaicin-sensitive neurons, it may modulate the sensitivity of TRPV1, possibly by forming heteromultimers (Smith et al. 2002). TRPV4 shows a wide spectrum of sensitivity including heat, arachidonic acid derivatives, endocannabinoids, and hypo-osmolar stimuli (Guler et al. 2002; Nilius et al. 2003; Suzuki et al. 2003; Watanabe et al. 2003). Animals lacking TRPV4 reportedly have a mild impairment in their mechanical nociception (Suzuki et al. 2003). Interestingly, hypo-osmolar stimuli, leading to swelling of neurons, have been used in culture to simulate mechanical stimuli (Viana et al. 2001), and cells responding to this stimulus express TRPV4 (Alessandri-Haber et al. 2003).

TRP channels have also been identified as the crucial molecules in cold sensation (Jordt et al. 2003). TRPM8 is found in a small percentage of sensory neurons in the trigeminal and dorsal root ganglia. In heterologous expression studies, TRPM8 is activated by a small temperature decrease and is sensitized by the cooling compound menthol (McKemy et al. 2002; Peier et al. 2002a). The properties of this channel suggest that it mediates the excitation of non-nociceptive cold-sensitive neurons that signal innocuous cold (Konietzny 1984). However, many sensory neurons in the skin are also excited by noxious cold stimuli, and it is generally thought that these neurons do not respond to menthol. Another cold-sensitive TRP channel, TRPA1, has many properties that make it a strong candidate for mediating the excitation of cold-sensitive nociceptors. They include a restricted distribution among DRG neurons that also express markers for nociceptors (Story et al. 2003), a cold activation threshold in the noxious temperature range (Story et al. 2003), and a response to the irritant mustard oil (Jordt et al. 2004), which specifically excites nociceptors (Reeh et al. 1986). While the percentage of neurons expressing TRPM8 and responding to small temperature changes in culture corresponds to the proportion of cold-sensitive fibers recorded in peripheral nerves, the relatively low prevalence of TRPA1 and high-threshold cold responses in cultured native sensory neurons contrasts with the higher percentage of cold-sensitive nociceptors studied in peripheral nerves. This finding could indicate that other transduction mechanisms of cold are important; reduction of potassium conductances has been implicated as an important mechanism for the activation of neurons by cold (Viana et al. 2002).

ALTERED SENSITIVITY OF NOCICEPTORS
DURING TISSUE INFLAMMATION

The properties of nociceptors change profoundly following tissue injury and inflammation. The release of inflammatory mediators usually activates nociceptors; protons, bradykinin, serotonin, and prostaglandins (Reeh and Kress 1995) are among the most potent substances that excite nociceptive terminals, whereas non-nociceptive afferents typically are not affected (Reeh and Kress 1995; Handwerker 1996; Raja et al. 1999).

While a persistent change in excitability undoubtedly is partly the consequence of the maintained availability of mediators, evidence also suggests that chronic inflammation leads to long-lasting changes in the receptive properties of nociceptors. Nerve growth factor (NGF) appears to play a prominent role in this process of acute and long-term sensitization. The tissue concentration of NGF increases rapidly in inflammatory lesions (Donnerer et al. 1993; McMahon and Bennett 1997) or after application of proinflammatory cytokines, notably interleukin 1β or tumor necrosis factor α (Safieh-Garabedian et al. 1995; Woolf et al. 1997). Moreover, application of NGF to rodents results in profound hyperalgesia (Lewin and Mendell 1993). In the adult nervous system, many nociceptors express receptors for NGF. While all small-diameter sensory neurons require NGF during early development (Crowley et al. 1994), only a subpopulation of peptidergic neurons continues to express the NGF receptors trkA and p75 throughout adult life. Nonpeptidergic neurons express the receptor elements for the transforming growth factor β (TGFβ)-related neurotrophic factor, glial cell line-derived neurotrophic factor (GDNF), ret, and the GDNF-family receptor GFRα (Snider and McMahon 1998; Airaksinen et al. 1999). This finding suggests that NGF could sensitize the subpopulation of peptidergic (but not the nonpeptidergic) nociceptors.

During tissue inflammation, the hallmarks of an altered excitability of polymodal nociceptors are ongoing activity and strong sensitization to thermal, but usually not to mechanical, stimuli. At the onset of inflammation, the excitation of mechanically insensitive nociceptors appears to be particularly important for signaling some aspects of mechanical hyperalgesia (Schmidt et al. 1994; Schmelz et al. 2000; Koltzenburg et al. 2002). The intensity of the ongoing discharge of these nociceptors correlates with the magnitude of persistent pain and hyperalgesia to heat in humans (Treede et al. 1992; Koltzenburg 1995). Electrophysiological recordings of the receptive properties of thin myelinated and unmyelinated nociceptors innervating normal hairy skin or carrageenan-inflamed skin have shown a close correlation between nociceptor excitability and NGF (Koltzenburg et al. 1999). Following carrageenan inflammation, about half the nociceptors displayed ongoing activity that was only rarely observed in nociceptors innervating non-inflamed skin. Spontaneously active fibers were sensitized to heat, and a standard noxious heat stimulus provoked more than a two-fold increase in their discharge, but the same fibers showed no changes following mechanical stimuli. Furthermore, the number of nociceptors responding to the algesic mediator bradykinin increased significantly. When the NGF-neutralizing molecule trkA-IgG was co-administered with carrageenan at the onset of inflammation, primary afferent nociceptors did not sensitize and displayed essentially normal response properties, although the inflammation developed normally, as evidenced by tissue edema. Thus, endogenous NGF is an important factor in the sensitization of nociceptors, and it is tempting to suggest that the nociceptors that developed NGF-mediated ongoing activity are peptidergic neurons that express the trkA receptor. Studies of cultured DRG cells have extended these findings and have shown that NGF regulates capsaicin and bradykinin sensitivity (Bevan and Winter 1995; Petersen et al. 1998; Nicholas et al. 1999).

Several studies investigating the relative contribution of both NGF receptors have shown that the relative importance of trkA or p75 may depend on the functional context. Whereas p75-knockout mice develop a normal acute heat hyperalgesia to systemic injection of recombinant human NGF (Bergmann et al. 1998), DRG cells from these animals do not show the upregulation of bradykinin-binding sites that normally can be induced by NGF (Petersen et al. 1998). In contrast, several studies suggest that trkA mediates the acute effects of NGF that result in heat hyperalgesia (Lewin and Barde 1996). TRPV1 is an essential component for the behavioral manifestation of heat hyperalgesia, because mice lacking TRPV1 show a complete abolition of the behavioral correlates of hyperalgesia to heat, but not to mechanical stimuli (Caterina et al. 2000; Davis et al. 2000). The strong link between TRPV1 and inflammatory mediators for the generation of heat hyperalgesia is also apparent on a cellular level, and this interaction has at least two possible explanations that are not mutually exclusive. In the model of bradykinin-induced hyperalgesia, it appears that the activation of bradykinin type 2 receptors leads to the membrane translocation of protein kinase C epsilon (PKC-ε) (Cesare et al. 1999) and subsequent phosphorylation of TRPV1. Another possibility that may explain TRPV1 sensitization is the diminution of plasma membrane phosphatidylinositol-biphosphate through hydrolysis mediated by phospholipase C (PLC). Thus, the excitatory PKC-ε effects and the disinhibition mediated by PLC would in aggregate result in the sensitization of TRPV1 and hence of nociceptors.

In conclusion, increasing evidence implicates TRP channels as the key foundation for the different functional properties seen in a subpopulation of sensory neurons. While several TRP channels of the vanilloid family appear to be important for the signaling of normal heat, TRPM8 and possibly TRPA1 are cold sensors. TRPV1 and TRPA1 mediate the pungency of many irritant chemicals, including capsaicin and mustard oil. The role of TRP channels for mechanotransduction is less clear, although some studies have implicated TRPV4 for this important function. The specific and crucial involvement of TRPV1 in the generation of heat hyperalgesia demonstrates its important role in pathological conditions that lead to chronic pain.

REFERENCES

Adriaensen H, Gybels J, Handwerker HO, Van Hees J. Latencies of chemically evoked discharges in human cutaneous nociceptors and of the concurrent subjective sensations. *Neurosci Lett* 1980; 20:55–59.

Adriaensen H, Gybels J, Handwerker HO, Van Hees J. Response properties of thin myelinated (A-delta) fibers in human skin nerves. *J Neurophysiol* 1983; 49:111–122.

Airaksinen MS, Titievsky A, Saarma M. GDNF family neurotrophic factor signaling: four masters, one servant? *Mol Cell Neurosci* 1999; 13:313–325.

Alessandri-Haber N, Yeh JJ, Boyd AE, et al. Hypotonicity induces TRPV4-mediated nociception in rat. *Neuron* 2003; 39:497–511.

Beise RD, Carstens E, Kohlloffel LU. Psychophysical study of stinging pain evoked by brief freezing of superficial skin and ensuing short-lasting changes in sensations of cool and cold pain. *Pain* 1998; 74:275–286.

Bennett DLH, Koltzenburg M, Priestley JV, Shelton DL, McMahon SB. Endogenous nerve growth factor regulates the sensitivity of nociceptors in the adult rat. *Eur J Neurosci* 1998;10:1282–1291.

Bergmann I, Reiter R, Toyka KV, Koltzenburg M. Nerve growth factor evokes hyperalgesia in mice lacking the low-affinity neurotrophin receptor p75. *Neurosci Lett* 1998; 255:87–90.

Bevan S, Winter J. Nerve growth factor (NGF) differentially regulates the chemosensitivity of adult rat cultured sensory neurons. *J Neurosci* 1995; 15:4918–4926.

Bini G, Cruccu G, Hagbarth K-E, Schady W, Torebjörk E. Analgesic effect of vibration and cooling on pain induced by intraneural electrical stimulation. *Pain* 1984; 18:239–248.

Booth CS, Hahn JF. Thermal and mechanical stimulation of type II receptors and field receptors in the cat. *Exp Neurol* 1974; 44:49–59.

Burton H, Terashima S-I, Clark J. Response properties of slowly adapting mechanoreceptors to temperature stimulation in cats. *Brain Res* 1972; 45:401–416.

Cain DM, Khasabov SG, Simone DA. Response properties of mechanoreceptors and nociceptors in mouse glabrous skin: an in vivo study. *J Neurophysiol* 2001; 85:1561–1574.

Campero M, Serra J, Ochoa JL. C-polymodal nociceptors activated by noxious low temperature in human skin. *J Physiol* 1996; 497(Pt 2):565–572.

Campero M, Serra J, Bostock H, Ochoa JL. Slowly conducting afferents activated by innocuous low temperature in human skin. *J Physiol* 2001; 535:855–865.

Casey DE, Hahn JF. Thermal effects on response of cat touch corpuscle. *Exp Neurol* 1970; 28:35–45.

Caterina MJ. Vanilloid receptors take a TRP beyond the sensory afferent. *Pain* 2003; 105:5–9.

Caterina MJ, Julius D. The vanilloid receptor: a molecular gateway to the pain pathway. *Annu Rev Neurosci* 2001; 24:487–517.

Caterina MJ, Schumacher MA, Tominaga M, et al. The capsaicin receptor: a heat-activated ion channel in the pain pathway. *Nature* 1997; 389:816–824.

Caterina MJ, Rosen TA, Tominaga M, Brake AJ, Julius D. A capsaicin-receptor homologue with a high threshold for noxious heat. *Nature* 1999; 398:436–441.

Caterina MJ, Leffler A, Malmberg AB, et al. Impaired nociception and pain sensation in mice lacking the capsaicin receptor. *Science* 2000; 288:306–313.

Cesare P, Dekker LV, Sardini A, Parker PJ, McNaughton PA. Specific involvement of PKC-epsilon in sensitization of the neuronal response to painful heat. *Neuron* 1999; 23:617–624.

Chung MK, Lee H, Caterina MJ. Warm temperatures activate TRPV4 in mouse 308 keratinocytes. *J Biol Chem* 2003; 278:32037–32046.

Clapham DE. TRP channels as cellular sensors. *Nature* 2003; 426:517–524.

Clapham DE, Montell C, Schultz G, Julius D. International Union of Pharmacology. XLIII. Compendium of voltage-gated ion channels: transient receptor potential channels. *Pharmacol Rev* 2003; 55:591–596.

Craig AD, Reiman EM, Evans A, Bushnell MC. Functional imaging of an illusion of pain. *Nature* 1996; 384:258–260.

Crowley C, Spencer SD, Nishimura MC. Mice lacking nerve growth factor display perinatal loss of sensory and sympathetic neurons yet develop basal forebrain cholinergic neurons. *Cell* 1994; 76:1001–1011.

Davis JB, Gray J, Gunthorpe MJ, et al. Vanilloid receptor-1 is essential for inflammatory thermal hyperalgesia. *Nature* 2000; 405:183–187.

Davis KD. Cold-induced pain and prickle in the glabrous and hairy skin. *Pain* 1998; 75:47–57.

Dodt E, Zotterman Y. The discharge at specific cold fibres at high temperatures. (The paradoxical cold). *Acta Physiol Scand* 1952; 26:358–365.

Donnerer J, Schuligoi R, Stein C, Amann R. Upregulation, release and axonal transport of substance P and calcitonin gene-related peptide in adjuvant inflammation and regulatory function of nerve growth factor. *Regul Pept* 1993; 46:150–154.

Duclaux R, Kenshalo DR. The temperature sensitivity of the type I slowly adapting mechanoreceptors in cats and monkeys. *J Physiol (Lond)* 1972; 224:647–664.

Fleischer E, Handwerker HO, Joukhadar S. Unmyelinated nociceptive units in two skin areas of the rat. *Brain Res* 1983; 267:81–92.

Guler AD, Lee H, Iida T, et al. Heat-evoked activation of the ion channel, TRPV4. *J Neurosci* 2002; 22:6408–6414.

Gybels J, Handwerker HO, Van Hees J. A comparison between the discharges of human nociceptive nerve fibres and the subject's ratings of his sensations. *J Physiol (Lond)* 1979; 292:193–206.

Hamalainen H, Vartiainen M, Karvanen L, Jarvilehto T. Paradoxical heat sensations during moderate cooling of the skin. *Brain Res* 1982; 251:77–81.

Handwerker HO. Sixty years of C-fiber recordings from animal and human skin nerves: historical notes. *Prog Brain Res* 1996; 113:39–51.

Harrison JL, Davis KD. Cold-evoked pain varies with skin type and cooling rate: a psychophysical study in humans. *Pain* 1999; 83:123–135.

Hellon RF, Hensel H, Schafer K. Thermal receptors in the scrotum of the rat. *J Physiol* 1975; 248:349–357.

Hensel H, Schafer K. Effects of calcium on warm and cold receptors. *Pflügers Arch* 1974; 352:87–90.

Hensel H, Andres KH, von During M. Structure and function of cold receptors. *Pflügers Arch* 1974; 352:1–10.

Iggo A. Cutaneous thermoreceptors in primates and subprimates. *J Physiol (Lond)* 1969; 200:402–430.

Jordt SE, McKemy DD, Julius D. Lessons from peppers and peppermint: the molecular logic of thermosensation. *Curr Opin Neurobiol* 2003; 13:487–492.

Jordt SE, Bautista DM, Chuang HH, et al. Mustard oils and cannabinoids excite sensory nerve fibres through the TRP channel ANKTM1. *Nature* 2004; 427:260–265.

Koltzenburg M. The stability and plasticity of the encoding properties of peripheral nerve fibres and their relationship to provoked and ongoing pain. *Semin Neurosci* 1995; 7:199–210.

Koltzenburg M, Handwerker HO. Differential ability of human cutaneous nociceptors to signal mechanical pain and to produce vasodilatation. *J Neurosci* 1994; 14:1756–1765.

Koltzenburg M, Stucky CL, Lewin GR. Receptive properties of mouse sensory neurons innervating hairy skin. *J Neurophysiol* 1997; 78:1841–1850.

Koltzenburg M, Bennett DL, Shelton DL, McMahon SB. Neutralization of endogenous NGF prevents the sensitization of nociceptors supplying inflamed skin. *Eur J Neurosci* 1999; 11:1698–1704.

Koltzenburg M, Handwerker HO, Koerber HR. The differential effect of nociceptor subtypes for generating chronic pain. *Proceedings of the 10th World Congress on Pain,* Progress in Pain Research and Management, Vol. 24. Seattle: IASP Press, 2003, pp 141–153.

Konietzny F. Peripheral neural correlates of temperature sensation in man. *Hum Neurobiol* 1984; 3:21–32.

Kress M, Koltzenburg M, Reeh PW, Handwerker HO. Responsiveness and functional attributes of electrically localized terminals of cutaneous C-fibers in vivo and in vitro. *J Neurophysiol* 1992; 68:581–595.

LaMotte RH, Torebjörk HE, Robinson CJ, Thalhammer JG. Time-intensity profiles of cutaneous pain in normal and hyperalgesic skin: a comparison with C-fiber nociceptor activities in monkey and human. *J Neurophysiol* 1984; 51:1434–1450.

Leem JW, Willis WD, Chung JM. Cutaneous sensory receptors in the rat foot. *J Neurophysiol* 1993; 69:1684–1699.

Lewin GR, Barde Y-A. Physiology of the neurotrophins. *Ann Rev Neurosci* 1996; 19:289–317.

Lewin GR, Mendell LM. Nerve growth factor and nociception. *Trends Neurosci* 1993; 16:353–359.

Lewin GR, Mendell LM. Regulation of cutaneous C-fiber heat nociceptors by nerve growth factor in the developing rat. *J Neurophysiol* 1994; 71:941–949.

Long RR. Sensitivity of cutaneous cold fibers to noxious heat: paradoxical cold discharge. *J Neurophysiol* 1977; 40:489–502.

Lynn B, Carpenter SE. Primary afferent units from the hairy skin of the rat hindlimb. *Brain Res* 1982; 238:29–43.

Lynn B, Shakhanbeh J. Properties of A delta high threshold mechanoreceptors in the rat hairy and glabrous skin and their response to heat. *Neurosci Lett* 1988; 85:71–76.

Mackenzie RA, Burke D, Skuse NF, Lethlean AK. Fibre function and perception during cutaneous nerve block. *J Neurol Neurosurg Psychiatry* 1975; 38:865–873.

McKemy DD, Neuhausser WM, Julius D. Identification of a cold receptor reveals a general role for TRP channels in thermosensation. *Nature* 2002; 416:52–58.

McMahon SB, Bennett DLH. Growth factors and pain. In: Dickenson A, Besson J-M (Eds). *The Pharmacology of Pain.* Berlin: Springer Verlag, 1997, pp 135–165.

Meyer RA, Campbell JN, Raja SN. Peripheral neural mechanisms of nociception. In: Wall PD, Melzack R (Eds). *Textbook of Pain.* Edinburgh: Churchill Livingstone, 1994, pp 13–44.

Minke B, Cook B. TRP channel proteins and signal transduction. *Physiol Rev* 2002; 82:429–472.

Nagy I, Rang H. Noxious heat activates all capsaicin-sensitive and also a sub-population of capsaicin-insensitive dorsal root ganglion neurons. *Neuroscience* 1999; 88:995–997.

Nicholas RS, Winter J, Wren P, Bergmann R, Woolf CJ. Peripheral inflammation increases the capsaicin sensitivity of dorsal root ganglion neurons in an nerve growth factor-dependent manner. *Neuroscience* 1999; 91(4):1425-1433.

Nilius B, Watanabe H, Vriens J. The TRPV4 channel: structure-function relationship and promiscuous gating behaviour. *Pflügers Arch* 2003; 446:298–303.

Peier AM, Moqrich A, Hergarden AC, et al. A TRP channel that senses cold stimuli and menthol. *Cell* 2002a;108:705–715.

Peier AM, Reeve AJ, Andersson DA, et al. A heat-sensitive TRP channel expressed in keratinocytes. *Science* 2002b; 296(5575):2046–2049.

Petersen M, Segond von Banchet G, Heppelmann B, Koltzenburg M. Nerve growth factor regulates the expression of bradykinin binding sites on adult sensory neurons via the neurotrophin receptor p75. *Neuroscience* 1998; 83:161–168.

Pierau FK, Torrey P, Carpenter DO. Afferent nerve fiber activity responding to temperature changes of scrotal skin of the rat. *J Neurophysiol* 1975; 601–612.

Raja SN, Meyer RA, Ringkamp M, Campbell JN. Peripheral neural mechanisms of nociception. In: Wall PD, Melzack R (Eds). *Textbook of Pain.* Edinburgh: Churchill Livingstone, 1999, pp 11–57.

Reeh PW, Kress M. Effect of classic algogens. *Semin Neurosci* 1995; 7:221–226.

Reeh PW, Kocher L, Jung S. Does neurogenic inflammation alter the sensitivity of unmyelinated nociceptors in the rat? *Brain Res* 1986; 384:42–50.

Safieh-Garabedian B, Poole S, Allchorne A, Winter J, Woolf CJ. Contribution of interleukin-1 beta to the inflammation-induced increase in nerve growth factor levels and inflammatory hyperalgesia. *Br J Pharmacol* 1995; 115:1265–1275.

Schmelz M, Schmid R, Handwerker HO, Torebjörk HE. Encoding of burning pain from capsaicin-treated human skin in two categories of unmyelinated nerve fibres. *Brain* 2000; 123:560–571.

Schmelz M, Schmidt R, Weidner C, et al. Chemical response pattern of different classes of C-nociceptors to pruritogens and algogens. *J Neurophysiol* 2003; 89:2441–2448.

Schmidt RF, Schaible H-G, Messlinger K, et al. 1994; Silent and active nociceptors: structure, functions and clinical implications. In: Gebhart GF, Hammond DL, Jensen TL (Eds). *Proceedings of the 7th World Congress on Pain*, Progress in Pain Research and Management, Vol. 2. Seattle: IASP Press, 1994, pp 213–250.

Schmidt R, Schmelz M, Forster C, et al. Novel classes of responsive and unresponsive C nociceptors in human skin. *J Neurosci* 1995; 15:333–341.

Schmidt R, Schmelz M, Torebjork HE, Handwerker HO. Mechano-insensitive nociceptors encode pain evoked by tonic pressure to human skin. *Neuroscience* 2000; 98:793–800.

Serra J, Campero M, Ochoa J, Bostock H. Activity-dependent slowing of conduction differentiates functional subtypes of C fibres innervating human skin. *J Physiol* 1999; 515 (Pt 3):799–811.

Simone DA, Kajander KC. Excitation of rat cutaneous nociceptors by noxious cold. *Neurosci Lett* 1996; 213:53–56.

Simone DA, Kajander KC. Responses of cutaneous A-fiber nociceptors to noxious cold. *J Neurophysiol* 1997; 77:2049–2060.

Smith GD, Gunthorpe MJ, Kelsell RE, et al. TRPV3 is a temperature-sensitive vanilloid receptor-like protein. *Nature* 2002; 418:186–190.

Snider WD, McMahon SB. Tackling pain at source: new ideas about nociceptors. *Neuron* 1998; 20:629–632.

Story GM, Peier AM, Reeve AJ, et al. ANKTM1, a TRP-like channel expressed in nociceptive neurons, is activated by cold temperatures. *Cell* 2003; 112:819–829.

Susser E, Sprecher E, Yarnitsky D. Paradoxical heat sensation in healthy subjects: peripherally conducted by A delta or C fibres? *Brain* 1999; 122(Pt 2):239–246.

Suzuki M, Mizuno A, Kodaira K, Imai M. Impaired pressure sensation in mice lacking TRPV4. *J Biol Chem* 2003; 278:22664–22668.

Torebjörk HE, Hallin RG. Perceptual changes accompanying controlled preferential blocking of A and C fibre responses in intact human skin nerves. *Exp Brain Res* 1973; 16:321–332.

Treede R-D, Meyer RA, Raja SN, Campbell JN. Peripheral and central mechanisms of cutaneous hyperalgesia. *Prog Neurobiol* 1992; 38:397–421.

Trost C, Bergs C, Himmerkus N, Flockerzi V. The transient receptor potential, TRP4, cation channel is a novel member of the family of calmodulin binding proteins. *Biochem J* 2001; 355:663–670.

Van Hees J, Gybels J. C nociceptor activity in human nerve during painful and non painful skin stimulation. *J Neurol Neurosurg Psychiatry* 1981; 44:600–607.

Viana F, de la Pena E, Pecson B, Schmidt RF, Belmonte C. Swelling-activated calcium signalling in cultured mouse primary sensory neurons. *Eur J Neurosci* 2001; 13:722–734.

Viana F, de la Pena E, Belmonte C. Specificity of cold thermotransduction is determined by differential ionic channel expression. *Nat Neurosci* 2002; 5:254–260.

Vriens J, Watanabe H, Janssens A, et al. Cell swelling, heat, and chemical agonists use distinct pathways for the activation of the cation channel TRPV4. *Proc Natl Acad Sci USA* 2004; 101:396–401.

Wahren LK, Torebjork E, Jorum E. Central suppression of cold-induced C fibre pain by myelinated fibre input. *Pain* 1989; 38:313–319.

Wasner G, Schattschneider J, Binder A, Baron R. Topical menthol—a human model for cold pain by activation and sensitization of C nociceptors. *Brain* 2004; 127(Pt 5):1159–1171.

Watanabe H, Vriens J, Prenen J, et al. Anandamide and arachidonic acid use epoxyeicosatrienoic acids to activate TRPV4 channels. *Nature* 2003; 424:434–438.

Werner G, Mountcastle VB. Neural activity in mechanoreceptive cutaneous afferents: stimulus-response relations, Weber functions, and information transmission. *J Neurophysiol* 1965; 28:359–397.

Woolf CJ, Allchorne A, Safieh-Garabedian B, Poole S. Cytokines, nerve growth factor and inflammatory hyperalgesia: the contribution of tumour necrosis factor alpha. *Br J Pharmacol* 1997; 121:417–424.

Xu H, Ramsey IS, Kotecha SA, Moran MM, et al. TRPV3 is a calcium-permeable temperature-sensitive cation channel. *Nature* 2002; 418:181–186.

Yarnitsky D, Ochoa JL. Release of cold-induced burning pain by block of cold-specific afferent input. *Brain* 1990; 113:893–902.

Correspondence to: Martin Koltzenburg, Dr. med, FRCP, Neural Plasticity Unit, Institute of Child Health, University College London, 30 Guilford Street, London WC1N 1EH, United Kingdom. Email: m.koltzenburg@ich.ucl.ac.uk.

The Pain System in Normal and Pathological States:
A Primer for Clinicians, Progress in Pain Research
and Management, Vol. 31, edited by Luis Villanueva,
Anthony Dickenson, and Hélène Ollat, IASP Press,
Seattle, © 2004.

3

Peripheral Mechanisms of Allodynia and Other Forms of Hyperalgesia in Human Skin

Hermann O. Handwerker[a] and Martin Schmelz[b]

[a]Department of Physiology and Experimental Pathophysiology, University of Erlangen/Nürnberg, Erlangen, Germany; [b]Department of Anesthesiology, Mannheim Clinic, University of Heidelberg, Mannheim, Germany

Primary nociceptive afferents are unique among sensory receptors in their capacity to become sensitized following exposure to noxious stimuli. Consequences of sensitization are increased spike discharges to stimulation and decreased thresholds. These phenomena may be formally conceptualized as a leftward shift of the stimulus-response function. Hyperalgesia was traditionally seen as the perceptual correlate of sensitization, and indeed, it encompasses decreased pain threshold and increased pain responses to suprathreshold stimuli, together with spontaneous pain. However, the simple concept of hyperalgesia as a linear corollary of sensitization of a uniform nociceptor population is inadequate, given the complexity of the phenomenon.

DIFFERENT FORMS OF HYPERALGESIA

Hyperalgesias fall into two categories with regard to pathophysiology. *Hyperalgesias in neuropathies* are a consequence of pathological alterations in the function and structure of the primary afferent neuron, whereas *hyperalgesias in inflammatory diseases* are due to the reactive adaptations of the nociceptor terminals to pathological processes in the surrounding tissue. Remarkably, similar forms of hyperalgesias may arise under both conditions. Thus, a second differentiation that is even more important concerns the modality and quality of stimuli to which nociceptors become sensitized. A third important distinction is that between *primary* and *secondary*

45

hyperalgesias, which has not uniformly been made in the literature. The term "primary" often labels forms of hyperalgesia assumed to be due to sensitization of primary afferent nociceptors, and the term "secondary" labels forms in which the neuronal correlate is thought to be plasticity of central synaptic processes. However, lack of proof of the neuronal mechanisms of hyperalgesia means that the labels "primary" and "secondary" may lead to circular arguments. It appears more practical to attach "primary" to all forms of hyperalgesia that are confined to the area of the pathological process—the primary zone. "Secondary" hyperalgesias are those observed in the primary zone and also in unaffected areas outside the inflamed area or the innervation territory of a neuropathic nerve.

EXPERIMENTAL MODELS FOR APPLICATION IN HUMAN SKIN

Experimental models for application in human skin have been developed to study cutaneous hyperalgesias in the absence of the confounding aspects of disease. In one such model capsaicin is topically applied to a small patch of skin to mimic the sensitization of nociceptors by inflammatory processes (Kilo et al. 1994). A localized burn served the same purpose in other studies (Moiniche et al. 1993). For a more sustained form of inflammation, Kilo et al. (1994) briefly exposed small patches of skin to freezing. Psychophysical methods have been used, sometimes in combination with the assessment of vascular reactions (Koppert et al. 1999, 2000), to study the intensity and time course of the different forms of hyperalgesia. In addition, the technique of microneurography (the percutaneous recording of single nerve fibers) has made it possible to study nociceptor plasticity directly in alert human subjects (Torebjörk et al. 1996). Three decades ago, Torebjörk and Hallin (1970) first adapted this technique to recordings of human afferent C fibers. Since that time, other studies have extensively used this technique to study the discharge patterns of human cutaneous, and to a lesser extent, of muscle C-fiber nociceptors (Marchettini et al. 1996). The development of a refined "marking technique" that employs the post-excitatory slowing of unmyelinated axons for identification and characterization made it possible to study for many hours the spike responses from single C-fiber units in healthy subjects (Schmidt et al. 1995). This approach has now been extended to studies of patients suffering from neuropathies (Campero et al. 1998; Orstavik et al. 2003). Comparing the responses of alert subjects with their nociceptor discharges gives a much clearer picture of the contribution of peripheral and central mechanisms to different forms of hyperalgesia.

HYPERALGESIA TO THERMAL STIMULI

Numerous psychophysical and microneurographic experiments have studied hyperalgesia to heating. This form of hyperalgesia gave rise to the concept of hyperalgesia as a perceptual correlate of peripheral sensitization of primary nociceptive afferents. In addition, the "spontaneous pain" from inflamed tissue can be interpreted as a drop of nociceptor thresholds to the range of ambient (or slightly increased) temperature in the inflamed tissue (Liang et al. 2001). Alleviation of inflammatory pain by cooling supports this concept. Microneurographic studies have proven that the development of heat hyperalgesia runs parallel with sensitization of polymodal, mechano-heat-responsive, mostly unmyelinated nociceptors (LaMotte et al. 1982; Torebjörk et al. 1984). Interestingly, no clear secondary heat hyperalgesia has been observed (Ali et al. 1996). Likewise, C-mechano-heat and mechano-insensitive nociceptors in the skin surrounding a trauma are generally not sensitized. In human skin, a study of nociceptor units with widely spaced branches showed that sensitization of one branch did not induce changes in others of the same unit (Schmelz et al. 1996).

The recent discovery of the TRPV1 membrane receptor, also known as the capsaicin receptor, offers a hypothetical molecular mechanism of sensitization to heating. This cation channel contributing to the depolarization of the nociceptor terminals by heating may dramatically lower their thresholds when phosphorylated by protein kinases A or C, which are activated by G proteins coupled to membrane receptors of vaso-neuroactive substances such as prostaglandins and bradykinin (Kress and Zeilhofer 1999).

HYPERALGESIA TO COLD

Hyperalgesia to cold is a clinically important phenomenon because it is characteristic of certain forms of neuropathies. However, its mechanism is still enigmatic. The evidence for peripheral sensitization of nociceptive afferents is sparse, perhaps because only a few studies have investigated the peripheral encoding of noxious cold stimuli (Campero et al. 1996; Simone and Kajander 1997). The assumption is that there is central sensitization to non-nociceptive cold-fiber input or central disinhibition by selective loss of a sensory channel specific for non-noxious cold that normally exerts a tonic inhibition of nociceptive channels (Wahren et al. 1989; Yarnitsky and Ochoa 1990; Craig and Bushnell 1994).

HYPERALGESIA TO MECHANICAL STIMULI

Studies have described various forms of mechanical hyperalgesia based on the type of stimulus applied. Increased pain sensitivity occurs at the site of injury with *blunt mechanical pressure* applied for several seconds (pressure hyperalgesia), and also with brief *impact stimulation* by small plastic bullets shot toward a skin site (Kohlloffel et al. 1991; Kilo et al. 1994). Both forms of hyperalgesia are restricted to the site of an experimental trauma and thus may be largely due to peripheral sensitization of nociceptors. However, microneurographic studies have not revealed a convincing sensitization to mechanical stimulation in the largest nociceptor population, the mechano-heat-responsive C nociceptors (CMH units) (Schmelz et al. 1996, 2000b). However, mechanically insensitive C nociceptors can be sensitized by repetitive noxious stimulation; they then respond readily to subsequent mechanical stimuli (Schmidt et al. 1995; Schmelz et al. 2000b). This phenomenon has prompted the poetic label "sleeping nociceptors," although these nociceptors often initially respond to chemical irritants and to heating (Schmidt et al. 1995; Schmelz et al. 2000b). These units in human skin nerves have been named CMi for mechanoinsensitive C units. A similar type was previously described in monkey skin and named Mia for mechano-sensitive afferents (Meyer et al. 1991). Some Aδ fibers also may contribute to the increased population response in inflamed tissue, and suprathreshold responses to mechanical stimuli might be enhanced in certain mechano-sensitive polymodal nociceptors (Andrew and Greenspan 1999). Recruitment of mechano-insensitive nociceptive afferents will lead to enhanced synaptic input in the central nervous system by spatial summation. Both blunt pressure and impact stimuli induce only primary hyperalgesia in the models using capsaicin and freezing, as mentioned above (Kilo et al. 1994).

Two other forms of mechanical hyperalgesia are not restricted to the primary zone: *hyperalgesia to pinprick* and to *stroking the skin with a soft brush or a swab of cotton wool* (LaMotte et al. 1991). Pinprick excites a few nociceptors in a very restricted area. Aδ units, with their more extended terminal branching and their higher discharge rates, might be more relevant for this type of input than are C-fiber nociceptors. Nonsensitized mechano-insensitive nociceptors are not excited by pinprick. In contrast, stroking the skin with a soft brush excites only sensitive mechanoreceptors with fast-conducting Aβ axons. Brush-evoked hyperalgesia has thus been named "allodynia," i.e., hyperalgesia to another form of input, namely activation of the "touch" channel.

Both pinprick and brush hyperalgesia have been observed in extended skin areas in the experimental models described above. The former type usually covers a broader area and persists longer after a trauma (LaMotte et al. 1991; Kilo et al. 1994). Table I summarizes the types of hyperalgesia occurring in the experimental models using capsaicin and freezing.

NEURONAL MECHANISMS OF SECONDARY HYPERALGESIA

The brush and pinprick forms of secondary hyperalgesia show one remarkable difference. In the capsaicin model, but also in certain forms of neuropathies (Koltzenburg et al. 1992; Ochoa and Yarnitsky 1993), hyperalgesia elicited by stroking or brushing depends on continuous input from sensitized C-fiber nociceptors in the traumatized area. Because this input probably constitutes burning pain, a close correlation between ongoing pain and the extension of brush hyperalgesia is not surprising (Koltzenburg et al. 1994). Cooling an inflamed or capsaicin-treated skin area alleviates the burning pain and abolishes brush hyperalgesia. In a microneurographic study, Torebjörk et al. (1992) demonstrated that microstimulation of a mechanosensitive A-fiber-induced touch sensation in normal skin. However, the same input induced pain when the expanding secondary zone after intracutaneous capsaicin injection reached the "perceptive field" to which the stimulated A fiber projected. As soon as the capsaicin effect leveled off and the expanding zone of secondary hyperalgesia shrank, the sensory quality evoked by stimulating this A-fiber mechanosensor switched back to touch (Torebjörk et al. 1992). This experiment shows clearly that brush hyperalgesia is induced by A-fiber input that is gated into the pain pathway by continuous afferent barrage of C nociceptors from a traumatic focus.

Table I
Forms of hyperalgesia in two experimental models

Form of Hyperalgesia/Pain	Capsaicin	Freezing
Heat hyperalgesia	Primary zone	Primary zone
Pressure hyperalgesia	Primary zone	Primary zone
Impact hyperalgesia	–	Primary zone
Brush hyperalgesia	Primary and secondary zones	–
Hyperalgesia to punctate stimuli	Primary and secondary zones	Primary and secondary zones
Background pain	Ongoing	–

Source: Adapted from Kilo et al. (1994).
Note: Capsaicin was topically applied to the skin at the volar side of the lower arm to a patch of about 1 cm^2. It induced burning pain and hyperalgesia for less than 1 hour. Freezing a skin patch of similar size lead to hyperalgesia, but no ongoing pain was prominent 24 hours after the trauma.

Pinprick hyperalgesia does not depend in the same way on continuous input from a traumatized region. The units responsible are capsaicin-insensitive Aδ nociceptors (Meyer et al. 1998; Ziegler et al. 1999; Magerl et al. 2001). Notably, hyperalgesia to punctate stimuli involves facilitation of a nociceptive input that is painful even in normal skin; this form of pain is a quantitative rather than a qualitative phenomenon. Perceived pain increases with no remarkable change in quality of perception, which does not require cross-talk of a non-nociceptive input into nociceptive pathways as in brush hyperalgesia (allodynia). Nevertheless, in the case of punctate hyperalgesia, we must also assume that the Aδ input from the secondary zone is gated by processes of synaptic plasticity induced by the nociceptive input from the traumatized region. Table II summarizes the hypotheses regarding the neuronal mechanisms of different forms of mechanical hyperalgesias in two experimental models.

PERIPHERAL FLARE RESPONSES AND ZONES OF SECONDARY HYPERALGESIA

Topical application of capsaicin to a patch of skin not larger than 1 cm^2, or intracutaneous injection of a few microliters of capsaicin solution, may

Table II
Different forms of mechanical hyperalgesia and their hypothetic neuronal mechanism

Stimulus	Models	Location	Primary Afferents	Possible Neural Mechanisms
Blunt pressure	Capsaicin, freeze	Primary zone	Sensitization of mechano-insensitive nociceptors	Peripheral sensitization and recruitment, spatial summation at central neurons
Impact stimuli	Freeze	Primary zone	Nociceptors (mainly mechano-insensitive C fibers)	Peripheral sensitization and recruitment, spatial summation at central neurons
Brush, stroking with cotton swab	Capsaicin	Primary and secondary zones	Low threshold mechano-sensitive Aβ afferent units	Central plasticity, induced and sustained by persistent peripheral nociceptor activity in the primary zone
Punctate stimuli	Capsaicin, freeze	Primary and secondary zones	Nociceptors (Aδ fibers)	Central plasticity, induced, but not dependent on further peripheral nociceptor input

Source: Adapted from Kilo et al. (1994).

induce extended flare reactions in the surrounding skin. The areas are often very similar to the area of brush hyperalgesia arising simultaneously (Simone et al. 1989). Therefore, it is tempting—although probably misleading—to assume a direct link between the two phenomena (Serra et al. 1998).

The flare response is caused by release of vasoactive neuropeptides (calcitonin gene-related peptide and substance P) from axon collaterals that are antidromically invaded from axon branches affected by the capsaicin. In microneurographic experiments we were able to prove that the flare reaction largely depends on the excitation of mechano-insensitive C fibers (Schmelz et al. 2000a) and that the size of the flare is comparable to the extended receptive fields of these nerve fibers in human skin (Schmidt et al. 2002). This fiber class has a higher electrical threshold to percutaneous stimulation compared to the more common mechano-heat-responsive (polymodal) nociceptors (Weidner et al. 1999), and we were able to induce a flare response electrically only by stimuli sufficiently strong to recruit mechano-insensitive C-units. To test whether brush and pinprick hyperalgesias can be induced by a peripheral, axon-reflex-related mechanism in such an experiment, we blocked the spike propagation in cutaneous axon collaterals by

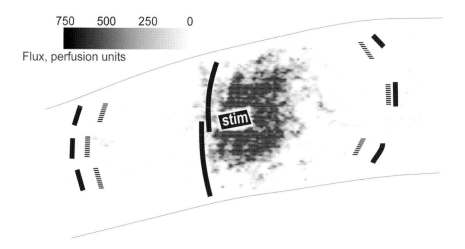

Fig. 1. Blockade of the neurogenic flare response, but not of the extension of mechanical hyperalgesia, by an anesthetic strip. Flare and secondary mechanical hyperalgesia were induced by electrical excitation of mechano-insensitive nociceptors (stim) on the volar side of the lower forearm of a human subject while lidocaine was perfused through two intracutaneous microdialysis membranes (diameter 0.4 mm, cut-off 3 MDa). The extension of the flare response was assessed using a laser Doppler scanner. The extension of touch hyperalgesia (hatched lines) and to pinprick hyperalgesia (solid lines) was determined. While the anesthetic strip effectively stopped the spread of the axon reflex flare, it did not alter the distribution of the mechanical hyperalgesias, proving their "secondary" nature and central origin (for details see Klede et al. 2003).

lidocaine perfusion through a microdialysis membrane. This localized anesthetic strip effectively stopped the expansion of the axon reflex flare measured by laser-Doppler scanning, but did not affect the extension of the areas of secondary hyperalgesia to brush and pinprick (Klede et al. 2003; see Fig. 1).

We may assume that the extension of the flare response reflects the extension of peripheral receptive fields, i.e., of the peripheral branching of primary afferent mechano-insensitive nociceptor units. The areas of secondary hyperalgesia, however, are related to the much more complex receptive areas of central neurons with their normally mixed excitatory and inhibitory input.

CONCLUSIONS

Hyperalgesia cannot be explained by one single peripheral or central mechanism. Different forms of hyperalgesia are mediated by quite different peripheral and probably also central mechanisms. In clinical studies it is important to distinguish between hyperalgesias according to: (1) neuropathic or inflammatory origin; (2) extension only to the primary zone of a trauma or also into a secondary zone; (3) stimulus modality and quality, e.g., thermal or mechanical; and (4) stimulus form and dynamics.

Experimental models applied to human volunteers have shown that different forms of trauma induce different patterns of hyperalgesia. Microneurographic experiments allow a differentiation of the sensory input in skin nerves leading to these different forms of neuropathy. These results have led to hypotheses on the neuronal mechanisms underlying hyperalgesia that may now be used to develop new therapeutic strategies.

ACKNOWLEDGMENT

The work of the authors has been supported by the Deutsche Forschungs gemeinschaft and by the BMBF Network for Neuropathic Pain.

REFERENCES

Ali Z, Meyer RA, Campbell JN. Secondary hyperalgesia to mechanical but not heat stimuli following a capsaicin injection in hairy skin. *Pain* 1996; 68:401–411.
Andrew D, Greenspan JD. Mechanical and heat sensitization of cutaneous nociceptors after peripheral inflammation in the rat. *J Neurophysiol* 1999; 82:2649–2656.
Campero M, Serra J, Ochoa JL. C-polymodal nociceptors activated by noxious low temperature in human skin. *J Physiol* 1996; 497(Pt 2):565–572.

Campero M, Serra J, Marchettini P, Ochoa JL. Ectopic impulse generation and autoexcitation in single myelinated afferent fibers in patients with peripheral neuropathy and positive sensory symptoms. *Muscle Nerve* 1998; 21:1661–1667.

Craig AD, Bushnell MC. The thermal grill illusion: unmasking the burn of cold pain. *Science* 1994; 265:252–255.

Kilo S, Schmelz M, Koltzenburg M, Handwerker HO. Different patterns of hyperalgesia induced by experimental inflammations in human skin. *Brain* 1994; 117:385–396.

Klede M, Handwerker HO, Schmelz M. Central origin of secondary mechanical hyperalgesia. *J Neurophysiol* 2003; 90:353–359.

Kohlloffel LU, Koltzenburg M, Handwerker HO. A novel technique for the evaluation of mechanical pain and hyperalgesia. *Pain* 1991; 46:81–87.

Koltzenburg M, Lundberg LE, Torebjörk HE. Dynamic and static components of mechanical hyperalgesia in human hairy skin. *Pain* 1992; 51:207–219.

Koltzenburg M, Torebjörk HE, Wahren LK. Nociceptor modulated central sensitization causes mechanical hyperalgesia in acute chemogenic and chronic neuropathic pain. *Brain* 1994; 117:579–591.

Koppert W, Zeck S, Blunk JA, et al. The effects of intradermal fentanyl and ketamine on capsaicin-induced secondary hyperalgesia and flare reaction. *Anesth Analg* 1999; 89:1521–1527.

Koppert W, Ostermeier N, Sittl R, Weidner C, Schmelz M. Low-dose lidocaine reduces secondary hyperalgesia by a central mode of action. *Pain* 2000; 85:217–224.

Kress M, Zeilhofer HU. Capsaicin, protons and heat: new excitement about nociceptors. *Trends Pharmacol Sci* 1999; 20:112–118.

LaMotte RH, Thalhammer JG, Torebjörk HE, Robinson CJ. Peripheral neural mechanisms of cutaneous hyperalgesia following mild injury by heat. *J Neurosci* 1982; 2:765–781.

LaMotte RH, Shain CN, Simone DA, Tsai EFP. Neurogenic hyperalgesia psychophysical studies of underlying mechanisms. *J Neurophysiol* 1991; 66:190–211.

Liang YF, Haake B, Reeh PW. Sustained sensitization and recruitment of rat cutaneous nociceptors by bradykinin and a novel theory of its excitatory action. *J Physiol* 2001; 532:229–239.

Magerl W, Fuchs PN, Meyer RA, Treede RD. Roles of capsaicin-insensitive nociceptors in cutaneous pain and secondary hyperalgesia. *Brain* 2001; 124:1754–1764.

Marchettini P, Simone DA, Caputi G, Ochoa JL. Pain from excitation of identified muscle nociceptors in humans. *Brain Res* 1996; 740:109–116.

Meyer RA, Davis KD, Cohen RH, Campbell JN. Mechanically insensitive afferents (Mias) in cutaneous nerves of monkey. *Brain Res* 1991; 561:252–261.

Meyer RA, Magerl W, Campbell JN, Treede RD, Fuchs PN. Normal punctate hyperalgesia in capsaicin desensitized skin. *Soc Neurosci Abstr* 1998; 24:2086.

Moiniche S, Dahl JB, Kehlet H. Time course of primary and secondary hyperalgesia after heat injury to the skin. *Br J Anaesth* 1993; 71:201–205.

Ochoa JL, Yarnitsky D. Mechanical hyperalgesias in neuropathic pain patients: dynamic and static subtypes. *Ann Neurol* 1993; 33:465–472.

Orstavik K, Weidner C, Schmidt R, et al. Pathological C-fibres in patients with a chronic painful condition. *Brain* 2003; 126:567–578.

Schmelz M, Schmidt R, Ringkamp M, et al. Limitation of sensitization to injured parts of receptive fields in human skin C-nociceptors. *Exp Brain Res* 1996; 109:141–147.

Schmelz M, Michael K, Weidner C, et al. Which nerve fibers mediate the axon reflex flare in human skin? *Neuroreport* 2000a; 11:645–648.

Schmelz M, Schmidt R, Handwerker HO, Torebjörk HE. Encoding of burning pain from capsaicin-treated human skin in two categories of unmyelinated nerve fibres. *Brain* 2000b; 123:560–571.

Schmidt R, Schmelz M, Forster C, et al. Novel classes of responsive and unresponsive C nociceptors in human skin. *J Neurosci* 1995; 15:333–341.

Schmidt R, Schmelz M, Weidner C, Handwerker HO, Torebjörk HE. Innervation territories of mechano-insensitive C nociceptors in human skin. *J Neurophysiol* 2002; 88:1859–1866.

Serra J, Campero M, Ochoa J. Flare and hyperalgesia after intradermal capsaicin injection in human skin. *J Neurophysiol* 1998; 80:2801–2810.

Simone DA, Kajander KC. Responses of cutaneous A fiber nociceptors to noxious cold. *J Neurophysiol* 1997; 77:2049–2060.

Simone DA, Baumann TK, LaMotte RH. Dose-dependent pain and mechanical hyperalgesia in humans after intradermal injection of capsaicin. *Pain* 1989; 38:99–107.

Torebjörk HE, Hallin RG. C-fibre units recorded from human sensory nerve fascicles in situ: a preliminary report. *Acta Soc Med Ups* 1970; 75:81–84.

Torebjörk HE, LaMotte RH, Robinson CJ. Peripheral neural correlates of magnitude of cutaneous pain and hyperalgesia: simultaneous recordings in humans of sensory judgments of pain and evoked responses in nociceptors with C-fibers. *J Neurophysiol* 1984; 51:325–339.

Torebjörk HE, Lundberg LE, LaMotte RH. Central changes in processing of mechanoreceptive input in capsaicin-induced secondary hyperalgesia in humans. *J Physiol (Lond)* 1992; 448:765–780.

Torebjörk HE, Schmelz M, Handwerker HO. Functional properties of human cutaneous nociceptors and their role in pain and hyperalgesia. 1996; 349–369.

Wahren LK, Torebjörk HE, Jorum E. Central suppression of cold-induced C fibre pain by myelinated fibre input. *Pain* 1989; 38:313–319.

Weidner C, Schmelz M, Schmidt R, et al. Functional attributes discriminating mechano-insensitive and mechano-responsive C nociceptors in human skin. *J Neurosci* 1999; 19:10184–10190.

Yarnitsky D, Ochoa JL. Release of cold-induced burning pain by block of cold-specific afferent input. *Brain* 1990; 113:893–902.

Ziegler EA, Magerl W, Meyer RA, Treede RD. Secondary hyperalgesia to punctate mechanical stimuli—central sensitization to A-fibre nociceptor input. *Brain* 1999; 122:2245–2257.

Correspondence to: Prof. Hermann O. Handwerker, Dr med, Department of Physiology and Experimental Pathophysiology, University of Erlangen/Nürnberg, Universitätsstr. 17, D-91054 Erlangen, Germany. Tel: 9131-85-22400; Fax: 9131-85-22497; email: handwerker@physiologie1.uni-erlangen.de.

Part II

Dorsal Horn Plasticity following Injury

The Pain System in Normal and Pathological States:
A Primer for Clinicians, Progress in Pain Research
and Management, Vol. 31, edited by Luis Villanueva,
Anthony Dickenson, and Hélène Ollat, IASP Press,
Seattle, © 2004.

4

Molecular Approaches to the Study of Pain

Stephen P. Hunt

Department of Anatomy and Developmental Biology,
University College London, London, United Kingdom

Over the past few years we have begun to understand, using a variety of experimental approaches, the cellular and molecular mechanisms by which the flow of nociceptive information into the spinal cord is transmitted to higher centers of the brain and how this input is in turn regulated by descending pathways from the brainstem under the control of the forebrain. Researchers have gradually identified molecular changes within the dorsal horn of the spinal cord that may contribute to the increase in pain sensitivity that accompanies injury to the periphery and have come to a greater understanding of how the major pain pathways work together to ensure that nociception is appropriately regulated within the prevailing environmental context of the behaving animal. Yet chronic pain remains poorly understood (Besson 1999). This chapter considers molecular aspects of nociceptive signaling within the context of the neural systems that interact to synthesize the experience of pain.

PRIMARY AFFERENT TERMINATION WITHIN THE SPINAL CORD

Somatosensory information reaches the spinal cord and areas of the brainstem through primary afferent sensory fibers. Sensory fibers terminate within the 10 designated laminae (I–X) of the spinal cord in a highly reproducible and characteristic fashion depending upon their diameter, biochemical composition, and receptive field properties (Fig. 1) (Nagy and Hunt 1982; Hunt and Rossi 1985; Snider and McMahon 1998; Hunt and Mantyh 2001). Nociceptive information is relayed to spinal cord neurons throughout

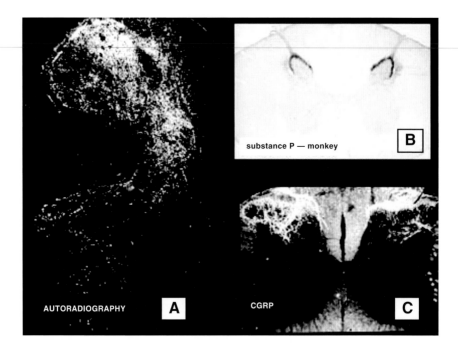

Fig. 1. (A) Titrated amino acid injection into the L4 dorsal root ganglion to show the extent of primary afferent termination within the spinal cord (Nagy and Hunt 1983). (B) Substance P immunoreactivity in the spinal cord of the rhesus monkey (unpublished). (C) Calcitonin gene-related peptide (CGRP) immunoreactivity in the rat spinal cord. The right sciatic nerve had been sectioned 7 days before perfusion.

the dorsal horn, particularly within laminae I–II and V–VII, but largely avoids populations of neurons within laminae III–IV, which receive, almost exclusively, non-nociceptive information from Aβ sensory afferents (Todd 2002). Neurons within laminae I–II and V–VI receive nociceptive information through unmyelinated C fibers and finely myelinated Aδ sensory afferents. C fibers, which form the major part of the sensory input to the dorsal horn, can be further divided into almost equal numbers of peptide-containing and nonpeptide-expressing neurons that stain for isolectin B4 (IB4) (Hunt and Rossi 1985) (Fig. 2). Nociceptive information from the skin is distributed between laminae I–II and V, while visceral, joint, and muscle input terminates largely within laminae I and V, avoiding lamina II (Nagy and Hunt 1982; De Groat 1986; Cervero and Laird 1999; Lawson 2002). However, while projection neurons in lamina I receive peptidergic C-fiber input from the whole of the body, neurons from laminae I and V, the origins of two of the major ascending pathways, potentially receive all types of nociceptive input (Craig 2002).

NOCICEPTIVE PATHWAYS FROM THE DORSAL HORN

Neurons that relay nociceptive information to the brain are located primarily in laminae I, III, V–VII, and X (Bernard and Bandler 1998; Todd 2002; Gauriau and Bernard 2004a). Considerable attention has recently focused on the pathway arising largely from lamina I neurons, and many of the functions once ascribed to the deeper pathways are now being reallocated to this

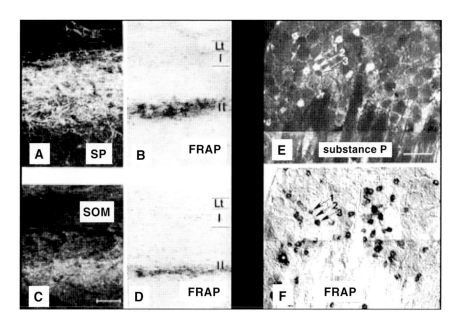

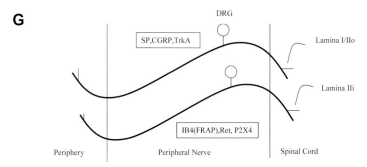

Fig. 2. Parasagittal sections of the spinal cord showing the distributions, generally only partially overlapping, of (A) substance P (SP), (B,D) fluoride-resistant acid phosphatase (FRAP), and (C) somatostatin (SOM) both within the dorsal horn (A–D) and dorsal root ganglion (E and F) (from Nagy and Hunt 1982). (G) The concept of two C-fiber pathways identified by different biochemical signatures and terminating within different areas of the dorsal horn but carrying similar nociceptive information (Hunt and Rossi 1985).

pathway arising from the most superficial layer of the dorsal horn. Retro-grade and anterograde pathway tracing techniques have greatly improved in sensitivity, prompting a reappraisal of the connections of spinal projection neurons (see Bernard and Gauriau, this volume). Species differences are also important, as is the level of the spinal cord at which the analysis is made; the cervical cord is very different from the lumbar cord, which has traditionally received more attention. However, there has also been a shift in the way that various functions have been allocated to particular pathways, particularly in terms of the affective, discriminative, and homeostatic dimensions of pain (Craig 2002; Gauriau and Bernard 2004a). Finally, chemical lesioning tech-niques have been introduced that specifically destroy subpopulations of lamina I neurons and effectively dissociate the lamina I projection from the deeper-lying nociceptive pathways that project upon the brainstem without disrupt-ing descending pathways (Mantyh et al. 1997; Nichols et al. 1999). This dissociation has permitted the behavioral assessment of the role played by particular pathways in nociceptive behavior and has led to a rethinking of the contribution of the different spinal projections to acute and chronic pain behaviors (see Dickenson et al., this volume).

The lamina I pathway has been repeatedly described in numerous stud-ies both in a variety of animals and in humans, where it is thought to have reached the highest degree of differentiation. Several sites of termination of the pathway have been described that hint at its function both in homeostatic regulation and in supplying information to areas of the brain concerned with discrimination, affect, and motor and autonomic regulation (Craig 2002; Gauriau and Bernard 2004a). Only a small percentage of superficial dorsal horn neurons are projection neurons (Todd 2002); they are found mainly in lamina I (Bester et al. 1997, 2000), but with a small contribution from laminae III and IV (Ding et al. 1995; Naim et al. 1997; Todd 2002). Strik-ingly, projection neurons, which comprise only 10% of the lamina I neuron population, are largely nociceptive, receiving input from C and Aδ nociceptors and responding to noxious thermal and mechanical stimulation (Bester et al. 2000; Lawson 2002). Up to 90% of these projection neurons express the substance P-preferring neurokinin-1 (NK1) receptor (Todd et al. 2002). These neurons, which have small receptive fields, receive nociceptive information from all areas of the body and have axons that terminate within the sympa-thetic preganglionic motor column of the thoracic cord, in the medulla, and throughout other regions of the brainstem as far rostral as the thalamus. These areas of termination can be broken down, somewhat artificially, into areas concerned with sympathetic regulation, affect, cognition, motor con-trol, and sensory discrimination. In a recent description of this pathway in rats using anterograde tracing techniques, termination was described predominantly in the parabrachial area (which subsequently projects upon the amygdala and hypothalamus) and in the posterior, mediodorsal, and ventrobasal thalamic nuclei. Subsequent thalamic projections innervate areas of the insular, premotor, and somatosensory cortices involved in affective, cognitive, and discriminative aspects of pain processing, respectively (Craig 2002; Gauriau and Bernard 2004a,b).

In contrast, the projections from the deeper dorsal horn, principally lamina V, terminate in brainstem areas notably associated with arousal and motor functions. Some of these deep projections synapse as far rostrally as the basal ganglia and within thalamic nuclei that project upon the motor cortex, emphasizing the role of this projection in arousal and in motor responses to injury rather than in discrimination. However, termination in areas of the thalamus related to the primary somatosensory cortex has been reported, particularly in primates (Willis et al. 2001). The division of function between the deep and superficial "pain" pathways thus may not be complete (for example in the posterior thalamus), and there may well be shared functional capacities. Similarly, many of the areas to which lamina V neurons project in the hindbrain subsequently project rostrally onto areas of the thalamus that receive direct lamina I projections from the spinal cord, further complicating any simple distinction between the contributions of the two spinal ascending projections to pain behavior (Villanueva et al. 1996, 1998; Monconduit et al. 2002). Recent evidence, however, supports the view that the lamina I pathway is crucial for the regulation of spinal cord excitability, and therefore pain behavior, primarily through privileged access to descending inhibitory and excitatory pathways from the brainstem (Suzuki et al. 2002).

IMMEDIATE EARLY GENE ACTIVATION
AND THE DORSAL HORN

Noxious stimulation results in the activation of a number of immediate early genes within discrete populations of neurons within the dorsal horn (Hunt et al. 1987; Herdegen et al. 1991a,b; Lanteri-Minet et al. 1993; Traub et al. 1993; Tolle et al. 1994; Honore et al. 1997; Besson 1999). Expression of c-fos mRNA and protein has been most intensively studied (particularly by the Besson group) and was shown to be largely a response to noxious stimulation alone, occurring within the immediately postsynaptic target neurons within the dorsal horn 2 hours following stimulation. Study of c-fos expression is a particularly effective way of monitoring the activity of the dorsal horn (and higher brain areas) in response to injury to the body.

Histochemistry of c-fos expression has been used extensively to map the response to different types of stimulation and the efficacy of various analgesics (Honore et al. 1997; Buritova and Besson 1998; Buritova et al. 1998; Le Guen et al. 1999; Gestreau et al. 2000). However, 2 hours after stimulation, the pattern of c-fos expression changes, and by 24 hours it has become bilateral and occurs predominantly in deeper neurons not directly innervated by nociceptive afferents (Williams et al. 1990, 1991). This finding implies that nociceptive processing evolves over time from the acute phase of nociceptive processing to the longer-term phase reflected by central sensitization and other physiological events that ensure increased pain sensitivity until the injury has been resolved (Fig. 3). In rats, c-fos histochemistry combined with noxious stimulation at a variety of deep and superficial sites in the body has indicated that NK1-positive neurons in lamina I are primarily concerned with the intensity of noxious stimulation rather than with the location or tissue of origin of the pain (Doyle and Hunt 1999a,b). Noxious stimulation of muscle, joint, or cutaneous targets resulted in extensive double labeling of NK1-positive neurons within lamina I in direct proportion to the total number of c-fos-labeled neurons within the dorsal horn (which was taken as a measure of stimulus intensity) (Fig. 4B).

LAMINA I PROJECTION NEURONS

One route toward understanding the underlying problem of chronic pain is to examine the molecular changes that occur at various stages in the pain pathway, and some progress has been made in this regard. The lamina I projection neuron of the dorsal horn has been identified as being pivotal in the control of pain sensitivity following a variety of peripheral injuries to the nerve or inflammation (Nichols et al. 1999). Lamina I projection neurons receive inputs from C and Aδ nociceptors and are largely nocispecific, although some also respond to temperature. Many of these primary sensory fibers co-release substance P (SP) and glutamate in response to tissue injury (Duggan and Hendry 1986; De Biasi and Rustioni 1988; Duggan et al. 1988). SP binds to its cognate receptor, now referred to as the neurokinin-1 (NK1) receptor, present on a small minority (5–10%) of lamina I neurons. Release of SP from nociceptor terminals induces activation and internalization of these receptors (Mantyh et al. 1997). While the ability of released SP to induce internalization of the NK1 receptor has allowed the mapping of sites of SP activity in the spinal cord (Abbadie et al. 1997; Honor et al. 1999), other work has shown that nearly all lamina I neurons that project to

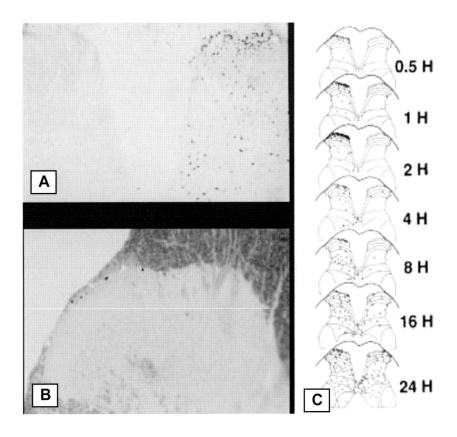

Fig. 3. The distribution of Fos-immunoreactive neurons that follows a brief noxious stimulus. (A) Ipsilateral Fos labeling 2 hours following ipsilateral injection of formalin into the hindpaw. (B) Brief noxious stimulation of muscle primarily results in lamina I staining (Hunt et al. 1987). (C) Over 24 hours following a brief noxious thermal stimulus there is a gradual loss of Fos staining dorsally from laminae I–II to expression in deeper laminae bilaterally within the spinal cord (Williams et al. 1990).

higher centers of the brain express the NK1 receptor and vice versa (although some studies describe considerably more NK1-expressing interneurons in lamina I; see Todd et al. 1998). This confirmation of the close correlation of projection and NK1-expressing neurons in lamina I was followed by reports showing that selective ablation of the NK1-expressing neurons (following intrathecal administration and subsequent internalization of an SP-toxin conjugate) markedly reduced the pain behavior produced in experimental inflammatory and neuropathic chronic pain models without compromising the animals' response to acute noxious stimulation (Nichols et al. 1999). More recently, several reports have shown that these NK1-expressing lamina I

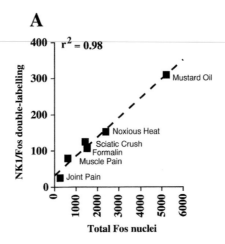

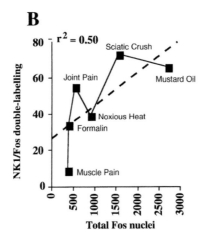

Fig. 4. NK1-positive neurons in superficial (A) or deep laminae (B) that costain for c-fos following various types of noxious stimulation. In lamina I, double labeling follows the intensity of the stimulus irrespective of tissue or stimulus (Doyle and Hunt 1999b). Examples of such neurons are given in Fig. 5.

neurons not only transmit pain to higher centers of the brain but have privileged access to brainstem neurons that provide the descending modulation of spinal cord activity (Suzuki et al. 2002). These reports suggest that NK1-expressing lamina I neurons not only are involved in the ascending conduction of pain but also are intimately involved in setting the basal level of inhibitory tone in spinal nociceptive circuits. In other words, it seems that chronic pain states are established and maintained by the lamina I pathway

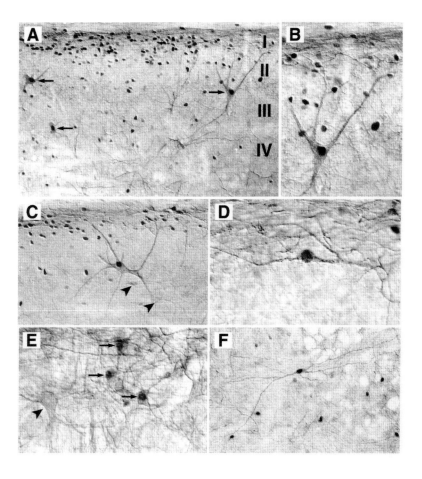

Fig. 5. NK1-positive neurons in superficial or deep laminae that costain for c-fos following various types of noxious stimulation. From Doyle and Hunt (1999b).

that projects to areas of the brainstem and forebrain concerned with discrimination, affect, and cognition. These brain areas are able to modulate the activity of descending excitatory and inhibitory pathways to the spinal cord from the brainstem. In contrast, Nichols et al. (1999) showed that acute discrimination of noxious stimulation is still possible in the absence of NK1-expressing neurons, either through the remaining neurons of the lamina I pathway or through other intact pathways originating principally from lamina V that project from the spinal cord to the brainstem and directly or indirectly to regions of the forebrain that are principally concerned with affect and with the complex behavioral responses that follow noxious stimulation.

THE NEUROBIOLOGY OF LAMINA I NEURONS:
SUBSTANCE P AND THE NK1 RECEPTOR

Given that lamina I neurons may be one key to understanding how pain sensitivity is controlled, it is necessary to ask whether primary afferent stimulation of these neurons results in long-term molecular changes that may outlive the period of stimulation and result in increased sensitivity to subsequent stimulation. Both molecular and physiological evidence suggests that this is indeed the case. The first events that follow noxious stimulation apart from internalization of the NK1 receptor (and presumably other G-protein-coupled receptors) include the rapid phosphorylation of cAMP-responsive element-binding protein (CREB) and mitogen-activated protein (MAP) kinase (Herdegen et al. 1997; Ji and Rupp 1997; Ji et al. 1999, 2002, 2003; Hoeger-Bement and Sluka 2003), both previously identified as members of signaling pathways crucial for long-term changes such as long-term potentiation (LTP) in the hippocampus (Ji et al. 2003). MAP kinase phosphorylation has been shown immunohistochemically to occur in NK1-positive neurons, although these were not identified as projection neurons. Evidence is insufficient to state unequivocally that CREB phosphorylation occurs in NK1-positive projection neurons, although it seems probable (Ji et al. 2002). We know little about the downstream events that follow CREB and MAP kinase activation, but it seems likely that the extensive immediate early gene (IEG) activation that occurs in superficial dorsal horn neurons is driven in part by these pathways. IEGs include *c-fos, zif 268* (which is crucial for the late phase of hippocampal LTP; Wisden et al. 1990; Jones et al. 2001; Ying et al. 2002), and many others. IEGs are largely transcription factors that direct downstream gene activation. While few target genes have been identified, evidence indicates that expression of the genes for DREAM and dynorphin may be regulated by noxious stimulation (Cheng et al. 2002; Vogt 2002).

Neurons within lamina I of the dorsal horn respond to SP through the NK1 receptor and respond to glutamate through N-methyl-D-aspartate (NMDA) receptors, α-amino-3-hydroxy-5-methyl-4-isoxazole propionate (AMPA) receptors, and metabotropic glutamate receptors (mGluR 1 and 5); they also respond to the inhibitory neurotransmitters γ-aminobutyric acid (GABA) and glycine, but they are largely devoid of μ-opioid receptors (Azkue et al. 2003; Ikeda et al. 2003; Muller et al. 2003). Unlike nonprojecting nociceptive lamina I neurons, NK1-receptor-activated signal transduction pathways and activation of low-threshold (T-type) voltage-gated calcium channels synergistically facilitate activity- and calcium-dependent long-term potentiation at synapses from nociceptive nerve fibers, suggesting that "memory traces" of painful events are retained (Ikeda et al. 2003). Additionally, recent work has shown that the loss of spinal inhibition in the dorsal horn of the spinal cord, which has been postulated to be a crucial substrate for chronic pain syndromes, involves a trans-synaptic reduction in the expression of the potassium-chloride exported-2 (KCC) channel in lamina I neurons (Coull et al. 2003). This event results in disruption of anion homeostasis in lamina I neurons, with the net result being an increase in excitability in lamina I neurons involved in the ascending conduction of pain. However, this change in KCC expression has not been directly demonstrated in lamina I projection neurons.

SUBSTANCE P, NK1, AND NOCICEPTION

The contribution of NK1 receptors to mediating postsynaptic LTP in lamina I projection neurons suggests that these receptors would be good analgesic targets. The most widely studied physiological aspect of SP is its role as a transmitter of nociceptive information. Given that painful stimuli bring about the release of SP onto dorsal horn neurons, SP was hypothesized to play an important role in pain transmission. Behavioral studies in animals supported this hypothesis, because intrathecal and intravenous administration of SP elicits scratching and biting of the abdomen, behaviors that are blocked by an NK1-receptor antagonist and by systemic morphine injection (Hylden and Wilcox 1981; Gamse and Saria 1986; Nance and Sawynok 1987; Sakurada et al. 1996; Inoue et al. 1999). Opiates inhibit the release of SP in the trigeminal nucleus induced by high potassium concentration and in the dorsal horn after stimulation of the primary afferents (Jessell and Iversen 1977; Yaksh et al. 1980; Abbadie et al. 1997; Honore et al. 2000). Noxious stimulation also brings about an increase in NK1 receptor protein, further supporting SP's involvement in the detection of pain (Abbadie et al. 1997; Honore et al. 2000).

However, early conclusions that SP was the "primary" pain transmitter have not been upheld by more recent findings (Hill 2000). Despite the anatomical evidence for a role of SP and the NK1 receptor in pain, they seem to have little influence on acute pain sensation, although responses to intense or inflammatory pain seem to engage NK1-receptor-dependent processes (Cao et al. 1998; De Felipe et al. 1998; Kidd et al. 2003). Hence, in the mouse, rat and guinea pig, NK1-receptor antagonists reduce SP-induced plasma extravasation (Grant and Brain 2001; Grant et al. 2002; Lever et al. 2003). Deletion of the NK1 receptor also attenuates hyperalgesia in models of chronic inflammatory and neuropathic pain, but with relatively few effects on

acute pain apart from intense heat, although this finding has not been repli-
cated in all strains of knockout mice (Cao et al. 1998; De Felipe et al. 1998;
Mansikka et al. 1999, 2000; Laird et al. 2000). Based on findings that NK1-
receptor antagonists can attenuate the increase in pain sensitivity that follows tissue or nerve injury, NK1 receptors might participate in the generation of central excitability. In support of this proposal, application of
NK1-receptor antagonists and receptor knockout block LTP and wind-up
(De Felipe et al. 1998; Laird et al. 2000; Weng et al. 2001; Khasabov et al.
2002; Suzuki et al. 2003), and NK1 immunoreactivity increases in persistent
pain states (Abbadie et al. 1997). Also, administration of NK1-receptor antagonists produces antinociception in studies that include acute pain models,
although somewhat variably. However, data from pharmacological studies
using NK1-receptor antagonists have been difficult to interpret due to con-
flicting reports that may arise from differences in the selectivity of the
compounds, as well as in their route of administration, dose, and modalities
tested. In humans, NK1-receptor antagonism has been disappointing in pain
studies (Hill 2000). One reason may be particular roles of the peptide in
certain modalities and intensities of pain stimuli.

Mice with genetic disruption of the NK1 or preprotachykinin-A gene
have normal acute pain behavior, apart from some difficulty in coding the
intensity of intermediate to very noxious thermal stimuli (Cao et al. 1998;
De Felipe et al. 1998). However, secondary pain states tend to be reduced
following gene knockout. For example, the hyperalgesia that develops after
inflammation following injection of complete Freund's adjuvant was attenuated by 4 days post-treatment in NK1-receptor knockout mice but not at 24
hours following treatment (Cao et al. 1998; De Felipe et al. 1998; Kidd et al.
2003). Hyperalgesia was similar to that in wild-type mice at shorter time points.

Secondary visceral nociception, second-phase formalin response, and
hyperalgesia induced by capsaicin were similarly depressed in NK1-receptor
knockout mice (De Felipe et al. 1998; Laird et al. 2000, 2001). Electrophysiological studies have revealed that although acute mechanical and thermal
nociception remained unaltered in knockout mice, these mice displayed was
less central sensitization following mustard oil application and less "wind-
up" of spinal neurons compared to wild-types. However, a second study
reported that these knockout mice displayed marked deficits in mechanical
and thermal coding in the noxious range of stimuli, as well as exhibiting
attenuated wind-up, thereby implicating NK1 receptors in the accurate intensity coding of suprathreshold stimuli (Suzuki et al. 2003; Weng et al. 2001).

Diffuse noxious inhibitory control (DNIC) was also substantially reduced in NK1-knockout mice (Fig. 6) (Bester et al. 2001). The concept of
DNIC is based on the observation that distant noxious stimuli applied

outside a neuron's receptive field can reduce the nociceptive impact of a noxious stimulus within the receptive field if applied simultaneously. DNIC has been demonstrated both electrophysiologically from recordings of lamina V neurons and with Fos histochemistry using simultaneous stimulation either of the forepaws and hindpaws or of the tail and hindpaws; it is thought to be mediated by descending inhibitory pathways (Dickenson and Le Bars 1987; Monconduit et al. 2002). The origin of these pathways is thought to be the both within the dorsal reticular nucleus and within the serotoninergic and nonserotoninergic neurons of the rostroventral medulla (RVM) (Lima 1998; Monconduit et al. 2002; Dugast et al. 2003). In wild-type mice, reduced Fos expression was seen within the lumbar spinal dorsal horn when stimulation was applied to the ipsilateral forepaw (Bester et al. 2001). However, in the raphe magnus and pallidus, Fos expression was elevated, implying that activity in raphe neurons was necessary to reduce lumbar cord Fos expression. In contrast, in NK1-knockout mice the same procedure elicited little change in Fos levels in the brain or spinal cord, again suggesting that many of the described changes in behavior such as reduced secondary hyperalgesia, decreased analgesic responsiveness to opiates, and reduced stress-induced analgesia can be explained by deficits in descending facilitation or inhibition of spinal processing through pathways originating in the brainstem. Surprisingly, NK1-receptor antagonists have been ineffective in the majority of clinical trials for analgesia, although a single trial showed that they reduced

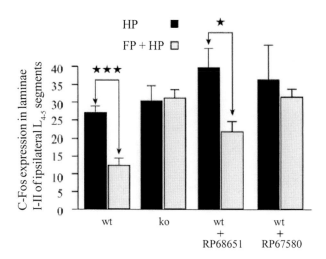

Fig. 6. C-fos histochemistry used to demonstrate diffuse inhibitory controls and their loss in NK1 knockout (ko) mice and in wild-type (wt) mice given the NK1 antagonist RP67580 but not the inactive enantiomer RP68651. C-fos expression in the lumbar cord following hindpaw (HP) was attenuated by a simultaneous noxious stimulus to the forepaw (FP) (from Bester et al. 2001).

postoperative pain after dental extraction (Hill 2000). Some success has been reported for patients with fibromyalgia, however (Russell 2002). It is possible that this apparent difference between humans and laboratory animals may denote a difference in NK1-receptor distribution, or perhaps it reflects targeting of inappropriate pain states.

ABLATION OF LAMINA I/NK1-EXPRESSING NEURONS

The importance of substance P in inducing LTP in lamina I neurons through the NK1 receptor and the deficits seen in NK1-receptor knockout

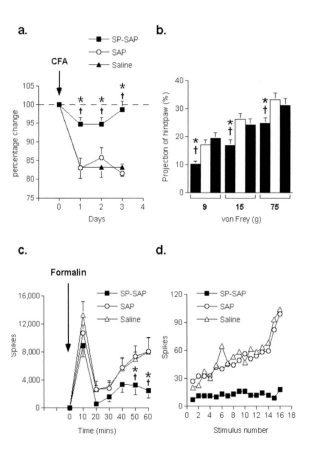

Fig. 7. The results of lesioning NK1-expressing lamina I projection neurons with substance P-saporin (SP-SAP) conjugates. (a) Attenuated hyperalgesia following intraplantar complete Freund's adjuvant (CFA); (b) reduced lamina V receptive field sizes in untreated rats; (c) reduced second-phase formalin response in lesioned rats; and (d) loss of wind-up from lamina V neurons (from Suzuki et al. 2002).

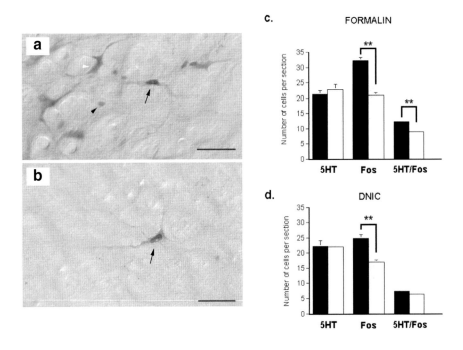

Fig. 8. Reduced activation of the raphe in lamina I ablated rats. (a,b) Rostroventral medulla (RVM) neurons labeled with antiserum against serotonin (cytoplasm) or c-fos (nuclei). Panels c and d show that while fos staining was generally reduced following formalin or heat stimulation concurrently administered to fore- and hindlimbs, only formalin stimulation showed a decline in numbers of fos-5HT-positive neurons; DNIC = diffuse noxious inhibitory control (from Suzuki et al. 2002).

mice indicate that complete loss of lamina I projection neurons could have similar but more substantial effects on pain processing. Using SP conjugated to the cytotoxin saporin to selectively ablate neurons expressing the NK1 receptor, Nichols et al. (1999) demonstrated a marked reduction of hyperalgesia following tissue and peripheral nerve injury, with no effect on acute behavioral nociceptive thresholds. This finding suggests that the lamina I projection neurons were crucial for hyperalgesia to develop. An electrophysiological study of rats with ablation of NK1-positive lamina I neurons also found a loss of central sensitization, as revealed by diminished wind-up and decreased formalin second-phase response in deeper-lying lamina V neurons (Khasabov et al. 2002; Suzuki et al. 2002) (Fig. 7). Fos histochemistry revealed that DNIC was also reduced: raphe Fos expression was relatively insensitive to concurrent stimulus of the hind- and forepaws, and no decrease in Fos expression was seen in the dorsal horn. To directly prove that descending pathways had been perturbed by the lamina I deletion, spinal 5HT$_3$ receptors were blocked with the selective antagonist ondansetron (Suzuki et al. 2002). Serotonin released from descending pathways originating in the raphe is excitatory at the 5HT$_3$ receptor. Application of ondansetron reproduced almost exactly the deficits seen electrophysiologically in deep dorsal horn neurons following ablation of lamina I projection neurons, confirming the suspicion that control of spinal excitability is mediated through the ascending spinal lamina I pathway and through the activation of descending facilitatory and inhibitory pathways that regulate nociceptive traffic (Urban and Gebhart 1999). The origin of these pathways is still unclear. Serotonin originating from axons of neurons that descend from the RVM is a strong possibility, although increased Fos expression in the RVM was only seen following formalin injection into the hind-paw and not following the DNIC protocol. The electrophysiological and behavioral responses to formalin injection are attenuated in animals with SP-saporin ablation of lamina I neurons (Figs. 7 and 8; see Dickenson et al., this volume).

CONCLUSIONS

Lamina I projection neurons that express the NK1 receptor are largely nociceptive specific, possess small receptive fields, support long-term potentiation, and are critical for the initiation of secondary pain states that accompany most injuries. Disruption of the lamina I pathway does not abolish acute pain sensation, implying that the lamina V ascending pain pathway is capable of mediating considerably more discriminative analysis of incoming nociceptive information than would have been predicted by its connections to regions of the brain concerned with motor and arousal behaviors. Moreover, the analysis of lamina V neuron receptive fields, which tend to be larger and of wide dynamic range, rely heavily upon an intact lamina I pathway for their plasticity in the face of injury to the periphery. Genetic deletion of the NK1 receptor replicates some of the deficits in pain processing that are seen with lamina I/NK1 neuron ablations but results in a milder phenotype with less dramatic influences on the changing pain sensitivity that follows injury. Analysis of both NK1 knockout mice and lamina I/NK1-lesioned animals indicated that both disruptions influence activity in descending excitatory and inhibitory pathways. It seems likely that pathology in these ascending-descending loops may underlie some aspects of chronic pain states.

REFERENCES

Abbadie C, Trafton J, Liu H, Mantyh PW, Basbaum AI. Inflammation increases the distribution of dorsal horn neurons that internalize the neurokinin-1 receptor in response to noxious and non-noxious stimulation. *J Neurosci* 1997; 17:8049–8060.

Azkue JJ, Liu XG, Zimmermann M, Sandkuhler J. Induction of long-term potentiation of C fibre-evoked spinal field potentials requires recruitment of group I, but not group II/III metabotropic glutamate receptors. *Pain* 2003; 106:373–379.

Bernard JF, Bandler R. Parallel circuits for emotional coping behaviour: new pieces in the puzzle. *J Comp Neurol* 1998; 401:429–436.

Besson JM. The neurobiology of pain. *Lancet* 1999; 353:1610–1615.

Bester H, Matsumoto N, Besson JM, Bernard JF. Further evidence for the involvement of the spinoparabrachial pathway in nociceptive processes: a c-Fos study in the rat. *J Comp Neurol* 1997; 383:439–458.

Bester H, Chapman V, Besson JM, Bernard JF. Physiological properties of the lamina I spinoparabrachial neurons in the rat. *J Neurophysiol* 2000; 83:2239–2259.

Bester H, De Felipe C, Hunt SP. The NK1 receptor is essential for the full expression of noxious inhibitory controls in the mouse. *J Neurosci* 2001; 21:1039–1046.

Buritova J, Besson JM. Dose-related anti-inflammatory/analgesic effects of lornoxicam: a spinal c-Fos protein study in the rat. *Inflamm Res* 1998; 47:18–25.

Buritova J, Besson JM, Bernard JF. Involvement of the spinoparabrachial pathway in inflammatory nociceptive processes: a c-Fos protein study in the awake rat. *J Comp Neurol* 1998; 397:10–28.

Cao YQ, Mantyh PW, Carlson EJ, et al. Primary afferent tachykinins are required to experience moderate to intense pain. *Nature* 1998; 392:390–394.

Cervero F, Laird JM. Visceral pain. *Lancet* 1999; 353:2145–2148.

Cheng HY, Pitcher GM, Laviolette SR, et al. DREAM is a critical transcriptional repressor for pain modulation. *Cell* 2002; 10831–10843.

Coull JA, Boudreau D, Bachand K, et al. Trans-synaptic shift in anion gradient in spinal lamina I neurons as a mechanism of neuropathic pain. *Nature* 2003; 424:938–942.

Craig AD. How do you feel? Interoception: the sense of the physiological condition of the body. *Nat Rev Neurosci* 2002; 3:655–666.

De Biasi S, Rustioni A. Glutamate and substance P coexist in primary afferent terminals in the superficial laminae of spinal cord. *Proc Natl Acad Sci USA* 1988; 85:7820–7824.

De Felipe C, Herrero JF, O'Brien JA, et al. Altered nociception, analgesia and aggression in mice lacking the receptor for substance P. *Nature* 1998; 392:394–397.

De Groat WC. Spinal cord projections and neuropeptides in visceral afferent neurons. *Prog Brain Res* 1986; 67:165–187.

Dickenson AH, Le Bars D. Supraspinal morphine and descending inhibitions acting on the dorsal horn of the rat. *J Physiol* 1987; 384:81–107.

Ding YQ, Takada M, Shigemoto R, Mizumo N. Spinoparabrachial tract neurons showing substance P receptor-like immunoreactivity in the lumbar spinal cord of the rat. *Brain Res* 1995; 674:336–340.

Doyle CA, Hunt SP. A role for spinal lamina I neurokinin-1-positive neurons in cold thermoreception in the rat. *Neuroscience* 1999a; 91:723–732.

Doyle CA, Hunt SP. Substance P receptor (neurokinin-1)-expressing neurons in lamina I of the spinal cord encode for the intensity of noxious stimulation: a c-Fos study in rat. *Neuroscience* 1999b; 89:17–28.

Dugast C, Almeida A, Lima D. The medullary dorsal reticular nucleus enhances the responsiveness of spinal nociceptive neurons to peripheral stimulation in the rat. *Eur J Neurosci* 2003; 18:580–588.

Duggan AW, Hendry IA. Laminar localization of the sites of release of immunoreactive substance P in the dorsal horn with antibody-coated microelectrodes. *Neurosci Lett* 1986; 68:134–140.

Duggan AW, Hendry IA, Morton CR, Hutchison WD, Zhao ZQ. Cutaneous stimuli releasing immunoreactive substance P in the dorsal horn of the cat. *Brain Res* 1988; 451:261–273.

Gamse R, Saria A. Nociceptive behavior after intrathecal injections of substance P, neurokinin A and calcitonin gene-related peptide in mice. *Neurosci Lett* 1986; 70:143–147.

Gauriau C, Bernard JF. A comparative reappraisal of projections from the superficial laminae of the dorsal horn in the rat: the forebrain. *J Comp Neurol* 2004a; 468:24–56.

Gauriau C, Bernard JF. Posterior triangular thalamic neurons convey nociceptive messages to the secondary somatosensory and insular cortices in the rat. *J Neurosci* 2004b; 24:752–761.

Gestreau C, Le Guen S, Besson JM. Is there tonic activity in the endogenous opioid systems? A c-Fos study in the rat central nervous system after intravenous injection of naloxone or naloxone-methiodide. *J Comp Neurol* 2000; 427:285–301.

Grant AD, Brain SD. Capsaicin-mediated neurogenic vasodilatation in neurokinin-1, NK 1, receptor knockout mice. *Scientific World Journal* 2001; 1(Suppl 1):26.

Grant AD, Gerard NP, Brain SD. Evidence of a role for NK1 and CGRP receptors in mediating neurogenic vasodilatation in the mouse ear. *Br J Pharmacol* 2002; 135:356–362.

Herdegen T, Kovary K, Leah J, Bravo R. Specific temporal and spatial distribution of JUN, FOS, and KROX-24 proteins in spinal neurons following noxious transsynaptic stimulation. *J Comp Neurol* 1991a; 313:178–191.

Herdegen T, Tolle TR, Bravo R, Zieglgansberger W, Zimmermann M. Sequential expression of JUN B, JUN D and FOS B proteins in rat spinal neurons: cascade of transcriptional operations during nociception. *Neurosci Lett* 1991b; 129:221–224.

Herdegen T, Blume A, Buschmann T, et al. Expression of activating transcription factor-2, serum response factor and cAMP/Ca response element binding protein in the adult rat brain following generalized seizures, nerve fibre lesion and ultraviolet irradiation. *Neuroscience* 1997; 81:199–212.

Hill R. NK1 (substance P) receptor antagonists—why are they not analgesic in humans? *Trends Pharmacol Sci* 2000; 21:244–246.

Hoeger-Bement MK, Sluka KA. Phosphorylation of CREB and mechanical hyperalgesia is reversed by blockade of the cAMP pathway in a time-dependent manner after repeated intramuscular acid injections. *J Neurosci* 2003; 23:5437–5445.

Honor P, Menning PM, Rogers SD, et al. Spinal substance P receptor expression and internalization in acute, short-term, and long-term inflammatory pain states. *J Neurosci* 1999; 19:7670–7678.

Honore P, Catheline G, Le Guen S, Besson JM. Chronic treatment with systemic morphine induced tolerance to the systemic and peripheral antinociceptive effects of morphine on both carrageenin induced mechanical hyperalgesia and spinal c-Fos expression in awake rats. *Pain* 1997; 71:99–108.

Honore P, Menning PM, Rogers SD, Nichols ML, Mantyh PW. Neurochemical plasticity in persistent inflammatory pain. *Prog Brain Res* 2000; 129:357–363.

Hunt SP, Mantyh PW. The molecular dynamics of pain control. *Nat Rev Neurosci* 2001; 2:83–91.

Hunt SP, Rossi J. Peptide- and non-peptide-containing unmyelinated primary afferents: the parallel processing of nociceptive information. *Philos Trans R Soc Lond B Biol Sci* 1985; 308:283–289.

Hunt SP, Pini A, Evan G. Induction of c-fos-like protein in spinal cord neurons following sensory stimulation. *Nature* 1987; 328:632–634.

Hylden JL, Wilcox GL. Intrathecal substance P elicits a caudally-directed biting and scratching behavior in mice. *Brain Res* 1981; 217:212–215.

Ikeda H, Heinke B, Ruscheweyh R, Sandkuhler J. Synaptic plasticity in spinal lamina I projection neurons that mediate hyperalgesia. *Science* 2003; 299:1237–1240.

Inoue M, Shimohira I, Yoshida A, et al. Dose-related opposite modulation by nociceptin/ orphanin FQ of substance P nociception in the nociceptors and spinal cord. *J Pharmacol Exp Ther* 1999; 291:308–313.

Jessell TM, Iversen LL. Opiate analgesics inhibit substance P release from rat trigeminal nucleus. *Nature* 1977; 268:549–551.

Ji RR, Rupp F. Phosphorylation of transcription factor CREB in rat spinal cord after formalin-induced hyperalgesia: relationship to c-fos induction. *J Neurosci* 1997; 17:1776–1785.

Ji RR, Baba H, Brenner GJ, Woolf CJ. Nociceptive-specific activation of ERK in spinal neurons contributes to pain hypersensitivity. *Nat Neurosci* 1999; 2:1114–1119.

Ji RR, Befort K, Brenner GJ, Woolf CJ. ERK MAP kinase activation in superficial spinal cord neurons induces prodynorphin and NK-1 upregulation and contributes to persistent inflammatory pain hypersensitivity. *J Neurosci* 2002; 22:478–485.

Ji RR, Kohno T, Moore KA, Woolf CJ. Central sensitization and LTP: do pain and memory share similar mechanisms? *Trends Neurosci* 2003; 26:696–705.

Jones MW, Errington ML, French PJ, et al. A requirement for the immediate early gene *Zif268* in the expression of late LTP and long-term memories. *Nat Neurosci* 2001; 4:289–296.

Khasabov SG, Rogers SD, Ghilardi JR. et al. Spinal neurons that possess the substance P receptor are required for the development of central sensitization. *J Neurosci* 2002; 22:9086–9098.

Kidd BL, Inglis JJ, Vetsika K, et al. Inhibition of inflammation and hyperalgesia in NK-1 receptor knock-out mice. *Neuroreport* 2003; 14:2189–2192.

Laird JM, Olivar T, Roza C, et al. Deficits in visceral pain and hyperalgesia of mice with a disruption of the tachykinin NK1 receptor gene. *Neuroscience* 2000; 98:345–352.

Laird JM, Roza C, De Felipe C, Hunt SP, Cervero F. Role of central and peripheral tachykinin NK1 receptors in capsaicin-induced pain and hyperalgesia in mice. *Pain* 2001; 90:97–103.

Lanteri-Minet M, de Pommery J, Herdegen T, et al. Differential time course and spatial expression of Fos, Jun, and Krox-24 proteins in spinal cord of rats undergoing subacute or chronic somatic inflammation. *J Comp Neurol* 1993; 333:223–235.

Lawson SN. Phenotype and function of somatic primary afferent nociceptive neurones with C-, A-delta- or A-alpha/beta-fibres. *Exp Physiol* 2002; 87:239–244.

Le Guen S, Catheline G, Besson JM. Effects of NMDA receptor antagonists on morphine tolerance: a c-Fos study in the lumbar spinal cord of the rat. *Eur J Pharmacol* 1999; 373:1–11.

Lever IJ, Grant AD, Pezet S, et al. Basal and activity-induced release of substance P from primary afferent fibres in NK1 receptor knockout mice: evidence for negative feedback. *Neuropharmacology* 2003; 45:1101–1110.

Lima D. Anatomical basis for the dynamic processing of nociceptive input. *Eur J Pain* 1998; 2:195–202.

Mansikka H, Shiotani M, Winchurch R, Raja SN. Neurokinin-1 receptors are involved in behavioral responses to high-intensity heat stimuli and capsaicin-induced hyperalgesia in mice. *Anesthesiology* 1999; 90:1643–1649.

Mansikka H, Sheth RN, DeVries C, et al. Nerve injury-induced mechanical but not thermal hyperalgesia is attenuated in neurokinin-1 receptor knockout mice. *Exp Neurol* 2000; 162:343–349.

Mantyh PW, Rogers SD, Honore P, et al. Inhibition of hyperalgesia by ablation of lamina I spinal neurons expressing the substance P receptor. *Science* 1997; 278:275–279.

Monconduit L, Desbois C, Villanueva L. The integrative role of the rat medullary subnucleus reticularis dorsalis in nociception. *Eur J Neurosci* 2002; 16:937–944.

Muller F, Heinke B, Sandkuhler J. Reduction of glycine receptor-mediated miniature inhibitory postsynaptic currents in rat spinal lamina I neurons after peripheral inflammation. *Neuroscience* 2003; 122:799–805.

Nagy JI, Hunt SP. Fluoride-resistant acid phosphatase-containing neurones in dorsal root ganglia are separate from those containing substance P or somatostatin. *Neuroscience* 1982; 7:89–97.

Nagy JI, Hunt SP. The termination of primary afferents within the rat dorsal horn: evidence for rearrangement following capsaicin treatment. *J Comp Neurol* 1983; 218:145–158.

Naim M, Spike RC, Watt C, Shehab SA, Todd AJ. Cells in laminae III and IV of the rat spinal cord that possess the neurokinin-1 receptor and have dorsally directed dendrites receive a major synaptic input from tachykinin-containing primary afferents. *J Neurosci* 1997; 17:5536–5548.

Nance PW, Sawynok J. Substance P-induced long-term blockade of spinal adrenergic analgesia: reversal by morphine and naloxone. *J Pharmacol Exp Ther* 1987; 240:972–977.

Nichols ML, Allen BJ, Rogers SD, et al. Transmission of chronic nociception by spinal neurons expressing the substance P receptor. *Science* 1999; 286:1558–1561.

Russell IJ. The promise of substance P inhibitors in fibromyalgia. *Rheum Dis Clin North Am* 2002; 28:329–342.

Sakurada T, Wako K, Sakurada C, et al. Spinally-mediated behavioural responses evoked by intrathecal high-dose morphine: possible involvement of substance P in the mouse spinal cord. *Brain Res* 1996; 724:213–221.

Snider WD, McMahon SB. Tackling pain at the source: new ideas about nociceptors. *Neuron* 1998; 20:629–632.

Suzuki R, Morcuende S, Webber M, Hunt SP, Dickenson AH. Superficial NK1-expressing neurons control spinal excitability through activation of descending pathways. *Nat Neurosci* 2002; 5:1319–1326.

Suzuki R, Hunt SP, Dickenson AH. The coding of noxious mechanical and thermal stimuli of deep dorsal horn neurones is attenuated in NK1 knockout mice. *Neuropharmacology* 2003; 45:1093–1000.

Todd AJ. Anatomy of primary afferents and projection neurones in the rat spinal dorsal horn with particular emphasis on substance P and the neurokinin 1 receptor. *Exp Physiol* 2002; 87:245–249.

Todd AJ, Spike RC, Polgar E. A quantitative study of neurons which express neurokinin-1 or somatostatin sst2a receptor in rat spinal dorsal horn. *Neuroscience* 1998; 85:459–473.

Todd AJ, Puskar Z, Spike RC, et al. Projection neurons in lamina I of rat spinal cord with the neurokinin 1 receptor are selectively innervated by substance p-containing afferents and respond to noxious stimulation. *J Neurosci* 2002; 22:4103–4113.

Tolle TR, Herdegen T, Schadrack J, et al. Application of morphine prior to noxious stimulation differentially modulates expression of Fos, Jun and Krox-24 proteins in rat spinal cord neurons. *Neuroscience* 1994; 58:305–321.

Traub RJ, Herdegen T, Gebhart GF. Differential expression of c-fos and c-jun in two regions of the rat spinal cord following noxious colorectal distention. *Neurosci Lett* 1993; 160:121–125.

Urban MO, Gebhart GF. Supraspinal contributions to hyperalgesia. *Proc Natl Acad Sci USA* 1999; 96:7687–7692.

Villanueva L, Bouhassira D, Le Bars D. The medullary subnucleus reticularis dorsalis (SRD) as a key link in both the transmission and modulation of pain signals. *Pain* 1996; 67:231–240.

Villanueva L, Desbois C, Le Bars D, Bernard JF. Organization of diencephalic projections from the medullary subnucleus reticularis dorsalis and the adjacent cuneate nucleus: a retrograde and anterograde tracer study in the rat. *J Comp Neurol* 1998; 390:133–160.

Vogt BA. Knocking out the DREAM to study pain. *N Engl J Med* 2002; 347:362–364.

Weng HR, Mansikka H, Winchurch R, Raja SN, Dougherty PM. Sensory processing in the deep spinal dorsal horn of neurokinin-1 receptor knockout mice. *Anesthesiology* 2001; 94:1105–1112.

Williams S, Evan GI, Hunt SP. Changing patterns of c-fos induction in spinal neurons following thermal cutaneous stimulation in the rat. *Neuroscience* 1990; 36:73–81.

Williams S, Evan G, Hunt SP. C-fos Induction in the spinal cord after peripheral nerve lesion. *Eur J Neurosci* 1991; 3:887–894.

Willis WD Jr, Zhang X, Honda CN, Giesler GJ Jr. Projections from the marginal zone and deep dorsal horn to the ventrobasal nuclei of the primate thalamus. *Pain* 2001; 92:267–276.

Wisden W, Errington ML, Williams S, et al. Differential expression of immediate early genes in the hippocampus and spinal cord. *Neuron* 1990; 4:603–614.

Yaksh TL, Jessell TM, Gamse R, Mudge AW, Leeman SE. Intrathecal morphine inhibits substance P release from mammalian spinal cord in vivo. *Nature* 1980; 286:155–157.

Ying SW, Futter M, Rosenblum K, et al. Brain-derived neurotrophic factor induces long-term potentiation in intact adult hippocampus: requirement for ERK activation coupled to CREB and upregulation of Arc synthesis. *J Neurosci* 2002; 22:1532–1540.

Correspondence to: Stephen P. Hunt, PhD, Department of Anatomy and Developmental Biology, University College London, Gower Street, London WC1E 6BT, United Kingdom. Email: hunt@ucl.ac.uk.

The Pain System in Normal and Pathological States:
A Primer for Clinicians, Progress in Pain Research
and Management, Vol. 31, edited by Luis Villanueva,
Anthony Dickenson, and Hélène Ollat, IASP Press,
Seattle, © 2004.

5

Balancing Excitations and Inhibitions in Spinal Circuits

Anthony H. Dickenson, Rie Suzuki, Elizabeth
A. Matthews, Wahida Rahman, Catherine Urch,
Lucinda Seagrove, and Lars Rygh

*Department of Pharmacology, University College London,
London, United Kingdom*

Studies on acute pain models in animals and humans make it clear that clinically important pains have distinct neurophysiological and pharmacological substrates. Thus, the transmission of impulses from the site of an injury into and through the central nervous system (CNS) can be altered. This plasticity, an ability of neuronal function to change after activity or injury-evoked dysfunction, leads to changes throughout the pathways involved in the perception of pain (Hunt and Mantyh 2001; Dickenson et al. 2002).

Much is known about the molecular and cellular mechanisms that contribute to the transduction of pain at peripheral levels, but numerous systems within the CNS can act at many levels to increase or decrease the incoming messages. Many of the pains that arise from damage to tissue, ranging from causes as varied as trauma, surgery, and arthritis, involve central changes, as do chronic neuropathic pains following lesions of the peripheral or central nervous system from causes such as diabetes and herpes zoster. The balance between modulating systems and excitatory function will determine the final sensation experienced by the patient. Analgesics can shift this balance—opioids increase inhibitions, whereas local anesthetics block excitations. At both peripheral and central sites, various mechanisms can amplify and prolong the painful stimulus, sometimes causing severe pain in the presence of relatively minor peripheral pathology. In fact, in pain conditions as diverse as arthritis, neuropathy, headache, and fibromyalgia, it is not uncommon to find increased responses to pain and a spread of pain to wider areas of the body (Staud et al. 2003a).

However, pain is not simply a sensation, and in addition to the sensory-discriminative aspects there are motor reflexes and the affective and emotional responses. Clearly, although the sensory and psychological aspects of pain are separable, the neural pathways that contribute to these aspects of pain are interlinked (Hunt and Mantyh 2001). This chapter examines some of the ways in which central inhibitory and excitatory systems can alter the level of pain and covers some new findings on the interactions between spinal and supraspinal systems that determine both the level of pain and the efficacy of drugs.

PERIPHERAL EXCITABILITY DRIVES THE SPINAL CORD

Primary afferent neurons, responding to sensory stimuli from the outside world, terminate in the dorsal horn of the spinal cord and are made up of distinct nerve fiber types (Millan 1999). The transmission of acute pain involves activation of sensory receptors on peripheral C and Aδ fibers, the nociceptors, which respond to noxious mechanical and thermal stimulation. The roles of the vanilloid receptors, part of the transient receptor potential (TRP) family of receptors, in heat and cold signals is covered by Drew and Wood (this volume), but once tissue damage and inflammation occur the production of chemical mediators in the damaged area of tissue becomes of great importance. Thus, prostanoids, bradykinin, protons, adenosine triphosphate (ATP), and 5-hydroxytryptamine (5HT, also known as serotonin) are released. Their actions on their excitatory receptors located on the peripheral C fibers play a major role in the sensitization and, at higher concentrations, the activation of C fibers during inflammation. The former action, *peripheral sensitization,* arises from these mediators acting to reduce the threshold of the sensory nerves so that they now respond to stimuli of lower intensity, the basis for the tenderness following injury to tissue. Other factors such as induction of, and changes in, agents such as nerve growth factor and cytokines are also important at the peripheral level (Dray and Urban 1996; see Fig. 1).

After damage to nerves, neuropathic pain is often characterized by both positive symptoms (abnormal spontaneous or evoked sensations) and negative symptoms (sensory deficits); intuitively, only the latter might be expected. Evidence indicates that altered somatosensory processing after partial nerve injury is set in motion by a number of changes in the peripheral nervous system. Studies after nerve section suggest that the generation of ectopic discharges within the neuroma and the dorsal root ganglia (DRG),

Peripheral events drive central systems

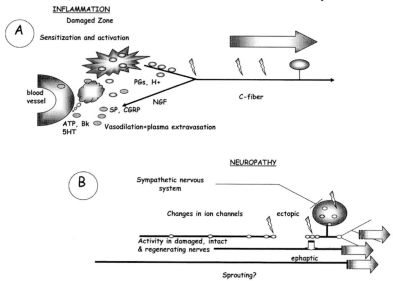

Fig. 1. Schematic diagrams showing the changes that occur in peripheral afferent fibers after (A) inflammation and (B) nerve injury. After inflammation, the actions of the peripheral mediators of pain such as prostanoids (PGs), adenosine triphosphate (ATP), serotonin (5HT), bradykinin (Bk), substance P (SP), calcitonin gene-related peptide (CGRP), nerve growth factor (NGF), and H+ on their receptors sensitize and activate C fibers. This event leads to action potentials running into the spinal cord and generates the axon reflex that causes vasodilation. These peripheral events underlie primary hyperalgesia. After neuropathy, changes occur within the nerves themselves that include ion channel expression and distribution, ectopic firing, and cross-talk between nerve fibers (ephaptic impulses). These combinations of activity in damaged and intact fibers leads to changes within the spinal cord that contribute to the pain of nerve injury.

cross-talk between damaged nerves (ephaptic transmission), and changes in both sodium and potassium channels occur in the damaged nerve fibers. Further, the sympathetic nervous system can sprout onto damaged nerve fibers and cell bodies (Suzuki and Dickenson 2000). Neurochemical changes also occur in the sensory nerves; Drew and Wood (this volume) discuss the roles of unique sodium channels in generating activity in small sensory nerves that have great potential as analgesic targets.

Neuronal hyperexcitability is a feature of epilepsy and both inflammatory and neuropathic pain. The M current ($I_{K(M)}$), a neuron-specific potassium current, plays a key role in regulating neuronal excitability, and neuronal KCNQ$_{2/3}$ potassium channel subunits, the molecular correlates of $I_{K(M)}$, are also present in nociceptive sensory systems. Retigabine, an opener of these currents, applied spinally, inhibited C- and Aδ-fiber-mediated responses of dorsal horn neurons evoked by natural or electrical afferent stimulation, and diminished "wind-up" after repetitive stimulation, in normal rats and in rats subjected to spinal nerve ligation. Retigabine also inhibited responses to intra-paw application of carrageenan in a rat model of chronic pain. It is suggested that $I_{K(M)}$ plays a key role in controlling the excitability of nociceptors and that $I_{K(M)}$ may represent a novel analgesic target (Passmore et al. 2003).

Despite the important peripheral changes that occur following nerve injury, neuropathic pain can only partly be explained by peripheral alterations. Simply stated, the fact that pain occurs in the face of marked sensory loss suggests that excitatory compensations within the nervous system are of major importance (Dickenson et al. 2002).

CENTRAL SPINAL MODULATORY EVENTS

Sensory information from nociceptors can be dramatically altered in the dorsal horn of the spinal cord by a remarkable number of excitatory and inhibitory systems, not only local to the spinal cord but also originating in the brain and descending to the dorsal horn. This complexity greatly complicates the study of pain and analgesia. Voltage-dependent calcium channels (VDCCs) on terminals and neurons are important both for transmitter release from peripheral afferents and for neuronal excitability. L-, N-, and P-type VDCC antagonists have distinct differential and time-dependent effects on acute, neuropathic, and inflammatory nociception (Vanegas and Schaible 2000; Matthews and Dickenson 2001a,b). However, the apparent specific upregulation of these channels in both pain states implies increases in transmitter release into the spinal cord.

Small afferent fibers release peptides, such as substance P and calcitonin gene-related peptide, and also glutamate. Together their many receptor actions allow the N-methyl-D-aspartate (NMDA) receptor for glutamate to be activated. Activation of the NMDA receptor underlies "wind-up," whereby the baseline response is amplified and prolonged even though the peripheral input remains the same (Dickenson et al. 2001). This increased responsiveness of dorsal horn neurons is probably the basis for *central hypersensitivity*. Activation of these processes not only increases the activity of the spinal neuron but also permits the neuron to become responsive to inputs normally too weak to excite the cell. Thus the receptive field area increases. As a consequence, both the degree and area of pain are enhanced by this spinal NMDA-receptor activation. This increase in the responsivity of the spinal cord is likely to underlie both the increased pain intensity and enlarged area of pain that are commonly observed after injury. The NMDA receptor is involved in persistent inflammatory and neuropathic pains, where it is critical for both the induction and subsequent maintenance of the enhanced pain state (Dickenson et al. 2001). Antagonists at multiple sites on the NMDA-receptor complex, including the licensed drug ketamine, are effective in a number of animal models and also in humans. Both volunteer and clinical studies support the ideas that have come from basic research to suggest that the dorsal horn NMDA receptor plays a key role in central hypersensitivity of inflammatory and neuropathic pains (Price et al. 1994; Sindrup and Jensen 1999).

Inhibitory controls are also active. There may be relatively little tonic activity in opioid systems, but opioid receptor activation by morphine provides a powerful inhibitory control. Until recently, there were three known receptors for the opioids, namely the μ-, δ-, and κ-opioid receptors. Additionally a fourth receptor, the ORL1 receptor, has now been characterized. Morphine acts on the μ-opioid receptor, as do most of the clinically used opioid drugs. The detailed structure of these receptors has been described, and we now have a reasonable understanding of their relative roles in physiological functions and in different pain states. The best understood sites of action of morphine are at spinal and brainstem/midbrain loci. The spinal actions of opioids and their mechanisms of analgesia involve (1) reduced release of peptides and glutamate from nociceptive C fibers so that spinal neurons are less excited by incoming painful messages and (2) postsynaptic inhibitions of neurons conveying information from the spinal cord to the brain. This dual action of opioids can result in a total block of sensory inputs as they arrive in the spinal cord and is the basis for their spinal analgesic effects. In the presence of inflammation, a peripheral site of action is revealed (Dickenson and Suzuki 1999).

At supraspinal sites, morphine can act to alter descending pathways from the brain to the cord involving norepinephrine and 5HT, and these pathways then act to reduce spinal nociceptive activity. In addition, these sites and transmitter systems form a link between emotions, depression, and anxiety and the level of pain and analgesia in a patient. Intriguing areas of research on opioids encompass the accumulating evidence for plasticity in opioid controls. The degree of effectiveness of morphine analgesia is subject to modulation by other transmitter systems in the spinal cord and by pathological changes induced by peripheral nerve injury. Thus in neuropathic states (pain after nerve injury), morphine analgesia can be reduced (but can still be effective); this reduced efficacy appears to partly result from increased levels of the anti-opioid peptide cholecystokinin (CCK) (Dickenson and Suzuki 1999).

Norepinephrine released from descending pathways and acting at α_2 adrenergic receptors, adenosine, and γ-aminobutyric acid (GABA) are all inhibitory systems that can modulate somatosensory pathways in the spinal cord. However, modulation by drugs is complicated by both sedative and cardiovascular events (Millan 2002).

Thus, both peripheral and central spinal changes occur in persistent pain, and much attention has quite rightly focused on tackling the induction and maintenance of these various mechanisms of hypersensitivity. However, recent evidence (Suzuki et al. 2002b, 2004) points to yet another type of facilitatory drive from within the brain that can further enhance spinal mechanisms of pain, independently but in concert with peripheral and central hypersensitivity. In a sense, the functioning of pain-facilitatory systems is most likely because following injury, most patients have pain. Even after neuropathy, when sensory loss is the predictable result of damage to peripheral sensory fibers, up to 30% of patients suffer pain. A recent study on patients with arthritis clearly showed increased responsiveness to pain in areas outside the arthritic area, indicative of central sensitization, but found that one type of descending inhibitory control was still normal, indicating that facilitations must have overcome inhibitions in these patients (Staud et al. 2003b).

VOLTAGE-DEPENDENT CALCIUM CHANNELS LINK PERIPHERAL EVENTS TO TRANSMITTER RELEASE

VDCCs are critical to sensory transmission. In response to membrane depolarization they mediate Ca^{2+} entry into numerous cell types and thus underlie synaptic transmission of sensory information from the periphery to the brain via the control of depolarization-coupled neurotransmitter release, neuronal excitability, and intracellular changes including gene induction (Fig. 2). Sensory neurons express a number of classes of VDCCs (L, N, P, Q, R, and T), distinguished by their electrophysiological and pharmacological profiles. Subsequent advances in molecular biology have identified 10 genes encoding the main pore-forming α_1 subunit, termed α_{1A} to α_{1I}, and a recently devised nomenclature groups these into three families, Ca_v1, 2, and 3, based upon structural and functional characteristics (Ertel et al. 2000).

The Ca_v2 VDCCs are widely expressed throughout the brain and spinal cord. Upon substantial membrane depolarization, such as that caused by impulses in peripheral fibers, they are activated and then mediate the release of excitatory neurotransmitters critical for neurotransmission, wind-up, and central sensitization. N-type ($Ca_v2.2$) and P/Q-type ($Ca_v2.1$) VDCCs have

Calcium channel structure and function

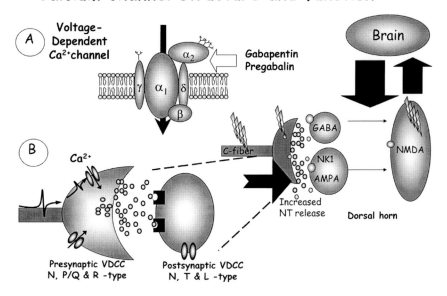

Fig. 2. (A) Structure of calcium channels. The α_1 subunit determines the type of channel (N, P/Q, R, T, or L) and contains the pore that allows calcium to enter the neuron or terminal when depolarized. Gabapentin and pregabalin bind to the $\alpha_2\delta$ subunit. (B) General location of these channels. N-, P/Q-, and R-type channels are found presynaptically on terminals, where they cause transmitter release as action potentials arrive from the peripheral nerve. N-, T-, and L-type channels on postsynaptic sites contribute to neuronal excitability, although L-type channels appear to have minimal roles in pain. The presynaptic channels cause release of glutamate and peptides such as substance P that act on their receptors (NK1 for substance P; AMPA, NMDA for glutamate) on spinal dorsal horn neurons to generate patterns of activity to send to the brain. Spinal activity is in turn controlled by local neurons (e.g., GABA-containing) and pathways that descend from the brain. Increased calcium channel activity is seen after both inflammation and nerve injury so that dorsal horn neurons are exposed to more primary afferent transmitters.

been extensively studied due to their established block by ω-conotoxin-GVIA and ω-agatoxin IVA, respectively. Only recently has SNX-482 been shown to specifically block $Ca_v2.3$ (α_{1E}, putatively R-type) VDCCs (Newcomb et al. 1998), and so this channel can now be more thoroughly investigated. Behavioral and electrophysiological nociceptive studies in animal models of acute and persistent pain have established the antinociceptive abilities of antagonists or blockers specific for the various VDCCs. These studies have highlighted the differential role each subtype plays in nociception, often dependent on the nature of the pain state (Vanegas and Schaible 2000; Matthews and Dickenson 2001a,b). Concentrated in laminae I and II of the superficial dorsal horn, where nociceptive primary afferents synapse, N-type VDCCs have a well-documented role in nociception that predominates over the other VDCCs because this channel assumes greater importance after both neuropathy and inflammation. Compensatory increases in peripheral and spinal neuronal activity after neuropathy may lead to a greater functional role of N-type VDCCs, resulting in an increase in neurotransmitter release and membrane depolarization, in turn promoting spinal mechanisms of hyperexcitability that contribute to the ensuing neuropathic syndromes. Indeed, spinal expression of the N-type VDCC α_{1B} subunit is increased in superficial L4 and L5 spinal segments after neuropathy (Cizkova et al. 2002), and mRNA and protein for the auxiliary $\alpha_2\delta$ subunit of VDCCs are also upregulated in the ipsilateral DRG and spinal cord of neuropathic rats (Luo et al. 2001, 2002). Additionally, knockout mice lacking the N-type VDCCs display reduced responses in persistent inflammatory conditions (Hatakeyama et al. 2001; Kim et al. 2001; Saegusa et al. 2001) and neuropathic pain signs (Saegusa et al. 2001). In contrast, P/Q-type channels appear to play a modest role in sensory transmission. They are implicated in the initiation of a facilitated pain state, especially inflammation, with little influence in the maintenance of neuropathy (Vanegas and Schaible 2000; Matthews and Dickenson 2001b; Ogasawara et al. 2001). To date there is little literature concerning the nociceptive role of R-type VDCCs, but preliminary data show they have some importance in sensory transmission at the level of the spinal cord in neuropathic conditions (E.A. Matthews, unpublished observations), and α_{1E} mutant mice show altered nociceptive behavior (Saegusa et al. 2000, 2002).

The importance of the enhanced role for N-type VDCCs after neuropathy is supported by clinical observations that intrathecal ziconotide (SNX-111, a potent, reversible N-type VDCC blocker) provides some pain relief in chronic pain patients (Brose et al. 1997; Atanassoff et al. 2000). Pharmacological targeting of these channels with toxin antagonists as a potential therapy for the treatment of chronic pain is hindered by the adverse systemic side effects (Penn and Paice 2000) and the inconvenient spinal route of administration. Perhaps conditions in which N-type channel function is of greater importance may minimize adverse effects, such that overactivity or expression of N-type VDCC function in the pathophysiological state is targeted, leaving normal physiological function intact.

L-type (Ca_v1) VDCCs appear to have a limited role in sensory transmission. Of the four L-type channels (selectively blocked by 1,4-dihydropyridines, for example), spinal cord neurons express $Ca_v1.2$ (α_{1C}) and $Ca_v1.3$ (α_{1D}) (Ahlijanian et al. 1990; Hell et al. 1993; Westenbroek et al. 1998); however, they seem to play little part in nociceptive transmission in both acute and more persistent pain states. T-type (Ca_v3) VDCCs are also present in the dorsal horn of the spinal cord and sensory ganglia. T-type channels are activated at voltages near the resting membrane potential. They allow Ca^{2+} influx when cells are at rest, thus regulating cell excitability and most likely influencing the depolarization required to activate high-voltage-activated N- and P/Q-type channels necessary for neurotransmission (Vanegas and Schaible 2000; Matthews and Dickenson 2001a,b). Ethosuximide, a relatively specific T-type VDCC antagonist (Coulter et al. 1989), is a clinically used anticonvulsant that inhibits nociceptive transmission in normal and neuropathic rats (Matthews and Dickenson 2001a; Dogrul et al. 2003; Todorovic et al. 2003). The parallels between epilepsy and pain, the likelihood of common causal mechanisms, and the ability of antiepileptic drugs to be effective in neuropathic pain states may merit assessment of ethosuximide for human pain management.

It is noteworthy that gabapentin and pregabalin, with analgesic efficacy in patients, may exert effects via binding to VDCCs. Gabapentin has been demonstrated to bind to the auxiliary $\alpha_2\delta$ subunit of VDCCs (Gee et al. 1996), where it is assumed to act as an antagonist (Taylor 1995). There is increased expression of $\alpha_2\delta$ in rat DRG that correlates with gabapentin-sensitive tactile allodynia only in neuropathies of mechanical and diabetic origin (Luo et al. 2001, 2002). Gabapentin may highlight the importance of VDCCs as targets in pain control (Vanegas and Schaible 2000; Matthews and Dickenson 2002).

Differences in the success of gabapentin in the clinic, as with many other drugs used for pain management, are observed even among patients with similar painful conditions and symptoms (Serpell 2002). It is becoming apparent that differences in drug sensitivity may be influenced by the nature of the insult and perhaps more importantly that the ensuing symptoms can vary by merit of recruitment of different neuronal systems; a number of different causal mechanisms are likely to underlie the basis of their diversity. Variability may also have a genetic component that relates to susceptibility to analgesic agents (at its simplest, gene polymorphisms coding for drug-binding sites), as well as to symptoms and severity of response to tissue and nerve damage, as demonstrated in extensive mouse behavioral studies (Mogil et al. 1999). For the future, extensive knowledge of human phenotypes may help predict susceptibility to pain, consequences of tissue and nerve damage, pharmacological sensitivity, and even optimal analgesia specific to the patient.

PROPERTIES OF LAMINA I AND V NEURONS
IN THE DORSAL HORN

The myelinated Aβ fibers terminate predominantly in laminae III–VI and transmit innocuous information in a fast and efficient manner. Thinly myelinated Aδ fibers, which terminate essentially in lamina I, transmit both innocuous and noxious information (Millan 1999). Unmyelinated C fibers, the slower nociceptive nerve fibers, terminate in lamina II_o of the dorsal horn, and to a smaller extent in lamina I (Millan 1999).

The dorsal horn is essentially divided into six distinct laminae, separated into five general areas. These are the marginal layer, substantia gelatinosa, nucleus proprius, the central canal and surrounding area, and finally the ventral horn. The marginal layer is the most dorsal layer of gray matter within the spinal cord; along with the substantia gelatinosa, it forms the superficial dorsal horn (Sorkin and Carlton 1997). The marginal layer is comprised mainly of small neurons and large, disk-shaped Waldeyer cells with protracted dendrites, extending throughout the rostrocaudal plane (Sorkin and Carlton 1997). The initial synapses in nociceptive transmission, from the point of noxious stimulation to supraspinal systems, lie within laminae I and II of the dorsal horn. This marginal layer is a fundamental component of the central representation of both pain and temperature and has major ascending outputs to the brain.

The primary ascending output from the superficial dorsal horn is via lamina I. Lamina I axons located in cats and primates project contralaterally in the lateral spinothalamic tract (STT) (Craig and Dostrovsky 2001). Crucial projections to spinal autonomic and brainstem homeostatic integration sites (Craig and Dostrovsky 2001) include the lateral periaqueductal gray (PAG), as well as the parabrachial (PB) area. Laminae IV–VI form the least densely packed layer in the dorsal horn and contain STT cell somas. The majority of lamina V neurons extend up toward the superficial lamina layers. Interestingly, some of the cell bodies located within lamina V form STT ascending pathways, as well as spinocervical tract and postsynaptic dorsal column ascending pathways to a lesser extent, and thus contribute to spinal nociceptive transmission (Sorkin and Carlton 1997).

Lamina I comprises modality-selective neurons (Craig and Dostrovsky 2001; Craig et al. 2001). There are three major physiological classes, in accordance with their responses to natural cutaneous stimuli: the nociceptive-specific (NS), polymodal, and thermoreceptive cells (Craig and Dostrovsky 2001; Craig et al. 2001). Most studies suggest that lamina I neurons receive sensory information mainly from high-threshold mechanoreceptors. However, reports of responses to mechanical, thermal, histamine, and cold stimuli indicate significant inputs from polymodal high-threshold nociceptors as well (Woolf and Fitzgerald 1983; Bester et al. 2000; Andrew and Craig 2001).

Although most work on lamina I neurons has focused on the response characteristics of STT lamina I neurons in the cat and monkey, recent work has also investigated the physiological properties of lamina I spinoparabrachial neurons in the rat (Bester et al. 2000). Interestingly, spino-PB neurons were composed predominantly of NS cells (75%) (Han et al. 1998; Bester et al. 2000). One of the most intriguing findings was that compared to deep dorsal horn neurons, which classically exhibit a wind-up response to repetitive noxious stimuli, lamina I spino-PB neurons do not exhibit wind-up (Dickenson et al. 1997; Bester et al. 2000), a characteristic feature of this neuronal population (Bester et al. 2000). These findings were in agreement with those found in electrophysiological characterizations of spinal lamina I neurons in the rat, whereby 61% of neurons were NS and 13% were NS with an additional response to cold based on their responses to natural mechanical and heat stimuli (Seagrove et al. 2004). However, in contrast, the majority (83%) of lamina V deep dorsal horn neurons are wide dynamic range (WDR) in response to mechanical and heat-evoked stimuli. These neurons had larger C-fiber and post-discharge response values and a clear wind-up response to evoked electrical stimuli (Fig. 3; Seagrove et al. 2004).

Interestingly, ablation of neurokinin-1 (NK1)-expressing lamina I neurons in the spinal cord, using a substance P and saporin conjugate (SP-SAP), results in behavioral deficits to noxious stimuli (Nichols et al. 1999) and reduced coding of both thermal and mechanical coding in deep dorsal horn neurons (Suzuki et al. 2002b). These studies imply a substantial control of lamina V coding and response properties mediated via superficial neurons with ascending projections.

Some of the differences between neurons in the superficial and deep spinal cord may result from their pharmacological makeup. Glutamate, the major excitatory neurotransmitter, is found abundantly throughout the mammalian CNS. Glutamate acts via ionotropic and metabotropic glutamate receptors (mGluRs) distributed throughout the spinal cord and the brain (Ozawa et al. 1998). Immunocytochemical staining studies show the presence of ionotropic glutamate receptor (iGlur) subunits 1–4 in laminae I–III of the spinal cord, implying a role for α-amino-3-hydroxy-5-methyl-4-isoxazole propionate (AMPA) receptors in sensory transmission at the spinal cord level (Furuyama et al. 1993; Yung 1998). Kainate receptor subunits (iGluR5–7) are also distributed within laminae I–III of the spinal cord (Furuyama et al. 1993; Yung 1998). DRG neurons contain functional kainate receptors, strongly suggesting a presynaptic control by kainate receptors of primary

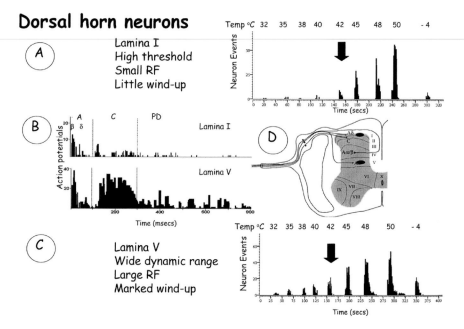

Fig. 3. Two main types of dorsal horn neuron respond to noxious stimuli. (A) Typical response of a high-threshold lamina I neuron with small receptive field (RF) to temperature; electrically evoked responses are shown in the upper part of panel B. The neuron fails to respond to temperatures below 42°C (marked by arrow). (B) Note the greater electrically evoked response in the lamina V neuron where wind-up plays a major role in amplifying the response. (C) Responses of a deep lamina V neuron that codes warm as well as noxious heat above 42°C. Both neurons (lamina I and V) respond to cold (final response in panels A, C). (D) Typical location of the two neuronal classes in lamina I and V of the dorsal horn.

afferent neurons in the superficial dorsal horn (Kerchner et al. 2001). Immunocytochemical studies in the rat have revealed subunits of the NMDA receptor, NMDAR1 and NMDAR2B, predominantly in laminae I–III (Yung 1998). Interestingly, NMDAR2A and NMDRAR2C subunits were not found in the dorsal horn, suggesting that these receptors play a minor role in nociceptive transmission at the spinal cord level (Furuyama et al. 1993; Yung 1998).

In vivo electrophysiological studies have suggested a role for the iGluRs (AMPA, kainate, and NMDA receptors) in both lamina I and lamina V dorsal horn neurons (Dickenson and Sullivan 1990; Seagrove et al. 2004). Although AMPA and kainate receptors have similar roles in both lamina I and lamina V neurons in that antagonists reduce electrically evoked neuronal responses, NMDA receptors have rather different roles in these two neuronal populations (Dickenson and Sullivan 1990; Seagrove et al. 2004).

Block of NMDA receptors has distinct inhibitory effects on wind-up, C-fiber-responses, and post-discharge responses in lamina V of the dorsal horn (Dickenson and Sullivan 1990). This effect is not seen in superficial dorsal horn neurons (Dickenson and Sullivan 1990). Thus, not only do lamina I neurons fail to show wind-up, but application of NMDA-receptor antagonists has minimal inhibitory effects on response properties of lamina I neurons (Seagrove et al. 2004). This lack of NMDA-receptor-mediated wind-up in superficial cells may explain their low excitability and high threshold properties.

CHANGES IN SPINAL CORD NEURONS IN AN ANIMAL MODEL OF BONE CANCER

Many studies over the years have examined how peripheral inflammation and nerve injury can change transmission through spinal neuronal systems (for reviews see Millan 1999, 2002; Dickenson et al. 2002). Pain from bone cancer is a major clinical problem (Mercadante 1997; Schwei et al. 1999). A recently developed rat model based on intratibial injection of mammary tumor cells has been used to mimic progressive cancer-induced bone pain. Stable behavioral changes (decreased thresholds to mechanical and cold stimuli) and bone destruction were coincident with a number of immunohistochemical changes that suggest features both common and distinct to neuropathy and nerve injury. In vivo electrophysiology was used to characterize the natural (mechanical, thermal, and cold) and electrical-evoked responses of both superficial and deep dorsal horn neurons in halothane-anesthetized rats. Receptive field size was significantly enlarged for superficial neurons in the rats injected with tumor cells. Superficial cells, as discussed previously, can be characterized as either NS or WDR. The ratio of WDR to NS cells altered radically between sham-operated rats (26%:74%) and rats with bone cancer (47%:53%). Although the NS cells showed no difference in their neuronal responses, superficial WDR neurons in rats with bone cancer had significantly increased responses to mechanical, thermal, and electrical stimuli (Urch et al. 2003). Thus, the spinal cord is significantly hyperexcitable; these changes in superficial dorsal horn neurons have not been seen in neuropathy or inflammation, which adds to the evidence that cancer-induced bone pain reflects a unique pain state. The implications of this change is that neurons in lamina I of the spinal cord have predominant projections to PB/PAG areas, whereas many deep cells project into the STT (Todd 2002). NMDA-receptor-dependent wind-up is clear and obvious in deep cells projecting to sensory areas of the brain and almost absent in lamina I neurons ascending to emotional areas (Dickenson et al. 1997; Rygh et al. 2000b; Ikeda et al. 2003). In this model of bone cancer, the shift from NS to WDR predominance in the superficial spinal cord may suggest that ascending information to the affective/emotional areas of the brain may include low-threshold information.

LONG-TERM POTENTIATION IN SPINAL NEURONS: ACUTE TO CHRONIC PAIN?

Longer-term changes than wind-up can be induced in spinal neurons. Bliss and Lomo (1973) showed that brief, high-frequency trains of electrical stimuli resulted in increased efficiency of transmission at synapses in the hippocampus that could last for hours. This phenomenon was named long-term potentiation (LTP) of synaptic transmission. It was also shown that synaptic transmission could be depressed for longer time periods (long-term depression; LTD). Since then LTP and LTD have become the most used experimental paradigms in modern neuroscience and are proposed to represent synaptic models for storage of information throughout the CNS.

With regard to pain, over the last decade LTP has also been shown by recording field potentials in the ventral (Randic et al. 1993) and the superficial dorsal horn (Liu and Sandkühler 1995), by recording evoked responses in deep single WDR neurons (Svendsen et al. 1997), and by patch-clamping superficial spino-PB neurons (Ikeda et al. 2003) in the spinal cord. It has been argued that LTP may underlie some forms of afferent-induced hyperalgesia (Sandkühler 2000), and there has been speculation as to whether central sensitization is a form of LTP or vice versa (Willis 1997, 2002).

Repetitive high-frequency electrical stimulation (HFS) of the sciatic nerve induces LTP of synaptic transmission in Aδ (Randic et al. 1993) and C fibers (Liu and Sandkühler 1995, 1997), both in vitro and in vivo. Furthermore, strong natural noxious stimuli such as skin burns, contusions, inflammation, and nerve injury also induce LTP in lamina II of the spinal cord, where most C fibers terminate (Sandkühler and Liu 1998). Simultaneous activation of multiple receptors such as the NMDA receptor, the NK1 receptor for substance P, and mGluRs are required for the induction of spinal LTP. The time course of spinal potentiation depends on the type and intensity of conditioning stimulation and on the activity of descending controls (Randic et al. 1993; Liu and Sandkühler 1995, 1997). After a brief electrical or mild natural noxious stimulus, the increased excitability can last only a few minutes (short-term potentiation), but it may last for at least 12 hours (LTP) following repetitive trains of high-frequency sciatic nerve stimulation

(Liu and Sandkühler 1995, 1997). LTD of synaptic strength at Aδ-fiber synapses in the superficial spinal dorsal horn has also been demonstrated following burst-like stimulation of Aδ fibers (Liu and Sandkühler 1998). However, selective stimulation of Aα/Aβ fibers did not affect synaptic strength at Aδ- or C-fiber synapses (Sandkühler et al. 1997; Liu and Sandkühler 1998). Thus in general, LTP can only be induced by activity in spino-PB projection neurons, thought to be part of the affective pain pathway, but not by activity in lamina I cells projecting to other areas (Ikeda et al. 2003). Thus, the conditioning stimuli that induce synaptic LTP in the superficial spinal dorsal horn are similar to those that trigger hyperalgesia. LTP is likely to occur in both the sensory and the affective pain pathways. Furthermore, spinal LTP and injury-induced hyperalgesia share the same signal transduction pathways, time course, and pharmacological profile, which makes use-dependent LTP an attractive model of injury-induced central sensitization and hyperalgesia.

If LTP at primary afferent C-fiber synapses in the superficial spinal dorsal horn are important for the development and maintenance of hyperalgesia, LTP should be found further along nociceptive transmission pathways. Interestingly, all major characteristics of LTP, originally shown at synapses in the superficial spinal dorsal horn, were confirmed by recording evoked C-fiber-mediated responses from WDR cells in the deep spinal dorsal horn (Svendsen et al. 1997; Rygh et al. 1999). The majority of these WDR cells project to the thalamus and constitute a large part of the STT, which is an important component of the sensory-discriminative pain pathway. Brief HFS of the sciatic nerve induced an increase in the C-fiber-evoked responses that outlasted the 6-hour recording period (Svendsen et al. 1997). Further, AMPA- and NMDA-receptor antagonists blocked the induction of LTP; while NMDA-receptor blockade could depotentiate the established LTP (Svendsen et al. 1998), AMPA-receptor blockade and opioid activation failed to do so (Svendsen et al. 1999b; Rygh et al. 2000a). In spinalized rats, where the descending controls are interrupted, HFS induced a greater LTP as compared to normal rats (Svendsen et al. 1999a; Gjerstad et al. 2001).

Surprisingly, LTP-inducing HFS evoked a long-lasting increase in hot-plate latencies in awake rats (Svendsen et al. 1999c). This finding has been interpreted as a masking of segmental facilitation by enhanced descending control, but could also partly be explained by the fact that the behavioral tests used are measuring thresholds for noxious heat, whereas LTP in WDR cells seems to be a suprathreshold phenomenon (Fig. 4).

Transmission at nociceptive synapses in the spinal cord can be potentiated following electrical and natural noxious peripheral stimulation. Generally,

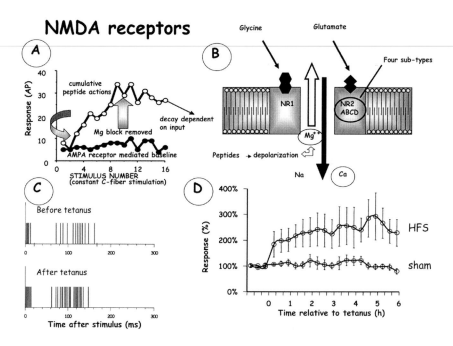

Fig. 4. Consequences of NMDA-receptor activation. (A) Wind-up, a brief increase in excitability when NMDA receptors on deep dorsal horn neurons are activated following repeated C-fiber stimulation. (B) Structure of the receptor with the glycine and glutamate binding sites on the NR1 and NR2 subunits. Variety in the NR2 subunit leads to four subtypes of the receptor. As the cumulative depolarizations produced by peptides such as substance P summate, the resting block of the NMDA-receptor channel by magnesium is removed and the receptor is activated. Sodium and calcium then enter the neuron, causing high levels of firing (A). The constant AMPA-receptor-mediated baseline now switches to a much greater number of action potentials (AP), i.e., wind-up. (C, D) Long-term potentiation (LTP) in spinal neurons. After a tetanic stimulus the C-fiber response in panel C above is increased to that shown in the lower panel. (D) LTP on a population of neurons in lamina V. A high-frequency stimulus (HFS) causes a sustained increase in activity that persists for 6 hours, whereas there is no change in the responses after a sham stimulus.

the greater the intensity of the noxious stimulation, the longer is the duration of the potentiation (Liu and Sandkühler 1995, 1997, 1998). Only extreme natural noxious stimulation induces LTP in intact animals (Rygh et al. 1999), whereas moderate to intense natural noxious stimulation induces LTP only in spinalized rats (Sandkühler and Liu 1998). Further, it seems rather convincing that descending inhibitory controls prevent LTP during and after most physiological noxious stimuli (Sandkühler and Liu 1998; Svendsen et al. 1999a). However, the activity in endogenous inhibitory systems can be modulated by the psychological state of a patient, e.g., by the level of vigilance or attention, by stress, and possibly by degree of depression and anxiety. Thus, under such unfavorable psychological states, the threshold for induction of LTP in pain pathways may be lowered. LTP is considered a cellular and synaptic model for learning and memory. The idea that memory traces of nociception and pain remain for long periods following noxious stimulation is attractive and may explain some forms of afferent-induced hyperalgesia. Indeed, as mentioned above, it has been hypothesized that LTP may be a form of central sensitization or vice versa (Willis 1997, 2002), which constitutes the most likely single phenomenon to explanation how acute pain may become chronic.

DESCENDING FACILITATION: A SPINOBULBOSPINAL LOOP

Peripheral and central spinal changes occur in persistent pain, and a great deal of attention has focused on tackling the induction and mainte- nance of these various mechanisms of hypersensitivity. In response to in- jury, spinal intrinsic mechanisms, together with peripheral inputs, can pro- duce a state of central sensitization, which may further amplify the pain response, as discussed above in terms of wind-up and LTP. More recently, another type of facilitatory drive of supraspinal origin has been identified. This descending excitatory pathway, which arises from the midbrain and brainstem, can further enhance the spinal mechanisms of pain, independent of, but in concert with, direct peripheral and spinal events (Urban and Gebhart 1999; Ossipov et al. 2000; Suzuki et al. 2002b).

SUPRASPINAL MODULATION OF SPINAL TRANSMISSION

Spinal transmission can be modulated from certain supraspinal sites, such as the PAG and rostral ventromedial medulla (RVM), to exert both facilitatory and inhibitory influences on the spinal cord (Urban and Gebhart 1999; Millan 2002). Earlier behavioral studies principally focused on the descending inhibitory influence of the PAG and RVM on the spinal cord, demonstrating a reduction in pain behavior following electrical stimulation or morphine injection (Basbaum et al. 1976). More recently, attention has turned toward the opposite function—the contribution of excitatory drives arising from these brainstem areas, in particular the RVM.

Mounting anatomical and pharmacological evidence attests to descend- ing facilitatory pathways and their role in the development and maintenance of central sensitization after injury (Urban and Gebhart 1999; Porreca et al. 2002). Following neuropathy, chemical inactivation of the RVM or selective ablation of μ-opioid-receptor-expressing RVM neurons time-dependently attenuated tactile and thermal hyperalgesia (Porreca et al. 2001; Burgess et al. 2002). Thus, an inappropriate activation of descending facilitatory influences may underlie some of the neuropathy-induced plasticity observed at the spinal level. In addition, administration of a CCK_B antagonist into the RVM reversed neuropathic pain behaviors, suggesting that tonic activity of CCK may have a role in modulating abnormal pain after nerve injury (Kovelowski et al. 2000). Recent evidence suggests that one such descending excitatory pathway requires 5HT as the key substrate. This transmitter is released into the spinal cord from pathways that originate in the RVM and exerts powerful excitatory effects by activating spinal $5HT_3$ receptors. $5HT_3$ receptors are predominantly localized in the superficial dorsal horn, where they are expressed on the nerve terminals of small-diameter afferents (Zeitz et al. 2002). Blockade of spinal $5HT_3$ receptors using the selective antagonist ondansetron, as well as genetic deletion of the receptor, has revealed a pronociceptive role of this receptor (Ali et al. 1996; Green et al. 1998; Zeitz et al. 2002).

DESCENDING FACILITATION DRIVEN BY NK1-EXPRESSING LAMINA I NEURONS

Lamina I neurons that express the NK1 receptor for substance P are predominantly projection neurons, i.e., they send ascending axons to a number of brainstem areas that are important in both sensory and affective aspects of nociceptive processing (Todd et al. 2000). A key supraspinal target is the parabrachial (PB) area, which receives a dense afferent projection from these cells. The PB in turn projects to brainstem areas such as the PAG and the ventrolateral medulla, which in turn project back to the spinal cord, forming complex loops that allow the brain to further regulate spinal activity.

NK1-expressing lamina I neurons play an important role in the central sensitization, allodynia, and hyperalgesia that underlie abnormal pain states (Nichols et al. 1999; Hunt and Mantyh 2001). Selective ablation of the lamina I NK1-receptor-expressing population of neurons, through the use of SP-SAP, markedly attenuates pain behavior in rats following intraplantar capsaicin injection, as well as in various models of inflammatory pain (carrageenan, formalin, or complete Freund's adjuvant) (Mantyh et al. 1997). Furthermore, SP-SAP treatment prevents nerve-injury-associated allodynia when given either before or after the development of neuropathic pain (Nichols et al. 1999). Electrophysiological recordings of spinal neurons in these animals revealed marked changes in the response characteristics of deeper dorsal horn neurons. These included a reduction in receptive field size; attenuation of mechanical and thermal evoked responses of spinal neurons; reduced responses to chemical (formalin) inflammation; and reduced central sensitization of deep dorsal horn neurons, as revealed by diminished wind-up.

Because these cells form part of an important ascending pathway to the brainstem (Todd et al. 2000), loss of the ascending lamina I–PB pathway was proposed to underlie these reduced pain responses, seen both behaviorally and in deep spinal neurons. Importantly, most of the effects of ablating these lamina I neurons were reproduced by blocking the pronociceptive $5HT_3$ receptor in the spinal cord using ondansetron in unlesioned animals, providing pharmacological evidence for a serotonergic descending facilitatory influence from the brainstem. Importantly, the only neuronal response unaffected by ondansetron was wind-up, although this effect was highly sensitive to SP-SAP treatment. Thus, wind-up is an intrinsic spinal phenomenon relying on lamina I–lamina V circuitry but not on descending excitations. Furthermore, c-Fos data for the raphe magnus—a nucleus of the RVM rich in 5HT-expressing neurons—showed reduced activation following peripheral formalin injection in SP-SAP-treated animals compared with the control group (Suzuki et al. 2002a). Taken together, these results provide evidence that NK1-lamina I projection neurons, which project to the PB and other areas implicated in emotional responses, are at the origin of a spinobulbospinal loop that involves the RVM, and that they control spinal excitability and pain sensitivity by activating a descending serotonergic pathway.

DESCENDING FACILITATORY SEROTONERGIC PATHWAYS AND PERIPHERAL NERVE INJURY

The hypothesis that the brain can amplify spinal pain processes through a serotonergic circuit is supported by our recent findings of enhanced efficacy of ondansetron after peripheral nerve injury compared to normal conditions (Suzuki et al. 2004). $5HT_3$-mediated descending pathways therefore not only are crucial for the full coding of polymodal peripheral inputs by spinal neurons, but also appear to be enhanced after neuropathy, showing a capacity for change in the spinobulbospinal loop. This finding suggests an active participation of supraspinal sites in driving sustained facilitatory influences on the spinal cord following neuropathy, in line with the previously reported role of these pathways in chronic pain states (Kovelowski et al. 2000; Ossipov et al. 2000; Burgess et al. 2002; Porreca et al. 2002). Interestingly, ondansetron produced a significantly greater effect on mechanical punctate-evoked responses compared with its effects on thermal responses in neuropathic animals. This observation, together with the finding that spinal transection (severing supraspinal circuits) blocks nerve-injury-induced tactile allodynia but not thermal nocifensive responses (Bian et al. 1998), may indicate strong descending facilitatory influences on allodynia.

The finding that SP-SAP-treated rats display a marked attenuation of mechanical allodynia following peripheral nerve injury (Nichols et al. 1999) led us to investigate whether the activity of gabapentin is altered in these animals. Remarkably, our electrophysiological recordings revealed that the sensitivity of spinal neurons to systemic gabapentin is completely lost in animals with nerve injury following pretreatment with SP-SAP (A.H. Dickenson et al., unpublished observations). This finding was in complete contrast to that seen in neuropathic SAP-pretreated control animals, where gabapentin produced robust inhibitions of mechanical and thermal responses. The (lamina I) spinobulbospinal loop is disrupted after SP-SAP treatment, so the lack of descending serotonergic facilitatory influence may explain the attenuated pain behavior following peripheral nerve injury and may contribute to the lack of effect of gabapentin on neuronal responses. Given the presynaptic localization of the $5HT_3$ receptor and VDCCs, one consequence of activation of this serotonergic system would be an interaction with drugs like gabapentin that alter transmitter release. We hypothesized, therefore, that an interaction exists between these two systems on terminals where they colocalize and that actions of gabapentin may depend on a functional $5HT_3$-mediated descending facilitatory pathway. The depolarizing effects of $5HT_3$-receptor activation could lead to a prolonged opening of VDCCs, thus allowing gabapentin to interact with VDCCs through the $\alpha_2\delta$ subunit, inhibiting transmitter release. This train of events may allow gabapentin to produce its injury-specific actions; thus, under pathological conditions where descending excitatory influences operate (e.g., inflammation or neuropathy), gabapentin can exert robust antinociceptive effects while it is totally ineffective in naive animals.

To further test the hypothesis that a facilitatory $5HT_3$-receptor drive is required to enable the antinociceptive and antiallodynic actions of gabapentin, spinal neurons of naive animals were pretreated with a spinal application of a $5HT_3$-receptor agonist, 2-methyl-5HT. The evoked responses of deep spinal neurons to peripheral mechanical and thermal stimuli were enhanced in the presence of 2-methyl-5HT, and subsequent systemic injection of gabapentin produced a robust inhibition of these responses, similar to that seen after nerve injury. Thus, these results confirmed our hypothesis that the effectiveness of gabapentin appears to be dependent on a possible presynaptic interaction of the excitatory $5HT_3$ receptor with VDCCs.

In conclusion, the behavioral and electrophysiological evidence for a descending facilitatory pathway originating from the RVM and driven by lamina I neurons is compelling (Fig. 5). Furthermore, findings support a differential supraspinal control of primary afferent input, which could allow the brain to exert submodality-dependent regulation of spinal neuronal responses. Under pathological conditions, such as neuropathy, descending facilitatory controls to the spinal cord are enhanced and excitatory influences predominate, resulting in increased central sensitization and possibly contributing to allodynia and hyperalgesia. Remarkably, activity in this circuit appears to be a factor that determines the efficacy of gabapentin through convergent interactions at the level of the peripheral terminals.

We believe that due to physiopathological changes in peripheral nerves caused by trauma, inflammation, and nerve injury, a wave of plasticity sweeps into the spinal cord. VDCCs become more active, pouring more transmitters onto spinal neurons, which then become hyperexcitable due to resultant

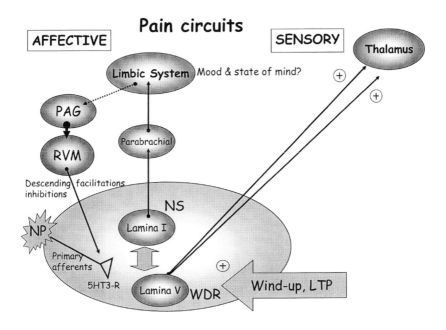

Fig. 5. A diagram of the lamina I projections to the "emotional" parts of the brain and the lamina V pathways to the thalamus and cortex that generate the affective and sensory components of pain. Wind-up and LTP can potentiate the output of lamina V. After neuropathy (NP), increases in descending facilitations driven by lamina I neurons and relaying through the periaqueductal gray (PAG) and rostral ventromedial medulla (RVM) activate spinal $5HT_3$ receptors that further enhance ascending activity from the dorsal horn. These pathways may be one of the ways in which mood can enhance the perception of pain and possibly also modify the effects of drugs on spinal activity.

wind-up of the deep dorsal horn neurons, and receptive fields expand. Continuing peripheral inputs maintain cells in a wound-up state. Higher-frequency peripheral stimuli can elicit LTP that endures for hours after the stimulus. However, neurons in lamina I of the spinal cord have projections to PB/PAG areas, whereas many deep cells project into the STT (Todd 2002). NMDA-receptor-dependent wind-up is clear and obvious in deep cells and almost absent in lamina I cells, although both neuronal types support LTP when high-frequency stimuli are given (Dickenson et al. 1997; Rygh et al. 2000b; Ikeda et al. 2003). This finding suggests that in pain states other than those activated by very high-frequency stimuli, spinothalamic inputs will be potentiated through wind-up-like mechanisms, whereas inputs to emotional areas will not. This situation may then lead to a dissociation between the emotional and sensory-discriminative aspects of pain. However, the lamina I high-threshold neurons can trigger descending facilitations mediated through PB-RVM connections, effects that are enhanced after neuropathy and that further enhance the activity of deep dorsal horn neurons, independently of wind-up. These loops, running through the emotional/affective areas, may become yet more active in patients with anxiety, fear, and negative affect, further driving the level of pain in the sensory-discriminative systems of the brain. Inhibitory controls are important, but the evidence favors the idea that facilitations dominate in many conditions.

With regard to induced inhibitory actions, opioids have identical dose-response curves for lamina I and V neurons, which would be consistent with their ability to modulate both the sensation of pain and the affective qualities. However, an added complexity regarding lamina V is that once wind-up is induced, opioid inhibitions fail to cope with the enhanced activity; when LTP is induced, morphine, at doses that completely suppress LTP, does not alter the underlying process. Thus, reversal of opioid inhibition only occurs to the post-LTP response level (Rygh et al. 2000a). We now think that the actions of gabapentin may be determined, to some extent, by the level of activity in the descending facilitatory loop. Peripheral inputs, the state of mind of the patient, and the efficacy of analgesic drugs have complex interactions with spinal and supraspinal mechanisms of hyperexcitability. Further exploration of this area could lead to useful clinical advances.

ACKNOWLEDGMENTS

We are funded by The Wellcome Trust and as part of the London Pain Consortium, the Medical Research Council, and Norwegian Research Council. We respectfully acknowledge our friends, colleagues, and collaborators

Steve Hunt, Frank Porreca, and John Wood. Jean-Marie Besson taught Anthony Dickenson a lot about pain and life and how science should be carried out. Prof. Dickenson in turn has taught his coauthors something of the same, and we now all teach each other. As a tribute to Jean-Marie this chapter considers how excitatory and inhibitory systems interact, through local and ascending and descending pathways, to alter the incoming painful messages. These are all areas where Jean-Marie and his colleagues made major contributions. Furthermore, Jean-Marie emphasized the importance of quantification in pain research and brought together scientists and clinicians from many countries in attempts to improve the understanding of pain and thereby its treatment. Salut Jean-Marie!

REFERENCES

Ahlijanian MK, Westenbroek RE, Catterall WA. Subunit structure and localization of dihydropyridine-sensitive calcium channels in mammalian brain, spinal cord, and retina. *Neuron* 1990; 4:819–832.

Ali Z, Wu G, Kozlov A, Barasi S. The role of 5HT3 in nociceptive processing in the rat spinal cord: results from behavioural and electrophysiological studies. *Neurosci Lett* 1996; 208:203-207.

Andrew D, Craig AD. Spinothalamic lamina I neurones selectively responsive to cutaneous warming in cats. *J Physiol* 2001; 537:489–495.

Atanassoff PG, Hartmannsgruber MW, Thrasher J, et al. Ziconotide, a new N-type calcium channel blocker, administered intrathecally for acute postoperative pain. *Reg Anesth Pain Med* 2000; 25:274–278.

Basbaum AI, Marley N, O'Keefe J. Spinal cord pathways involved in the production of analgesia by brain stimulation. In: Bonica JJ, Albe-Fessard DG (Eds). *Proceedings of the First World Congress on Pain,* Advances in Pain Research and Therapy, Vol. 1. New York: Raven Press, 1976, pp 511–515.

Bester H, Chapman V, Besson JM, Bernard JF. Physiological properties of the lamina I spinoparabrachial neurons in the rat. *J Neurophysiol* 2000; 83:2239–2259.

Bian D, Ossipov MH, Zhong C, et al. Tactile allodynia, but not thermal hyperalgesia, of the hindlimbs is blocked by spinal transection in rats with nerve injury. *Neurosci Lett* 1998; 241:79–82.

Bliss TV, Lomo T. Long-lasting potentiation of synaptic transmission in the dentate area of the anaesthetized rabbit following stimulation of the perforant path. *J Physiol* 1973; 232:331–356.

Brose WG, Gutlove DP, Luther RR, et al. Use of intrathecal SNX-111, a novel, N-type, voltage-sensitive, calcium channel blocker, in the management of intractable brachial plexus avulsion pain. *Clin J Pain* 1997; 13:256–259.

Burgess SE, Gardell LR, Ossipov MH, et al. Time-dependent descending facilitation from the rostral ventromedial medulla maintains, but does not initiate, neuropathic pain. *J Neurosci* 2002; 22:5129–5136.

Cizkova D, Marsala J, Lukacova N, et al. Localization of N-type Ca^{2+} channels in the rat spinal cord following chronic constrictive nerve injury. *Exp Brain Res* 2002; 147:456–463.

Coulter DA, Huguenard JR, Prince DA. Characterization of ethosuximide reduction of low-threshold calcium current in thalamic neurons. *Ann Neurol* 1989; 25:582–593.

Craig AD, Dostrovsky JO. Differential projections of thermoreceptive and nociceptive lamina I trigeminothalamic and spinothalamic neurons in the cat. *J Neurophysiol* 2001; 86:856–870.

Craig AD, Krout K, Andrew D. Quantitative response characteristics of thermoreceptive and nociceptive lamina I spinothalamic neurons in the cat. *J Neurophysiol* 2001; 86:1459–1480.

Dickenson AH, Sullivan AF. Differential effects of excitatory amino acid antagonists on dorsal horn nociceptive neurones in the rat. *Brain Res* 1990; 506:31–39.

Dickenson AH, Suzuki R. Function and dysfunction of opioid receptors in the spinal cord. In: Kalso E, McQuay H, Wiesenfeld-Hallin Z (Eds). *Opioid Sensitivity of Chronic Noncancer Pain,* Progress in Pain Research and Management, Vol. 14. Seattle: IASP Press, 1999, pp 17–44.

Dickenson AH, Chapman V, Green GM. The pharmacology of excitatory and inhibitory amino acid-mediated events in the transmission and modulation of pain in the spinal cord. *Gen Pharmacol* 1997; 28:633–638.

Dickenson AH, Matthews EA, Suzuki R. Central nervous system mechanisms of pain in peripheral neuropathy. In: Hansson PT, Fields HL, Hill RG, Marchettini P (Eds). *Neuropathic Pain: Pathophysiology and Treatment,* Progress in Pain Research and Management, Vol. 21. Seattle: IASP Press, 2001, pp 85–106.

Dickenson AH, Matthews EA, Suzuki R. Neurobiology of neuropathic pain: mode of action of anticonvulsants. *Eur J Pain* 2002; 6(Suppl A):51–60.

Dogrul A, Gardell LR, Ossipov MH, et al. Reversal of experimental neuropathic pain by T-type calcium channel blockers. *Pain* 2003; 105:159–168.

Dray A, Urban L. New pharmacological strategies for pain relief. *Annu Rev Pharmacol Toxicol* 1996; 36:253–280.

Ertel EA, Campbell KP, Harpold MM, et al. Nomenclature of voltage-gated calcium channels. *Neuron* 2000; 25:533–535.

Furuyama T, Kiyama H, Sato K, et al. Region-specific expression of subunits of ionotropic glutamate receptors (AMPA-type, KA-type and NMDA receptors) in the rat spinal cord with special reference to nociception. *Brain Res Mol Brain Res* 1993; 18:141–151.

Gee NS, Brown JP, Dissanayake VU, et al. The novel anticonvulsant drug, gabapentin (Neurontin), binds to the alpha2delta subunit of a calcium channel. *J Biol Chem* 1996; 271:5768–5776.

Gjerstad J, Tjolsen A, Hole K. Induction of long-term potentiation of single wide dynamic range neurones in the dorsal horn is inhibited by descending pathways. *Pain* 2001; 91:263–268.

Green GM, Scarth J, Dickenson AH. An excitatory role for 5-HT in spinal inflammatory nociceptive transmission; state-dependent actions via dorsal horn 5-HT3 receptors in the anaesthetised rat. *Pain* 2000; 89:81–88.

Han ZS, Zhang ET, Craig AD. Nociceptive and thermoreceptive lamina I neurons are anatomically distinct. *Nat Neurosci* 1998; 1:218–225.

Hatakeyama S, Wakamori M, Ino M, et al. Differential nociceptive responses in mice lacking the alpha(1B) subunit of N-type Ca(2+) channels. *Neuroreport* 2001; 12:2423–2427.

Hell JW, Westenbroek RE, Warner C, et al. Identification and differential subcellular localization of the neuronal class C and class D L-type calcium channel alpha 1 subunits. *J Cell Biol* 1993; 123:949–962.

Hunt SP, Mantyh PW. The molecular dynamics of pain control. *Nat Rev Neurosci* 2001; 2:83–91.

Ikeda H, Heinke B, Ruscheweyh R, Sandkühler J. Synaptic plasticity in spinal lamina I projection neurons that mediate hyperalgesia. *Science* 2003; 299:1237–1240.

Kerchner GA, Wilding TJ, Li P, et al. Presynaptic kainate receptors regulate spinal sensory transmission. *J Neurosci* 2001; 21:59–66.

Kim C, Jun K, Lee T, et al. Altered nociceptive response in mice deficient in the alpha(1B) subunit of the voltage-dependent calcium channel. *Mol Cell Neurosci* 2001; 18:235–245.

Kovelowski CJ, Ossipov MH, Sun H, et al. Supraspinal cholecystokinin may drive tonic descending facilitation mechanisms to maintain neuropathic pain in the rat. *Pain* 2000; 87:265–273.

Liu XG, Sandkühler J. Long-term potentiation of C-fiber-evoked potentials in the rat spinal dorsal horn is prevented by spinal N-methyl-D-aspartic acid receptor blockage. *Neurosci Lett* 1995; 191:43–46.

Liu X, Sandkühler J. Characterization of long-term potentiation of C-fiber-evoked potentials in spinal dorsal horn of adult rat: essential role of NK1 and NK2 receptors. *J Neurophysiol* 1997; 78:1973–1982.

Liu XG, Sandkühler J. Activation of spinal N-methyl-D-aspartate or neurokinin receptors induces long-term potentiation of spinal C-fibre-evoked potentials. *Neuroscience* 1998; 86:1209–1216.

Luo ZD, Chaplan SR, Higuera ES, et al. Upregulation of dorsal root ganglion (alpha)2(delta) calcium channel subunit and its correlation with allodynia in spinal nerve-injured rats. *J Neurosci* 2001; 21:1868–1875.

Luo ZD, Calcutt NA, Higuera ES, et al. Injury type-specific calcium channel alpha 2 delta-1 subunit up-regulation in rat neuropathic pain models correlates with antiallodynic effects of gabapentin. *J Pharmacol Exp Ther* 2002; 303:1199–1205.

Mantyh P, Rogers S, Honore P, et al. Inhibition of hyperalgesia by ablation of lamina I spinal neurons expressing the substance P receptor. *Science* 1997; 27:275–279.

Matthews EA, Dickenson AH. Effects of ethosuximide, a T-type Ca(2+) channel blocker, on dorsal horn neuronal responses in rats. *Eur J Pharmacol* 2001a; 415:141–149.

Matthews EA, Dickenson AH. Effects of spinally delivered N- and P-type voltage-dependent calcium channel antagonists on dorsal horn neuronal responses in a rat model of neuropathy. *Pain* 2001b; 92:235–246.

Matthews EA, Dickenson AH. A combination of gabapentin and morphine mediates enhanced inhibitory effects on dorsal horn neuronal responses in a rat model of neuropathy. *Anesthesiology* 2002; 96:633–640.

Mercadante S. Malignant bone pain: pathophysiology and treatment. *Pain* 1997; 69:1–18.

Millan MJ. The induction of pain: an integrative review. *Prog Neurobiol* 1999; 57:1–164.

Millan M. Descending control of pain. *Prog Neurobiol* 2002; 66:354–474.

Mogil JS, Wilson SG, Bon K, et al. Heritability of nociception I: responses of 11 inbred mouse strains on 12 measures of nociception. *Pain* 1999; 80:67–82.

Newcomb R, Szoke B, Palma A, et al. Selective peptide antagonist of the class E calcium channel from the venom of the tarantula *Hysterocrates gigas*. *Biochemistry* 1998; 37:15353–15362.

Nichols M, Allen B, Rogers S, et al. Transmission of chronic nociception by spinal neurons expressing the substance P receptor. *Science* 1999; 286:1558–1561.

Ogasawara M, Kurihara T, Hu Q, Tanabe T. Characterization of acute somatosensory pain transmission in P/Q-type Ca(2+) channel mutant mice, leaner. *FEBS Lett* 2001; 508:181–186.

Ossipov MH, Lai J, Malan TP Jr, Porreca F. Spinal and supraspinal mechanisms of neuropathic pain. *Ann NY Acad Sci* 2000; 909:12–24.

Ozawa S, Kamiya H, Tsuzuki K. Glutamate receptors in the mammalian central nervous system. *Prog Neurobiol* 1998; 54:581–618.

Passmore GM, Selyanko AA, Mistry M, et al. KCNQ/M currents in sensory neurons: significance for pain therapy. *J Neurosci* 2003; 23:7227–7236.

Penn RD, Paice JA. Adverse effects associated with the intrathecal administration of ziconotide. *Pain* 2000; 85:291–296.

Porreca F, Burgess SE, Gardell LR, et al. Inhibition of neuropathic pain by selective ablation of brainstem medullary cells expressing the mu-opioid receptor. *J Neurosci* 2001; 21:5281–5288.

Porreca F, Ossipov MH, Gebhart GF. Chronic pain and medullary descending facilitation. *Trends Neurosci* 2002; 25:319–325.

Price DD, Mao J, Frenk H, Mayer DJ. The N-methyl-D-aspartate receptor antagonist dextromethorphan selectively reduces temporal summation of second pain in man. *Pain* 1994; 59:165–174.

Randic M, Jiang MC, Cerne R. Long-term potentiation and long-term depression of primary afferent neurotransmission in the rat spinal cord. *J Neurosci* 1993; 13:5228–5241.

Rygh LJ, Svendsen F, Hole K, Tjolsen A. Natural noxious stimulation can induce long-term increase of spinal nociceptive responses. *Pain* 1999; 82:305–310.

Rygh LJ, Green M, Athauda N, et al. Effect of spinal morphine after long-term potentiation of wide dynamic range neurones in the rat. *Anesthesiology* 2000a; 92:140–146.

Rygh LJ, Kontinen VK, Suzuki R, Dickenson AH. Different increase in C-fibre evoked responses after nociceptive conditioning stimulation in sham-operated and neuropathic rats. *Neurosci Lett* 2000b; 288:99–102.

Saegusa H, Kurihara T, Zong S, et al. Altered pain responses in mice lacking alpha 1E subunit of the voltage-dependent Ca^{2+} channel. *Proc Natl Acad Sci USA* 2000; 97:6132–6137.

Saegusa H, Kurihara T, Zong S, et al. Suppression of inflammatory and neuropathic pain symptoms in mice lacking the N-type Ca^{2+} channel. *Embo J* 2001; 20:2349–2356.

Saegusa H, Matsuda Y, Tanabe T. Effects of ablation of N- and R-type Ca^{2+} channels on pain transmission. *Neurosci Res* 2002; 43:1–7.

Sandkühler J. Learning and memory in pain pathways. *Pain* 2000; 88:113–118.

Sandkühler J, Liu X. Induction of long-term potentiation at spinal synapses by noxious stimulation or nerve injury. *Eur J Neurosci* 1998; 10:2476–2480.

Sandkühler J, Chen JG, Cheng G, Randic M. Low-frequency stimulation of afferent A-delta-fibers induces long-term depression at primary afferent synapses with substantia gelatinosa neurons in the rat. *J Neurosci* 1997; 17:6483–6491.

Schwei MJ, Honore P, Rogers SD, et al. Neurochemical and cellular reorganization of the spinal cord in a murine model of bone cancer pain. *J Neurosci* 1999; 19:10886–10897.

Seagrove LC, Suzuki R, Dickenson AH. Electrophysiological characterisations of rat lamina I dorsal horn neurones and the involvement of excitatory amino acid receptors. *Pain* 2004;108:76–87.

Serpell MG. Gabapentin in neuropathic pain syndromes: a randomised, double-blind, placebo-controlled trial. *Pain* 2002; 99:557–566.

Sindrup SH, Jensen TS. Efficacy of pharmacological treatments of neuropathic pain: an update and effect related to mechanism of drug action. *Pain* 1999; 83:389–400.

Sorkin LS, Carlton SM. Spinal anatomy and pharmacology of afferent processing. In: Yaksh TL, Lynch C III, Zapol WM, et al. (Eds). *Anesthesia: Biologic Foundations*. Philadelphia: Lippincott-Raven, 1997, pp 577–609.

Staud R, Robinson ME, Vierck CJ, et al. Ratings of experimental pain and pain-related negative affect predict clinical pain in patients with fibromyalgia syndrome. *Pain* 2003a; 105:215–222.

Staud R, Robinson ME, Vierck CJ, Price DD. Diffuse noxious inhibitory controls (DNIC) attenuate temporal summation of second pain in normal males but not in normal females or fibromyalgia patients. *Pain* 2003b; 101:167–174.

Suzuki R, Dickenson AH. Neuropathic pain: nerves bursting with excitement. *Neuroreport* 2000; 11:R17–21.

Suzuki R, Morcuende S, Webber M, et al. Superficial NK1 expressing neurones control spinal excitability by activation of descending pathways. *Nat Neurosci* 2002a; 5:1319–1326.

Suzuki R, Morcuende S, Webber M, et al. Superficial NK1-expressing neurons control spinal excitability through activation of descending pathways. *Nat Neurosci* 2002b; 5:1319–1326.

Suzuki R, Rahman W, Dickenson AH. Descending facilitatory control of mechanically evoked responses is enhanced in deep dorsal horn neurones following peripheral nerve injury. *Brain Res* 2004; in press.

Svendsen F, Tjolsen A, Hole K. LTP of spinal A beta and C-fibre evoked responses after electrical sciatic nerve stimulation. *Neuroreport* 1997; 8:3427–3430.

Svendsen F, Tjolsen A, Hole K. AMPA and NMDA receptor-dependent spinal LTP after nociceptive tetanic stimulation. *Neuroreport* 1998; 9:1185–1190.

Svendsen F, Tjolsen A, Gjerstad J, Hole K. Long term potentiation of single WDR neurons in spinalized rats. *Brain Res* 1999a; 816:487–492.

Svendsen F, Tjolsen A, Rygh LJ, Hole K. Expression of long-term potentiation in single wide dynamic range neurons in the rat is sensitive to blockade of glutamate receptors. *Neurosci Lett* 1999b; 259:25–28.

Svendsen F, Tjolsen A, Rykkja F, Hole K. Behavioural effects of LTP-inducing sciatic nerve stimulation in the rat. *Eur J Pain* 1999c; 3:355–363.

Taylor CP. Gabapentin: mechanisms of action. In: Levy RH, Mattson RH, Meldrum BS (Eds). *Antiepileptic Drugs*. New York: Raven Press, 1995, pp 829–841.

Todd AJ. Anatomy of primary afferents and projection neurones in the rat spinal dorsal horn with particular emphasis on substance P and the neurokinin 1 receptor. *Exp Physiol* 2002; 87:245–249.

Todd AJ, McGill MM, Shehab SA. Neurokinin 1 receptor expression by neurons in laminae I, III and IV of the rat spinal dorsal horn that project to the brainstem. *Eur J Neurosci* 2000; 12:689–700.

Todorovic SM, Rastogi AJ, Jevtovic-Todorovic V. Potent analgesic effects of anticonvulsants on peripheral thermal nociception in rats. *Br J Pharmacol* 2003; 140:255–260.

Urban MO, Gebhart GF. Supraspinal contributions to hyperalgesia. *Proc Natl Acad Sci USA* 1999; 96:7687–7692.

Urch CE, Donovan-Rodriguez T, Dickenson AH. Alterations in dorsal horn neurones in a rat model of cancer-induced bone pain. *Pain* 2003;106:347–356.

Vanegas H, Schaible H. Effects of antagonists to high-threshold calcium channels upon spinal mechanisms of pain, hyperalgesia and allodynia. *Pain* 2000; 85:9–18.

Westenbroek RE, Hoskins L, Catterall WA. Localization of Ca^{2+} channel subtypes on rat spinal motor neurons, interneurons, and nerve terminals. *J Neurosci* 1998; 18:6319–6330.

Willis WD Jr. Is central sensitization of nociceptive transmission in the spinal cord a variety of long-term potentiation? *Neuroreport* 1997; 8:iii.

Willis WD. Long-term potentiation in spinothalamic neurons. *Brain Res Brain Res Rev* 2002; 40:202–214.

Woolf CJ, Fitzgerald M. The properties of neurones recorded in the superficial dorsal horn of the rat spinal cord. *J Comp Neurol* 1983; 221:313–328.

Yung KK. Localization of glutamate receptors in dorsal horn of rat spinal cord. *Neuroreport* 1998; 9:1639–1644.

Zeitz KP, Guy N, Malmberg AB, et al. The 5-HT3 subtype of serotonin receptor contributes to nociceptive processing via a novel subset of myelinated and unmyelinated nociceptors. *J Neurosci* 2002; 22:1010–1019.

Correspondence to: Anthony H. Dickenson, PhD, Department of Pharmacology, University College London, Gower Street, London WC1E 6BT, United Kingdom. Email: anthony.dickenson@ucl.ac.uk.

The Pain System in Normal and Pathological States:
A Primer for Clinicians, Progress in Pain Research
and Management, Vol. 31, edited by Luis Villanueva,
Anthony Dickenson, and Hélène Ollat, IASP Press,
Seattle, © 2004.

6

Brainstem Modulation of Pain after Inflammation

Ronald Dubner and Ke Ren

Department of Biomedical Sciences, University of Maryland Dental School,
Baltimore, Maryland, USA

HISTORICAL PERSPECTIVE

Recent major advances in the understanding of pain mechanisms can be subdivided into three areas: sensory coding, or how the nervous system extracts information about stimulus features from the environment; sensory or descending modulation, or how control systems in the brain modulate this incoming information; and activity-dependent plasticity, or how the increased barrage from the peripheral nervous system after injury leads to long-term changes in central nervous system function. Jean-Marie Besson and his colleagues contributed to our knowledge in all of these areas, but we would like to focus on the area of descending modulation, where their *major* findings have been the basis of considerable subsequent research.

Information about the condition of injured peripheral tissues enters the spinal cord and then ascends to higher centers in the brainstem, thalamus, and cerebral cortex, ultimately elaborated as a complex sensory experience. What we perceive not only depends on the features of the stimulus but is also related to its meaning based on previous exposure to pain, its influence on our emotional state, and its relevance to our survival. Descending modulation of pain refers to how the pain experience is modified at supraspinal sites in the brainstem and forebrain. It is an important component of the sensory processing of pain because it provides the neural networks by which attention, motivation, and cognition modify what we perceive.

Our knowledge of the existence of endogenous descending pain-modulatory systems spans at least three decades (for comprehensive reviews, see Fields and Basbaum 1999; Millan 2002). The first line of evidence to support endogenous pain control came from the study of Reynolds (1969), who demonstrated that focal brain stimulation of the periaqueductal gray (PAG) produced sufficient analgesia to allow surgery in rats without the use of chemical anesthetics. Liebeskind and colleagues quickly confirmed this finding and concluded that stimulation of the PAG activated a normal function of the brain—pain inhibition (Mayer et al. 1971; Mayer and Liebeskind 1974). An important descending modulatory site in the brainstem is the rostral ventromedial medulla (RVM), whose major component is the nucleus raphe magnus (NRM), which receives signals directly from the PAG and indirectly from forebrain sites such as the prefrontal cortex, the amygdala, and the anterior cingulate gyrus (Bandler and Shipley 1994). Besson and colleagues were the first to show that electrical stimulation of the NRM produced a powerful analgesia and suppressed behavioral responses to strong pinch of the tail or the limbs as well as modifying the threshold of the jaw-opening reflex (Oliveras et al. 1975).

BIDIRECTIONAL DESCENDING CONTROL

The early studies by Besson and others established the presence of a descending inhibitory pain-modulatory circuit linking the brainstem PAG and RVM with the spinal cord (for reviews, see Basbaum and Fields 1984; Gebhart 1986; Fields and Basbaum 1999; Millan 2002). However, we now know that there are parallel descending facilitatory mechanisms. Descending facilitation was not recognized in the early reports because it was often masked by the more intense electrical stimulation or higher drug doses used to produce descending inhibition. Brainstem descending pathways also facilitate nociceptive transmission at the spinal cord level. Excitation and inhibition of dorsal horn neurons can be produced by stimulating the dorsolateral funiculus of the spinal cord (Dubuisson and Wall 1979; McMahon and Wall 1988), the NRM (Dubuisson and Wall 1980), and the nucleus reticularis gigantocellularis (NGC) (Haber et al. 1980). In the NGC, low-intensity electrical stimulation or microinjection of neurotensin, a low dose of glutamate, or a high dose of baclofen, a $GABA_B$-receptor agonist, all facilitate spinal behavioral and dorsal horn neuronal responses to noxious stimulation (Zhuo and Gebhart 1992, 1997; Zhuo et al. 2002; Thomas et al. 1995; Urban and Gebhart 1997). RVM neurons may exert bidirectional control of nociception through descending serotoninergic and noradrenergic pathways (Zhuo and Gebhart 1991; Holden et al. 1999). In addition, vagal afferent stimulation produces facilitation and inhibition of the nociceptive tail-flick reflex and of dorsal horn nociceptive neuronal activity (Randich and Gebhart 1992).

In the RVM, two types of cells have been identified by Fields and colleagues (1991) as pain-modulatory neurons: on-cells are characterized by a sudden increase in activity before the initiation of a nocifensive behavior, in this case, a tail flick to a transient noxious heat stimulus. Off-cells exhibit a pause in activity just prior to the initiation of the tail flick. While off-cells are usually associated with the inhibition of nocifensive behaviors, on-cells are correlated with a facilitation of nocifensive behavior. A third type of cell, the neutral-cell, was also identified, but its activity was not correlated with nocifensive behavior in response to transient stimuli.

PERSISTENT PAIN AND DESCENDING MODULATION

The findings described above demonstrate the bimodal nature of descending modulation, often originating from the same sites. However, these earlier findings focused on the responses to acute or transient stimuli. Recent studies have examined the effects of descending modulation on persistent pain that lasts for hours, days, or longer following tissue damage or nerve injury (for reviews see Dubner and Ren 1999, 2002). Persistent pain is associated with prolonged functional changes in the nervous system and leads to hyperexcitability at the level of the spinal and medullary dorsal horns, also referred to as central sensitization (for reviews, see Dubner and Ruda 1992; Woolf and Salter 2000). Considerable evidence now indicates that descending inhibition is enhanced after inflammation at sites of *primary hyperalgesia* where the injury takes place. The descending inhibition appears to dampen the central sensitization that occurs at the level of the spinal cord (Schaible et al. 1991; Ren and Dubner 1996; Tsuruoka and Willis 1996; Wei et al. 1999). The source of the inhibition can be traced back to brainstem structures. Fig. 1 shows that focal lesions of the RVM in hindpaw-inflamed rats are associated with decreases in paw-withdrawal latency to a noxious stimulus, a measure of nocifensive behavior, as compared to naive animals. This finding suggests that the chemical lesion attenuates the increase in descending inhibition produced in a behavioral model of inflammation-induced primary hyperalgesia.

Descending facilitation also can be seen when other sites in the brainstem are activated. Fig. 2 shows that destruction of the NGC in the medulla leads to an increase in paw-withdrawal latency, suggesting that a descending facilitation has been attenuated. These behavioral changes after NRM and NGC lesions are accompanied by parallel changes in the excitability of the spinal dorsal horn, providing evidence that the behavioral effects are spinally mediated, at least in part (Wei et al. 1999). A dominant descending

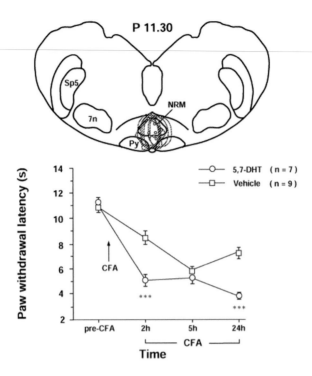

Fig. 1. Effects of a serotoninergic lesion to the nucleus raphe magnus (NRM) on inflammation-induced hyperalgesia. Upper panel: Schematic representation of 5,7-DHT microinjection sites and the extent of lesions (dotted lines) revealed by Nissl staining in the NRM. Small circles indicate the vehicle injection sites. Sp5 = spinal trigeminal nucleus; 7n = facial nucleus; Py = pyramidal tract. Lower panel: The effect of the NRM serotoninergic lesion on thermal hyperalgesia induced by complete Freund's adjuvant (CFA)-. Withdrawal latencies of the inflamed hindpaw in the lesioned animals were significantly shorter than those in corresponding vehicle-injected rats at 2 and 24 hours post-CFA (*** $P < 0.001$). Adapted from Wei et al. (1999).

facilitatory drive appears to contribute to other types of persistent pain, particularly those associated with secondary hyperalgesia outside the zone of inflammation or with nerve injury (see Porreca et al. 2002 for reviews).

DYNAMIC CHANGES IN DESCENDING MODULATION

Recent studies indicate that the enhancement of descending inhibition in response to peripheral tissue injury appears to build up gradually as inflammation persists (Schaible et al. 1991; Ren and Dubner 1996; Danziger et al. 1999; Dubner and Ren 1999; Hurley and Hammond 2000; Terayama et al. 2000). It appears that after inflammation, brainstem descending pathways

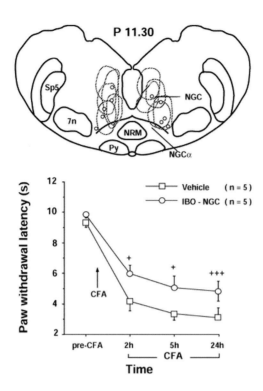

Fig. 2. Effects of lesions to the nucleus reticularis gigantocellularis (NGC) on inflamma-tion-induced hyperalgesia. Upper panel: The extent of lesions induced by ibotenic acid (IBO) is shown by dotted lines. Small circles indicate the vehicle injection sites. Lower panel: The hyperalgesia was significantly attenuated in IBO-lesioned rats 2–24 hours after the injection of CFA, compared to vehicle-injected controls (+ $P < 0.05$, +++ $P < 0.001$). Adapted from Wei et al. (1999).

become progressively more involved in modulating incoming sensory sig-nals from primary hyperalgesic zones. Descending inhibition dominates as time progresses. Injury-related primary afferent input is probably respon-sible for triggering this ascending-descending feedback circuit. This en-hancement of descending inhibition appears to be present when the animal is subject to continuous, persistent noxious stimulation.

We have studied the molecular, cellular, and neurochemical mecha-nisms that underlie these changes. We asked the following question: Are these changes merely a reflection of enhanced activity (i.e., activity-depen-dent plasticity) ascending from spinal cord levels to the brainstem, or is there also an increase in excitability at the RVM level (i.e., activity-depen-dent plasticity in the RVM)? The dynamic changes in descending inhibition after inflammation can be examined over time by monitoring nocifensive responses in lightly anesthetized rats during RVM stimulation (Terayama et al. 2000; Guan et al. 2002b). In these studies, we have demonstrated that persistent inflammation induces dramatic changes in the excitability of RVM pain-modulating circuitry, suggesting dynamic temporal changes in synaptic activation in the brainstem after inflammation. Early (within 3 hours) in the development of inflammation, descending facilitation increases (Urban and Gebhart 1999), which reduces the net effect of descending inhibition. Over time, the level of descending inhibition increases, or descending facilitation decreases, leading to a net enhancement of antinocifensive behavior. Direct stimulation of the dorsolateral funiculus that bypasses brain stem synaptic mechanisms does not produce a dynamic change in excitability, which indicates that the changes rely on mechanisms at the level of the RVM or higher.

What are the cellular mechanisms that underlie these changes? Excitatory amino acids (EAAs) mediate descending modulation in response to transient noxious stimulation and early inflammation (for reviews see Urban and Gebhart 1999; Heinricher et al. 1999), and they appear to be involved in the development of RVM excitability associated with inflammation and persistent pain (Terayama et al. 2000, 2002; Guan et al. 2002b; Miki et al. 2002). Fig. 3 shows that N-methyl-D-aspartate (NMDA), the prototype NMDA-receptor agonist, microinjected into the RVM, produced effects that are dependent upon the post-inflammatory time period. At 3 hours post-inflammation, low doses of NMDA facilitated the response to noxious heat of the inflamed hindpaw (and the non-inflamed hindpaw and tail, not shown), supporting previous findings that descending facilitatory effects are NMDA dependent and occur early after inflammation (Urban and Gebhart 1999). Higher doses of NMDA at 3 hours post-inflammation only produced inhibition. At 24 hours post-inflammation, NMDA produced only inhibition in a dose-dependent fashion. These effects were blocked by administration of NMDA-receptor antagonists. Fig. 3 shows that α-amino-3-hydroxy-5-methyl-4-isoxazole propionate (AMPA), a selective glutamate receptor agonist, produced dose-dependent and time-dependent levels of inhibition at all doses at 3 and 24 hours post-inflammation. These effects were blocked by an AMPA-receptor antagonist (not shown). The above findings indicate that there is a leftward shift of the dose-response curves of NMDA- and AMPA-produced inhibition at 24 hours post-inflammation as compared to 3 hours. The results suggest that the time-dependent functional changes in descending modulation are mediated, in part, by enhanced EAA neurotransmission and increased potency of EAA receptors.

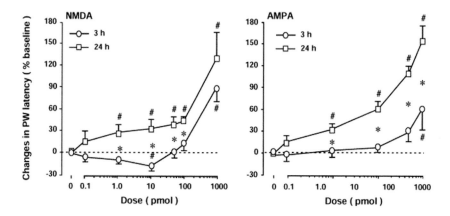

Fig. 3. The effects of microinjection of NMDA (left) and AMPA (right) into the rostral ventromedial medulla (RVM) on the paw-withdrawal latencies in inflamed rats at 3 and 24 hours post-inflammation. Changes in paw-withdrawal latencies are represented as a percentage change of the pre-drug baseline latencies. Cumulative dosing was performed in these experiments. Intra-RVM microinjection of NMDA produced a biphasic descending modulation on the paw-withdrawal latencies at 3 hours post-inflammation. NMDA significantly decreased the paw-withdrawal latencies, with 10 pmol indicating facilitation and a significant increase and 1000 pmol indicating inhibition. At 24 hours post-inflammation, NMDA produced only dose-dependent inhibition. AMPA produced a dose-dependent inhibition of the paw-withdrawal response at both 3 hours and 24 hours post-inflammation. Note a leftward shift of the dose-response curves at 24 hours after inflammation. Asterisks (*) denote significant differences between 3-hour and 24-hour groups; pound signs (#) indicate significant differences between the drug treatment and saline control group ($P < 0.05$–0.01). Each group consisted of 6–8 rats. From Guan et al. (2002b).

MOLECULAR MECHANISMS OF PLASTICITY IN THE RVM

What are the molecular and cellular mechanisms of this increased potency leading to enhanced synaptic activity and increases in descending net inhibition? Much is known about the role of NMDA and AMPA receptors in activity-dependent plasticity at the level of the spinal cord. Fig. 4 diagrams some of these changes (see Woolf and Salter 2000 for review). Transient pain, the normal response to acute noxious stimuli, is largely mediated by glutamate acting at its AMPA receptor on dorsal horn neurons, leading to fast synaptic transmission and activating the fast protective pain-warning system in the brain. The channel of this ionotropic receptor is selective mainly for sodium. If the injury persists, glutamate continues to be released from the central endings of nociceptive afferent neurons along with the

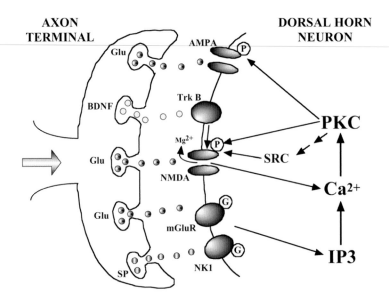

Fig. 4. Diagram illustrating cellular mechanisms of enhanced synaptic activity in the spinal dorsal horn after injury. BDNF = brain-derived neurotrophic factor; G = G protein; Glu = glutamate; IP3 = inositol triphosphate; mGluR = metabotropic glutamate receptor; NK1 = neurokinin-1 receptor; P = phosphorylation; PKC = protein kinase C; SP = substance P; trk B = tyrosine kinase B receptor.

neuropeptide substance P. The metabotropic glutamate receptor and the neurokinin 1 receptor, activated by glutamate and substance P, respectively, are G-protein-coupled receptors that lead to the activation of second-messenger systems, resulting in the release of calcium from intracellular stores. With the initiation of synaptic depolarization via the above receptors, the voltage-dependent magnesium block of the NMDA ion channel is removed, and glutamate release results in calcium flowing into the cell. Calcium is a critical player in this process because many protein kinases in the cell are dependent upon calcium for their activation. These protein kinases participate in the phosphorylation of membrane-bound receptors and ion channels. Finally, brain-derived neurotrophic factor (BDNF), a neurotrophin acting at a tyrosine kinase receptor (trk B), is released and activates other protein kinases. The NMDA receptor is the best characterized glutamate receptor, and its phosphorylation is a major factor in activity-dependent plasticity and the resulting hyperalgesia. Phosphorylation of the NMDA receptor increases the sensitivity of the receptor so that subsequent responsiveness to synaptically released glutamate is enhanced, increasing synaptic strength and resulting in subthreshold inputs reaching threshold levels. The outcome is an increased response to painful stimulation (hyperalgesia) and a perception of innocuous stimuli as painful (allodynia). These clinical signs are characteristic of many persistent pain conditions associated with tissue and nerve injury.

In recent studies we have examined whether transcriptional, translational, and post-translational changes occur in the RVM after inflammation and may underlie the changes in sensitivity we have observed. Increases in gene expression of subunits of the NMDA and AMPA receptors could lead to more receptors trafficking to the cell membrane and their participation in the sensitization. Changes in the affinity of the receptors for glutamate and other receptor agonists could occur due to the phosphorylation of receptor subunits. Examination of the mRNA expression of the NR1, NR2A, and NR2B subunits of the NMDA receptor in the RVM revealed an upregulation that parallels the time course of the RVM excitability changes (Miki et al. 2002). This upregulation is accompanied by an increase in NMDA-receptor protein. Western blot analysis also revealed a time-dependent increase in the AMPA receptor GluR1 subunit levels in the RVM at 5 hours and 24 hours post-inflammation as compared to naive animals (Guan et al. 2003). Western blots also demonstrated that GluR1 phosphoprotein levels were increased as early as 30 minutes post-inflammation and were time-dependent, suggesting that post-translational receptor phosphorylation may also contribute to the enhanced AMPA transmission (Guan et al. 2002a). More recently, we have also demonstrated an increase in phosphorylation of the NR2A subunit of the NMDA receptor in the RVM after inflammation (Turnbull et al. 2003). These findings support our hypothesis that activity-dependent plasticity takes place at the RVM level and involves both changes in EAA-receptor gene and protein expression and increased phosphorylation of these receptors.

This activity-induced plasticity in pain-modulating circuitry after inflammation complements the activity-dependent neuronal plasticity in ascending pain transmission pathways (Dubner and Ruda 1992). Inflammation leads to peripheral sensitization of nociceptors and central sensitization or activity-dependent plasticity of spinal nociceptive neurons. The spinal plasticity is dependent upon increased activation of nociceptors at the site of injury, and its initiation and maintenance is dependent upon transcriptional, translational, and post-translational modulation of EAA-receptor subunits. The increased neuronal barrage at the spinal level activates spinal projection neurons, leading to activation of glutamatergic, opioidergic, and GABAergic neurons at the brainstem level and causing a similar but not identical form of activity-dependent plasticity. It is likely that transmission sites at multiple levels in nociceptive pathways exhibit enhanced sensitivity in the face of a persistent neuronal barrage associated with tissue or nerve injury.

PHENOTYPIC CHANGES IN THE RVM AFTER INFLAMMATION

The time-dependent plasticity in descending pain-modulatory circuitry also involves changes in the response profiles of RVM neurons. We have used paw withdrawal as a behavioral correlate to assess the relationship between nocifensive behavior and RVM neural activity after inflammation (Miki et al. 2002). Similar to the findings of Fields and colleagues (1991), who correlated tail-flick responses to RVM neural activity after transient noxious thermal stimuli, we observed on-like, off-like, and neutral-like cells based on the relationship of their responses to paw-withdrawal behavior during the development of inflammation. Importantly, we found that some neutral-like cells changed their response profile and were reclassified as on-like or off-like cells during continuous recordings of 5 hours or more. The change in the response profile of RVM neurons correlated with the temporal changes in excitability in the RVM after inflammation (Terayama et al. 2000). To verify this phenotypic switch of RVM neurons, we performed a neuronal population study and noted a significant increase in the percentage of on-like and off-like cells and a decrease in the neutral-like cell population 24 hours after inflammation, supporting the observations in the long-term recording experiments. We also observed changes in the magnitude of the responses of on-like and off-like cells (Fig. 5). After inflammation, there was a greater increase in on-like responses before the onset of paw withdrawal as compared to on-like responses in naive controls, suggesting an increase in facilitatory activity in the RVM. In contrast, off-like responses were reduced after inflammation indicated by a lesser reduction in neuronal activity after the noxious stimulus, and a lack of a complete pause. The pause in off-like cell activity is associated with disinhibition, a form of activation; the loss of the pause and the lesser reduction in neuronal activity suggest an increase in inhibitory activity originating in the RVM. However, it is difficult to predict the net effect of descending facilitation and inhibition from changes in single neuronal activity without recording from very large populations of neurons. Further studies are required to identify the subclasses of RVM neurons that exhibit profile changes after inflammation and are also modulated by glutamatergic transmission.

CLINICAL IMPLICATIONS

Descending modulation and activity-dependent plasticity are normal functions of the brain; presumably they are activated to protect the organism from further environmental injury. We propose that the dynamic changes in

A. On-like cells B. Off-like cells

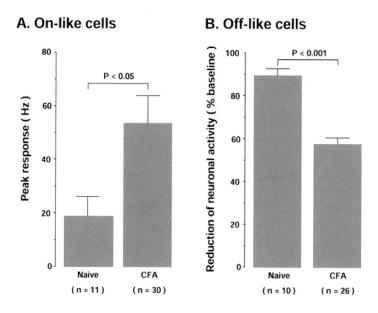

Fig. 5. Mean changes in responses of RVM on-like and off-like cells to the noxious thermal stimulus in noninflamed and CFA-inflamed rats. (A) Peak response frequency of on-like cells immediately prior to the onset of a withdrawal response in naive and CFA-inflamed rats. (B) Percentage reduction of neuronal activity of off-like cells before the onset of a withdrawal response. Note a nearly 90% reduction of activity in naive rats and only a less than 60% reduction of activity in CFA-inflamed rats. Adapted from Miki et al. (2002).

descending modulation after inflammation and primary hyperalgesia and allodynia are protective. The early facilitation may function to enhance nocifensive escape behavior whereas the dominant late inhibition may provide a mechanism by which movement of the injured site is suppressed or reduced to aid in healing and recuperation.

An imbalance between these modulatory pathways may also be one mechanism underlying variability in persistent or chronic pain conditions, especially those involving deep tissues such as muscle and viscera. Inputs from deep tissues produce more robust dorsal horn hyperexcitability and plasticity than do inputs from cutaneous tissues. Primary afferent and spinal neurons originating from muscle and viscera are often multimodal and responsive to innocuous as well as noxious stimuli. An imbalance of descending modulatory systems in which there is an increase in endogenous facilitation could lead to increases in and persistence of pain. For patients suffering from deep pains such as temporomandibular disorders, fibromyalgia, irritable bowel syndrome, and low back pain, the diffuse nature and amplification of persistent pain may partly be the result of a net increase in endogenous descending facilitation.

ACKNOWLEDGMENTS

The author's work has been supported by grants DA10275 and DE11964 from the National Institutes of Health, Bethesda, Maryland.

REFERENCES

Bandler R, Shipley MT. Columnar organization in the midbrain periaqueductal gray: modules for emotional expression? *Trends Neurosci* 1994; 17:379–389.

Basbaum AI, Fields HL. Endogenous pain control systems: brainstem spinal pathways and endorphin circuitry. *Annu Rev Neurosci* 1984; 7:309–338.

Danziger N, Weil-Fugazza J, Le Bars D, Bouhassira D. Alteration of descending modulation of nociception during the course of monoarthritis in the rat. *J Neurosci* 1999; 19:2394–2400.

Dubner R, Ren K. Endogenous mechanisms of sensory modulation. *Pain* 1999; Suppl 6:S45–53.

Dubner R, Ren K. Descending modulation in persistent pain: an update. *Pain* 2002; 100:1–6.

Dubner R, Ruda MA. Activity-dependent neuronal plasticity following tissue injury and inflammation. *Trends Neurosci* 1992; 15:96–103.

Dubuisson D, Wall PD. Medullary raphe influences on units in laminae 1 and 2 of cat spinal cord. *J Physiol (Lond)* 1979; 300:33P.

Dubuisson D, Wall PD. Descending influences on receptive fields and activity of single units recorded in laminae 1, 2 and 3 of cat spinal cord. *Brain Res* 1980; 199:283–298.

Fields, HL, Basbaum AI. Central nervous system mechanisms of pain modulation. Wall PD, Melzack R (Ed). *Textbook of Pain.* London: Churchill Livingstone, 1999, pp 309–329.

Fields HL, Heinricher MM, Mason P. Neurotransmitters in nociceptive modulatory circuits. *Annu Rev Neurosci* 1991; 14:219–245.

Gebhart GF. Modulatory effects of descending systems on spinal dorsal horn neurons. In: Yaksh TL (Ed). *Spinal Afferent Processing.* New York: Plenum, 1986, pp 391–416.

Guan Y, Guo W, Turnbach ME, Dubner R, Ren K. Changes in AMPA receptor phosphorylation in the rostral ventromedial medulla (RVM) after inflammation. *Neurosci Lett* 2004; in press.

Guan Y, Terayama R, Dubner R, Ren K. Plasticity in excitatory amino acid receptor-mediated descending pain modulation after inflammation. *J Pharmacol Exp Ther* 2002b; 300:513–520.

Guan Y, Guo W, Zou S-P, Dubner R, Ren K. Inflammation-induced upregulation of AMPA receptor subunit expression in brain stem pain modulatory circuitry. *Pain* 2003; 104:401–413.

Haber LH, Martin RF, Chung JM, Willis WD. Inhibition and excitation of primate spinothalamic tract neurons by stimulation in region of nucleus reticularis gigantocellularis. *J Neurophysiol* 1980; 43:1578–1593.

Heinricher MM, McGaraughty S, Farr DA. The role of excitatory amino acid transmission within the rostral ventromedial medulla in the antinociceptive actions of systemically administered morphine. *Pain* 1999; 81:57–65.

Holden JE, Schwartz EJ, Proudfit HK. Microinjection of morphine in the A7 catecholamine cell group produces opposing effects on nociception that are mediated by alpha1- and alpha2-adrenoceptors. *Neuroscience* 1999; 91:979–990.

Hurley RW, Hammond DL. The analgesic effects of supraspinal mu and delta opioid receptor agonists are potentiated during persistent inflammation. *J Neurosci* 2000; 20:1249–1259.

Mayer DJ, Liebeskind JC. Pain reduction by focal electrical stimulation of the brain: an anatomical and behavioral analysis. *Brain Res* 1974; 68:73–93.

Mayer DJ, Wolfle TL, Akil H, Carder B, Liebeskind JC. Analgesia from electrical stimulation in the brainstem of the rat. *Science* 1971; 174:1351–1354.

McMahon SB, Wall PD. Descending excitation and inhibition of spinal cord lamina I projection neurons. *J Neurophysiol* 1988; 59:1204–1219.

Miki K, Zhou QQ, Guo W, et al. Changes in gene expression and neuronal phenotype in brain stem pain modulatory circuitry after inflammation. *J Neurophysiol* 2002; 87:750–760.

Millan MJ. Descending control of pain. *Prog Neurobiol* 2002; 66:355–474.

Oliveras JL, Redjemi F, Guilbaud G, Besson JM. Analgesia induced by electrical stimulation of the inferior centralis nucleus of the raphe in the cat. *Pain* 1975; 1:139–145.

Porreca F, Ossipov MH, Gebhart GF. Chronic pain and medullary descending facilitation. *Trends Neurosci* 2002: 25:319–325.

Randich A, Gebhart GF. Vagal afferent modulation of nociception. *Brain Res Brain Res Rev* 1992; 17:77–99.

Ren K, Dubner R. Enhanced descending modulation of nociception in rats with persistent hindpaw inflammation. *J Neurophysiol* 1996; 76:3025–3037.

Reynolds DV. Surgery in the rat during electrical analgesia induced by focal brain stimulation. *Science* 1969; 164:444–445.

Schaible HG, Neugebauer V, Cervero F, Schmidt RF. Changes in tonic descending inhibition of spinal neurons with articular input during the development of acute arthritis in the cat. *J Neurophysiol* 1991; 66:1021–1032.

Terayama R, Guan Y, Dubner R, Ren K. Activity-induced plasticity in brain stem pain modulatory circuitry after inflammation. *Neuroreport* 2000; 11:1915–1919.

Terayama R, Dubner R, Ren K. The roles of NMDA receptor activation and nucleus reticularis gigantocellularis in the time-dependent changes in descending inhibition after inflammation. *Pain* 2002; 97:171–181.

Thomas DA, McGowan MK, Hammond DL. Microinjection of baclofen in the ventromedial medulla of rats: antinociception at low doses and hyperalgesia at high doses. *J Pharmacol Exp Ther* 1995; 275:274–284.

Tsuruoka M, Willis WD. Bilateral lesions in the area of the nucleus locus coeruleus affect the development of hyperalgesia during carrageenan-induced inflammation. *Brain Res* 1996; 726:233–236.

Turnbull ME, Guo W, Dubner R, Ren K. Inflammation induces tyrosine phosphorylation of the NR2A subunit and serine phosphorylation of the NR1 subunits in the rat rostral ventromedial medulla. *Soc Neurosci Abstr* 2003; 29.

Urban MO, Gebhart GF. Characterization of biphasic modulation of spinal nociceptive transmission by neurotensin in the rat rostral ventromedial medulla. *J Neurophysiol* 1997; 78:1550–1562.

Urban MO, Gebhart GF. Supraspinal contributions to hyperalgesia. *Proc Natl Acad Sci USA* 1999; 96:7687–7692.

Wei F, Dubner R, Ren K. Nucleus reticularis gigantocellularis and nucleus raphe magnus in the brain stem exert opposite effects on behavioral hyperalgesia and spinal Fos protein expression after peripheral inflammation. *Pain* 1999; 80:127–141.

Woolf CJ, Salter MW. Neuronal plasticity: increasing the gain in pain. *Science* 2000; 288:1765–1768.

Zhuo M, Gebhart GF. Spinal serotonin receptors mediate descending facilitation of a nociceptive reflex from the nuclei reticularis gigantocellularis and gigantocellularis pars alpha in the rat. *Brain Res* 1991; 550:35–48.

Zhuo M, Gebhart GF. Characterization of descending facilitation and inhibition of spinal nociceptive transmission from the nuclei reticularis gigantocellularis and gigantocellularis pars alpha in the rat. *J Neurophysiol* 1992; 67:1599–1614.

Zhuo M, Gebhart GF. Biphasic modulation of spinal nociceptive transmission from the medullary raphe nuclei in the rat. *J Neurophysiol* 1997; 78:746–758.

Zhuo M, Sengupta JN, Gebhart GF. Biphasic modulation of spinal visceral nociceptive transmission from the rostroventral medial medulla in the rat. *J Neurophysiol* 2002; 87:2225–2236.

Correspondence to: Ronald Dubner, DDS, PhD, Department of Biomedical Sciences, University of Maryland Dental School, 666 West Baltimore Street, Room 5E-14, Baltimore, MD 21201, USA. Fax: 410-706-0860; email: rnd001@dental.umaryland.edu.

Part III

Anatomical and Functional Organization of Ascending Pain Pathways

The Pain System in Normal and Pathological States: A Primer for Clinicians, Progress in Pain Research and Management, Vol. 31, edited by Luis Villanueva, Anthony Dickenson, and Hélène Ollat, IASP Press, Seattle, © 2004.

7

Molecular Approaches to Understanding the Anatomical Substrates of Nociceptive Processing

Allan I. Basbaum

Departments of Anatomy and Physiology and W. M. Keck Foundation Center for Integrative Neuroscience, University of California San Francisco, San Francisco, California, USA

THE ANATOMY OF NOCICEPTIVE PROCESSING

The traditional textbook view of the "pain" pathway illustrates an unmyelinated primary afferent C fiber, the nociceptor, contacting a second-order dorsal horn neuron that is at the origin of the spinothalamic or spinoreticular pathway. The third-order neuron projects to an as-yet unknown region in the cortex, ultimately producing pain. This view of a unitary pain transmission system is undoubtedly incorrect. We now recognize neurochemically distinct primary afferent nociceptors with cell bodies located in the trigeminal and dorsal root ganglia. The nociceptors can be broadly divided into two classes (Snider and McMahon 1998; Basbaum and Woolf 1999). One expresses pro-inflammatory peptides, including substance P (SP) and calcitonin gene-related peptide (CGRP). The second expresses fewer peptides, but can be identified by its binding of the IB4 lectin and its expression of a fluoride-resistant acid phosphatase. Although varying numbers of neurons within each subset express some of the same receptors, such as the capsaicin receptor (TRPV1), and channels, such as the TTX-resistant (TTX-r) Na^+ channel, they have many distinct features. For example, almost all of the peptide-expressing neurons, but only a subset of the IB4-binding population, synthesize CGRP. The peptide and IB4 populations, respectively, express the TrkA and *c-ret* neurotrophin receptors and respond to nerve growth factor and glial-derived neurotrophic factor, respectively. Furthermore, a subset of the IB4 population uniquely expresses the $P2X_3$ subtype of purinergic receptor, as well as a complex family of G-protein-linked receptors, whose function is just beginning to be studied (Dong et al. 2001; Lembo et al. 2002).

This remarkable heterogeneity of nociceptors offers good news and bad news. The good news is that these neurochemically and molecularly distinct features of nociceptors may be important as novel therapeutic targets. In particular, several of these molecularly distinct targets are only expressed in the primary afferent nociceptor, which may greatly increase the therapeutic window, which is the difference between the dose of drug that produces analgesic effects and that which produces adverse side effects. The side-effect profile of many analgesic drugs is to a great extent related to the widespread distribution of their target receptors throughout the central nervous system (CNS); in other words, the receptor is not just expressed in pain-related regions of the spinal cord and brain. The bad news, unfortunately, is that using highly targeted drugs for selective "removal" of the functional contribution of small subsets of nociceptors may not be sufficient to reduce nociceptive input to the spinal cord. The long-sought "magic bullet" may not be found. Rather, it may be necessary to reduce afferent drive more globally to achieve adequate pain relief. Of course, drug mixtures that target multiple sites can be used, but the development process for such approaches, and the potential side effects, are likely to be much more complicated.

Our studies have not only contributed to the growing appreciation of the complexity of the nociceptor, but also have shown that even the synaptic terminal of nociceptors is significantly more complex than previously assumed. David Julius and I have recently reviewed some of the molecules that define subsets of nociceptors (Julius and Basbaum 2001), so this chapter will focus on other features of the nociceptor that underscore their complexity. For example, the "traditional" nociceptor terminal contains two types of synaptic vesicle. The clear vesicle stores and releases glutamate, which is the major, if not exclusive, excitatory amino acid transmitter of the nociceptors. The synaptic terminal also contains dense core vesicles, which store a variety of molecules, notably the peptides CGRP and SP. CGRP regulates the enzymatic degradation of SP (Le Greves et al. 1985), an arrangement that raises the intriguing possibility that exocytosis of peptide from the terminal not only releases an excitatory pronociceptive peptide, but simultaneously evokes the release of a peptide that regulates the duration of action of the pronociceptive molecule. Other studies have shown that the dense core vesicle also contains brain-derived neurotrophic factor, which has multiple growth-promoting effects and may contribute to central sensitization (Kerr et al. 1999).

PRIMARY AFFERENT LOCALIZATION OF THE 5HT$_{1D}$ RECEPTOR

Studies of the molecular target of the triptan anti-migraine class of drugs have uncovered a further remarkable complexity of the dense core vesicle. We were studying the distribution of the 5HT$_{1D}$ receptor (Potrebic et al. 2003), one of the two likely targets of the triptans (the other being the 5HT$_{1B}$ receptor). We found that the 5HT$_{1D}$ receptor is expressed almost exclusively in small-diameter, unmyelinated afferents and that a very high percentage of dorsal root ganglion (DRG) neurons have colocalized SP and 5HT$_{1D}$ immunoreactivity. Not surprisingly, we also found that almost all 5HT$_{1D}$-immunoreactive terminals in the superficial dorsal horn were SP-immunoreactive.

Previous studies provided evidence that triptans exert their effects, at least in part, by reducing neurogenic inflammation, the process whereby stimulation of nociceptors evokes the release of peptides (SP and CGRP) from primary afferent terminals (Moskowitz 1993). The remarkably high colocalization of 5HT$_{1D}$ receptor and SP immunoreactivity in the primary afferent terminal suggests that the reduction of neurogenic inflammation results from a direct action of the triptans on the peripheral terminals of the nociceptors. Consistent with this hypothesis, we showed that the dural inner-vation is rich in 5HT$_{1D}$ -receptor immunoreactivity. Our observations could not determine whether the anti-migraine effects of the triptans also involve an action on the central terminal of the primary afferent nociceptor.

Subsequent electron microscopic analysis gave us a surprise: the 5HT$_{1D}$ receptor was not located on the plasma membrane of the afferent terminals. Instead, immunoreactivity was concentrated almost exclusively in dense core vesicles. Finding the receptor associated with the vesicle provided evidence that it is transported from the cell body, where it is synthesized, to the terminals. To reveal the location of the receptor with higher resolution, we turned to an immunogold procedure on tissue that had been fixed and rap-idly frozen prior to being embedded in plastic resin. This approach avoids the osmium fixation and extensive alcohol dehydration that occur with tradi-tional approaches, which undoubtedly decrease the sensitivity for detecting small amounts of antigen. Using this approach, we found that the receptor was still only detectable on the dense core vesicles. Moreover, when we simultaneously labeled both SP and 5HT$_{1D}$ with an electron microscope immunogold procedure (using two different size gold particles), we found that the same vesicle contained both the transmitter and the receptor that regulates its release, i.e., SP and 5HT$_{1D}$ receptor immunoreactivity, respec-tively.

This arrangement suggests several interesting features of the mechanism through which triptans could regulate the release of peptides from the terminals of primary afferent nociceptors. Because the receptor is not found on the plasma membrane, where it would be targeted by and accessible to exogenous administration of the triptan, it follows that triptans would not be effective without an ongoing release of SP or CGRP. During exocytosis of the dense core vesicles, the $5HT_{1D}$ receptor would be inserted into the membrane. (The extracellular part of the receptor, which binds the triptan, would only be exposed to the surface when the vesicle is inserted into the plasma membrane). The minimal expression of $5HT_{1D}$ on the plasma membrane under resting conditions may explain why triptans have little value in preventing the onset of a migraine attack. Rather, triptans are most efficacious when taken immediately after the attack begins, which should correspond to the time of greatest activity of the primary afferent nociceptors and maximal exocytosis of dense core vesicles. We recognize that our inability to detect plasma membrane expression of the receptor may be related to insufficient receptor concentrations (which may also explain why receptor expression is readily detectable in the dense core vesicle). Clearly, future studies should evaluate the targeting of the dense core vesicle to the membrane and may provide important new information concerning triptan regulation of peptide release and the relevance of this control to the anti-migraine action of triptans.

PRIMARY AFFERENT LOCALIZATION OF ENDOMORPHIN

In a parallel set of studies we examined the distribution of endomorphin, a tetrapeptide endogenous opioid that has remarkable affinity for the μ-opioid receptor (Zadina et al. 1997). In contrast to the enkephalins, which are concentrated in interneurons of the dorsal horn, endomorphin immunoreactivity predominates in primary afferents (Martin-Schild et al. 1997). We extended some of the earlier observations and found that endomorphin-2 immunoreactivity is highly concentrated in SP-containing primary afferents (Nydahl et al. 2004). Although some evidence suggested that this finding might be an artifact of endomorphin antibody cross-reactivity with SP or CGRP, our studies ruled out this possibility. First, we showed that endomorphin-2 immunoreactivity was not altered in tissue that was taken from preprotachykinin A mutant mice (Cao et al. 1998), in which SP is deleted. Second, the endomorphin immunoreactivity only colocalized in some neurons that were CGRP positive. As in our studies that examined the $5HT_{1D}$ receptor, in these studies we also used immunogold procedures to examine the distribution of endomorphin-2 at the ultrastructural level. We found that the endomorphin was also localized in the dense core vesicle and indeed colocalized with SP.

This result underscores the complexity of the dense core vesicle and raises the interesting possibility that endomorphin release from the primary afferent nociceptor provides a mechanism for feedback inhibition that comes into play during concurrent release of pronociceptive peptides. For example, during release of SP and CGRP, as occurs with injury-associated activation of nociceptors, endomorphins would be co-released. The postsynaptic neurons that express μ-opioid receptors are among the possible and likely targets of the primary-afferent-derived endomorphins. An action at this receptor would underlie a feed-forward inhibitory control of nociceptive processing. The endomorphins that are released from the nociceptor would also be in a position to target the presynaptic μ-opioid receptor. In this situation the primary afferent opioid receptor is an autoreceptor. This circuitry would underlie an inhibitory feedback mechanism for opioid control.

These studies illustrate that the primary afferent is far more complicated than previously assumed, with multiple ways to regulate transmission of nociceptive messages. Whether this new information can lead to better approaches to pain relief is not yet clear, but it is certain that new opportunities exist to regulate processing in the primary afferent nociceptor.

THE CIRCUIT MAP FOR THE TRANSMISSION OF NOCICEPTIVE MESSAGES

The two major classes of nociceptor can be distinguished neurochemically and also in their patterns of axon termination in the superficial dorsal horn. The peptide population terminates almost exclusively in the most superficial laminae (Snider and McMahon 1998), directly contacting lamina I projection neurons that transmit nociceptive messages (Carlton et al. 1990) as well as an extremely heterogeneous population of interneurons in lamina II (Grudt and Perl 2002). In contrast, the IB4 population primarily targets lamina II (Snider and McMahon 1998; Stucky and Lewin 1999) and is unlikely to make monosynaptic connections with lamina I projection neurons (Coimbra et al. 1974), which have dendrites largely restricted to lamina I itself (Light et al. 1979, 1993). These fundamental differences in the patterns of nociceptor termination argue strongly that primary afferent nociceptors engage a multiplicity of dorsal horn circuits. Unfortunately, the information about these circuits is extremely limited. In some cases, intracellular analyses have determined the physiological properties of morphologically distinct nociresponsive neurons (Light et al. 1979, 1993; Bennett et al. 1980; Hylden et al. 1986; Grudt and Perl 2002), at times in combination with electron microscopic studies (Ma et al. 1996), but the samples analyzed were extremely small. Finally, although studies that monitor Fos expression provide a much more extensive picture of populations of neurons activated by noxious stimuli (Presley et al. 1990), we have no information about the circuits that underlie Fos activation.

The identities of the neuronal populations immediately postsynaptic to the different nociceptors are inadequately specified, and the neurons and circuits that lie downstream of the first synapse in the dorsal horn are also largely uncharacterized. For example, morphologically and functionally distinct lamina I projection neurons (Lima and Coimbra 1989; Zhang and Craig 1997; Han et al. 1998) contact a variety of third-order neurons in the brainstem, thalamus, hypothalamus, and amygdala. However, the relationship is unclear between the particular afferent that contacts lamina I neurons and the identity of the third-order neurons to which the lamina I neurons project. Furthermore, regulation of the output of the projection neurons by interneurons in the substantia gelatinosa, in part via feed-forward connections from the primary afferent nociceptors, indicates that the circuit map is not merely a point-to-point connection between the nociceptor and the dorsal horn projection neuron. Although the afferent and the projection neurons certainly have some monosynaptic connections, the predominant circuitry engaged by the nociceptor involves dorsal horn interneurons. Unfortunately, the map of interneuronal circuits engaged by the nociceptor is largely unknown. For these reasons, our laboratory recently developed a novel approach to mapping complex circuits that arise from distinct subsets of neurons. With this approach, we hope to provide a much more detailed picture of the local and long-distance circuits (i.e., the wiring diagram) engaged by different classes of nociceptor and to understand how those circuits are altered after injury.

NEUROANATOMICAL TRACERS

Traditional tracers have proven immensely successful in neuroanatomical studies of neuronal connections. Unfortunately, many tracers have significant limitations (Kobbert et al. 2000; Vercelli et al. 2000). First, most tracers provide information only about the connections made by a single neuron, or by a population of neurons, with neurons immediately downstream (or upstream in the case of retrograde tracers) of the injection site. Second, most traditional approaches are hampered by the inevitable spread of the tracer at the site of injection. As a result it is often difficult, if not impossible, to determine the cells of origin of any particular projection pattern. This is true for all retrograde and anterograde tracers, including the enzyme tracers (e.g., horseradish peroxidase) and for dyes, radio-labeled amino acids, and some of the lectins and toxins that have replaced the traditional methods. Although the problem can be completely avoided through intracellular injections of dyes and other tracers into single cells, the number of cells from which conclusions can be drawn is extremely small. However, this approach is the best for correlating the projection pattern of physiologically identified neurons.

The development of transneuronal tracers that can be transferred from neuron to neuron, across synapses, was a big step forward, and recent modifications have provided important information about neurochemically distinct circuits. Our own laboratory has used viral tracers injected both into the periphery and into the CNS (Jasmin et al. 1997a,b). Those studies revealed novel features of the circuitry that transmits information from nociceptors to elements of the limbic system. However, the results were extremely difficult to interpret because effective viral tracers are often lytic and thus destroy the targeted neurons.

To develop neuroanatomical tools that will permit the mapping of circuits that are engaged by subsets of primary afferent nociceptors, we recently generated mice in which the transneuronal lectin tracer, wheat-germ agglutinin (WGA), is inducibly expressed in any neuron in the nervous system. Our work built on the studies of Yoshihara et al. (1999) and Zou et al. (2001), who developed transgenic mice in which WGA or barley lectin is driven off of a cell-specific promoter. Most importantly, in those studies the lectin not only was strongly expressed in first-order cells (which carry the transgene), but was also detectable in second- and third-order neurons downstream, i.e., following its transneuronal anterograde transport.

The tracer expression in the Yoshihara and Zou mice is under the control of neuron-specific promoters, so the circuits revealed are system specific. Yoshihara "drove" the WGA off of the L7 promoter, which induces very strong expression in cerebellar Purkinje cells and in bipolar neurons of the retina. The lectin is "on" from the time that the L7 promoter is on, and expression and transneuronal transport of the WGA begin in the embryo and continue throughout the life of the animal. Zou and colleagues, in contrast, were interested in the central circuits engaged by the very large family of G-protein-linked olfactory receptors. By inserting the barley lectin transgene into the locus of a particular olfactory receptor, the investigators were able to map the pathway from the receptor to the cerebral cortex. These elegant results, however, illustrate the limitation of the approach used in those two studies. The tracer was driven off of specific promoters, so the analysis was limited to these circuits. Investigation of a different circuit (e.g., one involved in pain processing) would require different mice.

To overcome this limitation, we generated mice that allowed us to study transneuronal labeling of circuits that arise from *any* region of the brain or spinal cord (Braz et al. 2002). The crucial feature of these mice is conditional expression of the WGA transgene; it is only induced when a particular molecular event occurs, namely excision of another gene. We refer to these mice as "ZW" mice. The "Z" denotes a "floxed" *lacZ* gene that is constitutively expressed in CNS neurons of the ZW mouse. The "W" refers to the WGA, which we induce by temporally and spatially controlling expression of Cre recombinase, a bacterial enzyme that recognizes specific sequences that determine a floxed gene, and then excises (cuts out) the intervening transgene. In the arrangement that we created, Cre excision of the Z deletes the *lacZ* gene, resulting in immediate induction of the WGA gene, which is located downstream of *lacZ,* but under the control of the same promoter that drove it. To date we have used a rather common promoter, chick β-actin, which drives expression in many CNS neurons.

In a typical WGA transneuronal tracing experiment, the lectin itself is injected into tissue (e.g., a peripheral nerve). The WGA is taken up by the nerve and transported to the DRG and from there transneuronally to terminals in the dorsal horn. Due to limited availability of the WGA, the extent of transport is limited. Only rarely are dorsal horn neurons labeled, presumably because the tracer rapidly degrades. In contrast, when WGA is genetically expressed, tracer is not limited. It continues to be expressed and is thus available for transport for the duration of the animal's life. This availability considerably facilitates the subsequent detection of the marker. Of course, lack of tracer synthesis in neurons downstream of those that express WGA limits the amount of tracer available for transneuronal transport in distant parts of the circuit. The half-life of the tracer in these neurons is not yet known.

Among the advantages of the genetic approach over conventional tracing techniques is the reproducibility of labeling between animals, the avoidance of uptake by axons of passage, which almost inevitably occurs when the tracer is microinjected into tissue, and the uniform labeling of cells that can be produced. Most importantly, the ability to restrict the expression of the tracer to a subpopulation of neurons makes it possible to study the circuits engaged by that subset only. To date we have used the ZW mice in a variety of systems, either after crossing the mice with others in which Cre is driven off of neuronal-specific promoters, or by microinjecting an adeno-associated virus that drives Cre expression (Kaspar et al. 2002) so that WGA can be "turned on" in particular brain regions. Those studies established the feasibility of our approach. We have now turned our attention specifically to questions relating to the development and adult configuration of the circuits engaged by primary afferent nociceptors, and to the plasticity of these circuits during injury. Below we illustrate how this novel transneuronal circuit-tracing method can be used to examine what is generally considered to be among the major contributors to persistent pain induced by nerve injury.

A NEW APPROACH TO STUDYING THE REORGANIZATION OF DORSAL HORN CIRCUITS AFTER PERIPHERAL TISSUE OR NERVE INJURY

The underlying hypothesis in these studies is that the development of tissue and nerve injury-induced persistent pain conditions results, in significant part, from a reorganization of CNS nociceptive circuitry, from phenotypic changes in the neurochemistry of primary afferent neurons after tissue injury (Neumann et al. 1996) or nerve injury (Noguchi et al. 1993, 1994; Hökfelt et al. 1994; Tsujino et al. 2000), and from the activation of novel descending control systems (Schaible et al. 1991; Ren and Dubner 1996). Reorganization occurs in several systems. For example, following the early studies of Liu and Chambers (1958), several laboratories reported that deafferentation of the spinal cord results in significant collateral sprouting of remaining afferents (Lekan et al. 1996) and that this reorganization has pathophysiological and electrophysiological consequences (Basbaum and Wall 1976). More recently, intra-axonal (Woolf et al. 1992) and transganglionic tracing studies (Woolf et al. 1995; Bennett et al. 1996) demonstrated that large-diameter primary afferent fibers, which normally terminate in laminae III and IV of the dorsal horn, sprout into overlying laminae I and II after peripheral nerve injury. This sprouting may contribute to the development of Aβ-mediated mechanical allodynia. The theory, of course, is not without controversy. For example, Shehab et al. (2004) argued that minimal large-diameter sprouting occurs after peripheral nerve injury, and Tong et al. (1999) suggested that the sprouting may, in part, have resulted from the de novo uptake of the B fragment of cholera toxin (the tracer in these studies) by injured unmyelinated afferents. To what extent the appearance of Aβ-fiber projections to lamina II after injury recapitulates a transient developmental pattern (Fitzgerald et al. 1994) is also controversial (Woodbury et al. 2000, 2001).

Despite the controversy as to the magnitude of the changes observed in the adult, development studies have reported compelling evidence for plasticity of afferent innervation in the setting of injury. For example, inflammation in the neonatal rat dramatically alters the central projections of small-diameter afferents that are transganglionically labeled with WGA-HRP (Ruda et al. 2000). Most importantly, these changes are associated with functional changes in the properties of dorsal horn nociresponsive neurons (Fitzgerald et al. 1994). After injury to the skin (removal of a patch of skin at birth), Torsney and Fitzgerald (2002) found dramatic increases in receptive field size, which they attributed to large and permanent alterations in synaptic connectivity, rather than to subtle changes in the biophysical properties of nociceptors or in the properties of the postsynaptic neurons. Thus, although expansion of receptive field size and decreased threshold for the firing of nociresponsive neurons could reflect a sensitization of dorsal horn neurons that is independent of anatomical reorganization, it is likely that anatomical changes are major contributors to the behavioral phenotypes observed.

These anatomical studies demonstrated profound anatomical rearrangement of primary afferent terminals, but they cannot provide information on the circuits that are altered following injury. For example, sprouting can manifest as movement of terminals into a novel terminal field (such as sprouting of Aβ afferents dorsally into the superficial dorsal horn), but may also represent increased arborization of axons within their normal zone of termination (as occurs for small-diameter afferents following tissue injury). In either case, the functional consequences of injury-induced sprouting depend not only and perhaps not so much upon the number of new terminals, but rather on the new connections made by the sprouts. Unfortunately, these studies rarely assess (largely due to lack of adequate methods) the identity of the new contacts at postsynaptic neurons.

In distinct contrast to what can be discerned from existing methods, the use of genetically induced transneuronal tracers and light microscopy allow the identification of large populations of the target neurons for new connections. We can characterize additional functional properties of the circuits by double-labeling the cell bodies to which the tracer has been transneuronally transported (e.g., with retrograde tracer to define projection neurons, or with cytochemical markers to define neurochemistry), or by using noxious-stimulus-induced Fos expression. The ideal technique, of course, would permit the triggering of the tracer when neurons are active. For example, it may be possible to use calcium-sensitive mechanisms that regulate gene expression to selectively activate WGA in nociceptors that are active under particular stimulus conditions. The difficulty in many of the experiments is a relatively high background activity associated with the normal spontaneous activity of the particular neuron system being studied.

To circumvent some of these problems, we are developing methods that will allow us to trigger the synthesis and transneuronal transport of WGA in primary afferent nociceptors with a transected peripheral branch. We can specify when WGA synthesis begins after injury, and thus follow the development and elaboration of novel circuits that are made by the modified central branch of the nociceptor. In these experiments, we will combine constitutive ZW expression in DRG cells with nerve-injury-induced expression of a modified estrogen receptor Cre construct (ER-Cre) (Vallier et al., 2001), under the control of an immediate early gene promoter (*c-jun* or ATF3 (Buschmann et al. 1998; Tsujino et al. 2000) that is induced in primary afferent neurons, but *only* after peripheral nerve injury. We are also considering a modification of the approach that builds upon the observation that neuropeptide Y (NPY) is induced in large-diameter afferents after nerve injury (Landry et al. 2000). Specifically, it should be possible to take advantage of the selectivity of NPY molecular expression to drive selective expression of the transneuronal tracer in a subset of primary afferents. These studies should provide some direct answers to questions concerning the reorganization of large-diameter primary afferents after nerve injury, including the particular circuits that are engaged during the establishment of novel connections.

Approaches such as these offer a new opportunity to dissect the complex nociceptive circuits that originate with the primary afferent nociceptor, and illustrate a novel approach to characterizing the development, adult expression, and modification of these circuits, which occurs after tissue or nerve injury. Through the use of promoters that induce Cre recombinase expression selectively in small-diameter primary afferents, such as the peripherin promoter (Zhou et al. 2002), it should be possible to induce selective expression of WGA in these afferents. This advance will make it possible to study the organization and injury-induced reorganization of central circuits engaged by unmyelinated afferents, most of which are nociceptors. Alternatively, we envision even more selectivity by using promoters that drive expression in neurochemically distinct subsets of nociceptors. This type of analysis is not limited to local circuits in the spinal cord. The WGA is transneuronally transported across several synapses, and studies using genetically engineered transneuronal tracers should provide information on circuit organization and reorganization, not only in the dorsal horn, but also at higher centers.

BUILDING ON THE BESSON FOUNDATION

Jean-Marie Besson has made a series of seminal observations that have influenced how we think about the processing of "pain" messages. Interestingly, although many of his studies were revolutionary when first published, few remember their origin. Besson's observations are now part of the textbook picture of pain generation and pain processing, which is a sign of utmost respect. Among the observations for which Besson and his laboratory deserve credit are the early studies of inhibitory effects of opiates on nociceptive processing in the spinal cord, the demonstration of the importance of the nucleus raphe magnus to descending control and stimulation-produced analgesia (SPA), including the report of the effects of naloxone in reversing SPA, and the more recent use of Fos immunocytochemistry to reveal the differential effects of various classes of analgesic agent. Finally, members of his laboratory have provided the most convincing evidence for a contribution of the parabrachial-amygdala pathway to the processing of nociceptive information.

Our own laboratory has often followed in Besson's footsteps, building upon his initial observations. The studies of endogenous pain control systems and the substrates for descending control that Howard Fields and I worked together on for many years were influenced strongly by Besson's observations on the critical contribution of the nucleus raphe magnus. Without question, our efforts to develop the transneuronal tracing methods outlined above were driven by our interest in understanding how distinct populations of nociceptive afferents engage the different ascending pathways that carry nociceptive information, with the spino-trigemino-parabrachial amygdala pathway among the most important.

ACKNOWLEDGMENTS

This work was supported by the National Institutes of Health (NS14627, 21445, and DE08973). I am indebted to Jean-Marie, not only for the intellectual stimulation that I derived from our numerous interactions (in both English and French), but also for his incredibly warm friendship. The year that I spent on sabbatical in Paris in his laboratory was among the most memorable of my scientific life, and without question the Dahlem Conference meeting that Jean-Marie and I co-organized, which unexpectedly began in Berlin the day after the wall came down, will remain one of my most cherished memories. Merci, Jean-Marie.

REFERENCES

Basbaum AI, Wall PD. Chronic changes in the response of cells in adult cat dorsal horn following partial deafferentation: the appearance of responding cells in a previously non-responsive region. *Brain Res* 1976; 116:181–204.

Basbaum AI, Woolf CJ. Pain. *Curr Biol* 1999; 9:R429–431.

Bennett GJ, Abdelmoumene M, Hayashi H, Dubner R. Physiology and morphology of substantia gelatinosa neurons intracellularly stained with horseradish peroxidase. *J Comp Neurol* 1980; 194:809–827.

Bennett DL, French J, Priestley JV, McMahon SB. NGF but not NT-3 or BDNF prevents the A fiber sprouting into lamina II of the spinal cord that occurs following axotomy. *Mol Cell Neurosci* 1996; 8:211–220.

Braz JM, Rico B, Basbaum AI. Transneuronal tracing of diverse CNS circuits by Cre-mediated induction of wheat germ agglutinin in transgenic mice. *Proc Natl Acad Sci USA* 2002; 99:15148–15153.

Buschmann T, Martin-Villalba A, Kocsis JD, et al. Expression of Jun, Fos, and ATF-2 proteins in axotomized, explanted and cultured adult rat dorsal root ganglia. *Neuroscience* 1998; 84:163–176.

Cao YQ, Mantyh PW, Carlson EJ, et al. Primary afferent tachykinins are required to experience moderate to intense pain. *Nature (Lond)* 1998; 392:390–394.

Carlton SM, Westlund KN, Zhang DX, et al. Calcitonin gene-related peptide containing primate afferent fibers synapse on primary spinothalamic tract cells. *Neurosci Lett* 1990; 109:76–81.

Coimbra A, Sodre-Borges BP, Magalhaes MM. The substantia gelatinosa Rolandi of the rat: fine structure, cytochemistry (acid phosphatase) and changes after dorsal root section. *J Neurocytol* 1974; 3:199–217.

Dong X, Han S, Zylka MJ, Simon MI, Anderson DJ. A diverse family of GPCRs expressed in specific subsets of nociceptive sensory neurons. *Cell* 2001; 106:619–632.

Fitzgerald M, Butcher T, Shortland P. Developmental changes in the laminar termination of A fibre cutaneous sensory afferents in the rat spinal cord dorsal horn. *J Comp Neurol* 1994; 348:225–233.

Grudt TJ, Perl ER. Correlations between neuronal morphology and electrophysiological features in the rodent superficial dorsal horn. *J Physiol* 2002; 540:189–207.

Han ZS, Zhang ET, Craig AD. Nociceptive and thermoreceptive lamina I neurons are anatomically distinct. *Nat Neurosci* 1998; 1:218–225.

Hökfelt T, Zhang X, Wiesenfeld HZ. Messenger plasticity in primary sensory neurons following axotomy and its functional implications. *Trends Neurosci* 1994; 17:22–30.

Hylden JLK, Hayashi H, Dubner R, Bennett GJ. Physiology and morphology of the lamina I spinomesencephalic projection. *J Comp Neurol* 1986; 247:505–515.

Jasmin L, Carstens E, Basbaum AI. Interneurons presynaptic to rat tail-flick motoneurons as mapped by transneuronal transport of pseudorabies virus: few have long ascending collaterals. *Neuroscience* 1997a; 76:859–876.

Jasmin L, Burkey AR, Card JP, Basbaum AI. Transneuronal labeling of a nociceptive pathway, the spino-(trigemino-) parabrachio-amygdaloid, in the rat. *J Neurosci* 1997b; 17:3751–3765.

Julius D, Basbaum AI. Molecular mechanisms of nociception. *Nature (Lond)* 2001; 413:203–210.

Kaspar BK, Vissel B, Bengoechea T, et al. Adeno-associated virus effectively mediates conditional gene modification in the brain. *Proc Natl Acad Sci USA* 2002; 99:2320–2325.

Kerr BJ, Bradbury EJ, Bennett DL, et al. Brain-derived neurotrophic factor modulates nociceptive sensory inputs and NMDA-evoked responses in the rat spinal cord. *J Neurosci* 1999; 19:5138–5148.

Kobbert C, Apps R, Bechmann I, et al. Current concepts in neuroanatomical tracing. *Prog Neurobiol* 2000; 62:327–351.

Landry M, Holmberg K, Zhang X, Hökfelt T. Effect of axotomy on expression of NPY, galanin, and NPY Y1 and Y2 receptors in dorsal root ganglia and the superior cervical ganglion studied with double-labeling in situ hybridization and immunohistochemistry. *Exp Neurol* 2000; 162:361–384.

Le Greves P, Nyberg F, Terenius L, Hökfelt T. Calcitonin gene-related peptide is a potent inhibitor of substance P degradation. *Eur J Pharmacol* 1985; 115:309–311.

Lekan HA, Carlton SM, Coggeshall RE. Sprouting of A beta fibers into lamina II of the rat dorsal horn in peripheral neuropathy. *Neurosci Lett* 1996; 208:147–150.

Lembo PM, Grazzini E, Groblewski T, et al. Proenkephalin A gene products activate a new family of sensory neuron-specific GPCRs. *Nat Neurosci* 2002; 5:201–209.

Light AR, Trevino DL, Perl ER. Morphological features of functionally identified neurons in the marginal zone and substantia gelatinosa of the spinal dorsal horn. *J Comp Neurol* 1979; 186:325–330.

Light AR, Sedivec MJ, Casale EJ, Jones SL. Physiological and morphological characteristics of spinal neurons projecting to the parabrachial region of the cat. *Somatosens Mot Res* 1993; 10:309–325.

Lima D, Coimbra A. Morphological types of spinomesencephalic neurons in the marginal zone (Lamina I) of the rat spinal cord, as shown after retrograde labelling with cholera toxin subunit B. *J Comp Neurol* 1989; 279:327–339.

Ma W, Ribeiro-Da-Silva A, De Koninck Y, et al. Quantitative analysis of substance P-immunoreactive boutons on physiologically characterized dorsal horn neurons in the cat lumbar spinal cord. *J Comp Neurol* 1996; 376:45–64.

Martin-Schild S, Zadina JE, Gerall AA, Vigh S, Kastin AJ. Localization of endomorphin-2-like immunoreactivity in the rat medulla and spinal cord. *Peptides* 1997; 18:1641–1649.

Moskowitz MA. Neurogenic inflammation in the pathophysiology and treatment of migraine. *Neurology* 1993; 43:S16–20.

Neumann S, Doubell TP, Leslie T, Woolf CJ. Inflammatory pain hypersensitivity mediated by phenotypic switch in myelinated primary sensory neurons. *Nature (Lond)* 1996; 384:360–364.

Noguchi K, De Leon M, Nahin RL, Senba E, Ruda MA. Quantification of axotomy-induced alteration of neuropeptide mRNAs in dorsal root ganglion neurons with special reference to neuropeptide Y mRNA and the effects of neonatal capsaicin treatment. *J Neurosci Res* 1993; 35:54–66.

Noguchi K, Dubner R, De LM, Senba E, Ruda MA. Axotomy induces preprotachykinin gene expression in a subpopulation of dorsal root ganglion neurons. *J Neurosci Res* 1994; 37:596–603.

Nydahl K, Skinner K, Julius D, Basbaum AI. Co-localization of endomorphin-2 and substance P in primary afferent nociceptors and effects of injury: a light and electron microscopic study in the rat. *Eur J Neurosci* 2004; 19:1789–1799.

Potrebic S, Ahn AH, Skinner K, Fields HL, Basbaum AI. Peptidergic nociceptors of both trigeminal and dorsal root ganglia express serotonin 1D receptors: implications for the selective antimigraine action of triptans. *J Neurosci* 2003; 23:10988–10997.

Presley RW, Ménétrey D, Levine JD, Basbaum AI. Systemic morphine suppresses noxious stimulus-evoked Fos protein-like immunoreactivity in the rat spinal cord. *J Neurosci* 1990; 10:323–335.

Ren K, Dubner R. Enhanced descending modulation of nociception in rats with persistent hindpaw inflammation. *J Neurophysiol* 1996; 76:3025–3037.

Ruda MA, Ling QD, Hohmann AG, Peng YB, Tachibana T. Altered nociceptive neuronal circuits after neonatal peripheral inflammation. *Science* 2000; 289:628–631.

Schaible HG, Neugebauer V, Cervero F, Schmidt RF. Changes in tonic descending inhibition of spinal neurons with articular input during the development of acute arthritis in the cat. *J Neurophysiol* 1991; 66:1021–1031.

Shehab SA, Spike RC, Todd AJ. Do central terminals of intact myelinated primary afferents sprout into the superficial dorsal horn of rat spinal cord after injury to a neighboring peripheral nerve? *J Comp Neurol* 2004; 474:427–437.

Snider WD, McMahon SB. Tackling pain at the source: new ideas about nociceptors. *Neuron* 1998; 20:629–632.

Stucky CL, Lewin GR. Isolectin B(4)-positive and -negative nociceptors are functionally distinct. *J Neurosci* 1999; 19:6497–6505.

Tong YG, Wang HF, Ju G, et al. Increased uptake and transport of cholera toxin B-subunit in dorsal root ganglion neurons after peripheral axotomy: possible implications for sensory sprouting. *J Comp Neurol* 1999; 404:143–158.

Torsney C, Fitzgerald M. Age-dependent effects of peripheral inflammation on the electrophysiological properties of neonatal rat dorsal neurons. *J Neurophysiol* 2002; 87:1311–1317.

Tsujino H, Kondo E, Fukuoka T, et al. Activating transcription factor 3 (ATF3) induction by axotomy in sensory and motoneurons: a novel neuronal marker of nerve injury. *Mol Cell Neurosci* 2000; 15:170–182.

Vallier L, Mancip J, Markossian S, et al. An efficient system for conditional gene expression in embryonic stem cells and in their in vitro and in vivo differentiated derivatives. *Proc Natl Acad Sci USA* 2001; 98:2467–2472.

Vercelli A, Repici M, Garbossa D, Grimaldi A. Recent techniques for tracing pathways in the central nervous system of developing and adult mammals. *Brain Res Bull* 2000; 51:11–28.

Woodbury CJ, Ritter AM, Koerber HR. On the problem of lamination in the superficial dorsal horn of mammals: a reappraisal of the substantia gelatinosa in postnatal life. *J Comp Neurol* 2000; 417:88–102.

Woodbury CJ, Ritter AM, Koerber HR. Central anatomy of individual rapidly adapting low-threshold mechanoreceptors innervating the "hairy" skin of newborn mice: early maturation of hair follicle afferents. *J Comp Neurol* 2001; 436:304–323.

Woolf CJ, Shortland P, Coggeshall RE. Peripheral nerve injury triggers central sprouting of myelinated afferents. *Nature (Lond)* 1992; 355:75–78.

Woolf CJ, Shortland P, Reynolds M, et al. Reorganization of central terminals of myelinated primary afferents in the rat dorsal horn following peripheral axotomy. *J Comp Neurol* 1995; 360:121–134.

Yoshihara Y, Mizuno T, Nakahira M, et al. A genetic approach to visualization of multisynaptic neural pathways using plant lectin transgene. *Neuron* 1999; 22:33–41.

Zadina JE, Hackler L, Ge LJ, Kastin AJ. A potent and selective endogenous agonist for the mu-opiate receptor. *Nature (Lond)* 1997; 386:499–502.

Zhang ET, Craig AD. Morphology and distribution of spinothalamic lamina I neurons in the monkey. *J Neurosci* 1997; 17:3274–3284.

Zhou L, Nepote V, Rowley DL, et al. Murine peripherin gene sequences direct Cre recombinase expression to peripheral neurons in transgenic mice. *FEBS Lett* 2002; 523:68–72.

Zou Z, Horowitz LF, Montmayeur JP, et al. Genetic tracing reveals a stereotyped sensory map in the olfactory cortex. *Nature (Lond)* 2001; 414:173–179.

Correspondence to: Allan I. Basbaum, PhD, Department of Anatomy, University of California San Francisco, 513 Parnassus Avenue, Box 0452, San Francisco, CA 94143, USA. Tel: 415-476-5270; Fax: 415-476-4845; email: aib@phy.ucsf.edu.

The Pain System in Normal and Pathological States: A Primer for Clinicians, Progress in Pain Research and Management, Vol. 31, edited by Luis Villanueva, Anthony Dickenson, and Hélène Ollat, IASP Press, Seattle, © 2004.

8

Brainstem and Pain: A Complementary Role with Regard to the Thalamus?

Jean-François Bernard and Caroline Gauriau

Faculty of Medicine Pitié-Salpêtrière, INSERM U-288, Paris, France

The caudal thalamus is generally considered the primary brain center for pain processing. As a direct consequence, the spinothalamic tract is often viewed as the main pain pathway for conveying nociceptive messages from the spinal cord to the thalamus. In this chapter, primarily based on data obtained in the rat, we point out that the role of the brainstem in ascending pain processing has been strongly underestimated. The brainstem plays a unique role complementary to the thalamus in directly conveying a strong nociceptive input to the hypothalamus and the amygdala. It probably has a more extensive role than the spinothalamic tract for conveying nociceptive input to the medial thalamus. Two regions in the dorsal horn of the spinal cord, the superficial and the deep laminae, play a key role in conveying nociceptive messages from the periphery to brain nociceptive centers. We found a dramatic difference between ascending projections originating from deep laminae versus those arising from lamina I of the dorsal horn.

Superficial laminae (I and II) are important in nociceptive processing because this region is the main recipient for Aδ- and C-fiber monosynaptic input. Lamina I neurons constitute the main output of this superficial layer. The lamina I neurons are primarily nociceptive, and most are nociceptive specific (Christensen and Perl 1970; Bester et al. 2000). In addition, some lamina I neurons can encode specifically innocuous thermal stimuli (Light et al. 1993; Craig et al. 2001).

Electrophysiology has demonstrated the involvement of deep laminae (V and VI and the adjacent laminae VII and X). This region contains numerous wide-dynamic-range neurons that have a great ability to encode cutaneous stimuli from clearly innocuous to frankly nociceptive magnitudes (Besson and Chaouch 1987; Willis and Coggeshall 1991). This region's anatomical link to primary nociceptive projections is less clear: deep laminae receive some collateral projections from Aδ and C fibers, but the main nociceptive input might be conveyed indirectly via superficial laminae (Willis and Coggeshall 1991).

Although this chapter draws on numerous electrophysiological studies of the brainstem, it is primarily based on studies in our laboratory that allowed us to make a comparative anatomical examination of the projections from nociceptive layers of the dorsal horn of the spinal cord to the brainstem and the thalamus (Bernard et al. 1995; Raboisson et al. 1996; Gauriau and Bernard 2004). This anatomical investigation required anterograde tracers with high resolution, such as *Phaseolus vulgaris* leukoagglutinin (PHA-L) or tetramethyl-rhodamine-dextran (RHO-D). These tracers have numerous unique properties: (1) PHA-L injections are sufficiently small and efficient to separately investigate projections from different layers of the dorsal horn; (2) PHA-L labeling is Golgi-like and provides an unambiguous view of the density of terminal labeling; and (3) the PHA-L anterograde strategy permitted us to compare, in the same animal, the projections from a few spinal layers to different brain areas. Thus, we were able to demonstrate separately and comparatively the projections of superficial and deep nociceptive laminae of the dorsal horn upon the brainstem and the thalamus.

PROJECTIONS ORIGINATING FROM THE SUPERFICIAL LAMINAE IN THE BRAINSTEM

We studied the ascending projections of lamina I neurons in the rat by injecting PHA-L only to laminae I–II of the dorsal horn. Anatomical studies using axonal retrograde transport show that lamina II neurons do not project substantially to the supraspinal level, so labeled projections observed with superficial injections chiefly originated from lamina I.

Lamina I axons ascend, close to laminae IV–VII axons, along the contralateral lateral funiculus of the spinal cord (see also Craig 1991; Zhang et al. 2000). As shown in Fig. 1 from caudal to rostral, lamina I neurons terminate chiefly in five brainstem sites as follows: the ventrolateral medulla (VLM), the subnucleus reticularis dorsalis (SRD) (including the adjacent portion of cuneate and solitary tract nuclei), the lateral parabrachial area (PBl), the periaqueductal gray matter (PAG), and the deep layers of the superior colliculus (DpSC) (Bernard et al. 1995; Craig 1995a; Villanueva et al. 1995). One target, the PBl, drew our attention because it receives many more extensive labeled projections than do the other sites in the brainstem (Fig. 2A,B). Importantly, we found a second extensive projection from lamina I in the caudal portion of the lateral thalamus (Fig. 2A,C) (Gauriau and Bernard 2004; see also Giesler et al. 1979).

The parabrachial (PB) area is a group of neurons that surround the brachium conjunctivum, dorsally, at the pontomesencephalic junction. Within the PB area, only the PB1 receives projections from lamina I neurons of the dorsal horn. The projections from the PB1 are especially interesting because they do not target both the thalamus and the cortex, but primarily reach two other important structures—the amygdala and the hypothalamus (Bernard et al. 1993; Bester et al. 1997). PHA-L injections in the PB1 permitted us to demonstrate the great predominance of amygdaloid and hypothalamic projections and to analyze their organization. In the amygdala, the "nociceptive" projections from the pontine PB1 area primarily target the lateral capsular division and to a lesser extent the lateral division of the central nucleus (Bernard et al. 1993; Jasmin et al. 1997). Another substantial projection reaches the lateral division of the bed nucleus of the stria terminalis. We recently demonstrated that the lateral capsular division of the central nucleus, the "nociceptive amygdala," sends most of its projections to the substantia innominata dorsalis (Bourgeais et al. 2001a). These areas, which all belong to the central division of the extended amygdala, probably contribute to specific components of aversive emotions, for example, anxiety, fear-evoked avoidance learning, antinociception, and autonomic adjustments that occur during dangerous or painful situations. In the hypothalamus, the "nociceptive" projections from the mesencephalic PB area target the ventromedial nucleus and the retrochiasmatic, periventricular, and median preoptic areas. Lighter projections also reach the paraventricular nucleus (Bester et al. 1997). The ventromedial hypothalamic nucleus corresponds to the satiety center and is also a major center for rage and aggressive behaviors. Thus, the PB1-hypothalamic tract could play an important role in motivational aspects of pain, such as defense, aggression, flight, and feeding responses (Malick et al. 2001). The projections to periventricular, paraventricular, median preoptic, and ventrolateral preoptic nuclei suggest an additional involvement in pain-related neuroendocrine functions, in awakening, and in alteration of homeostatic functions in response to pain such as blood fluid balance and thermoregulation.

These anatomical data provide strong support for the existence of spino-parabrachio-amygdaloid and hypothalamic nociceptive pathways. Electrophysiological studies have demonstrated the involvement of these pathways in nociceptive processing. Indeed, most PB1-projecting lamina I neurons are markedly excited by noxious stimuli. More interestingly, a high proportion (~60%) of PB1 neurons projecting to either the amygdala or the hypothalamus are strongly and specifically excited by noxious stimuli from very low spontaneous activity (Bernard and Besson 1990; Bernard et al. 1994, 1996; Bester et al. 1995; Menendez et al. 1996). Using electrical stimuli, we

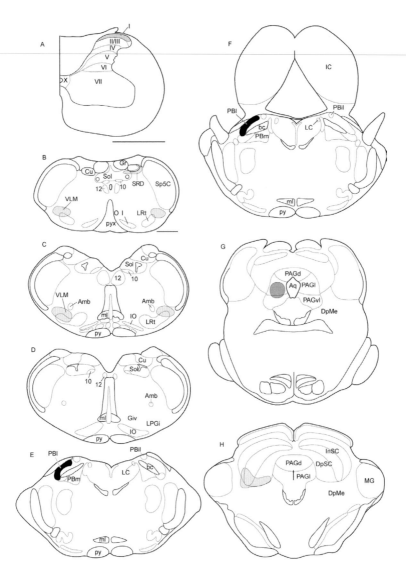

Fig. 1. Projections from the lamina I of the dorsal horn of the spinal cord. (A) cervical enlargement of the spinal cord, hatched area: lamina I projecting neurons; (B–D) medulla; (E) pons; (F–H) mesencephalon. Black, medium, and light gray; high, medium, and low density of projections, respectively. For abbreviations, see Table I. Scale bars in A and B (applies to B–H) = 1 mm.

demonstrated that these PBl neurons are driven by Aδ and C fibers (Fig 3A). The PBl nociceptive neurons encode thermal, mechanical, and visceral stimuli within the whole noxious range (Fig. 3B,C). Their responses to

Table I
List of abbreviations

I–X = laminae I–X of the spinal cord	opt = optic tract
10 = dorsal motor nucleus of vagus	PAG = periaqueductal gray matter
12 = hypoglossal nucleus	PAGd = periaqueductal gray, dorsal
Amb = ambiguus nucleus	PAGl = periaqueductal gray, lateral
APT = anterior pretectal nucleus	PAGvl = periaqueductal gray, ventrolateral
Aq = aqueduct (Sylvius)	PB = parabrachial area
ar = acoustic radiation	Pbil = internal lateral parabrachial nucleus
bc = brachium conjunctivum	PBl = lateral parabrachial nucleus
BL = basolateral amygdaloid nucleus	PBm = medial parabrachial nucleus
Ce = central amygdaloid nucleus	PC = paracentral thalamic nucleus
CL = central lateral thalamic nucleus	PHA-L = leukoagglutinin of *Phaseolus vulgaris*
CM = central medial thalamic nucleus	PIL = posterior intralaminar thalamic nucleus
Cpu = caudate putamen	Po = posterior thalamic group
Cu = cuneate nucleus	PoT = posterior thalamic group, triangular part
DM = dorsomedial hypothalamic nucleus	py = pyramidal tract
DpMe = deep mesencephalic nucleus	pyx = pyramidal decussation
DpSC = deep layers of the superior colliculus	RHO-D = tetramethyl-rhodamine-dextran
Eth = ethmoid thalamic nucleus	SG = suprageniculate nucleus
f = fornix	Sol = solitary tract nucleus
Gi = gigantocellular reticular nucleus	Sp5C = spinal trigeminal nucleus, caudal part
Giv = gigantocellular reticular nucleus, ventral	SPF = subparafascicular nucleus
Gr = gracile nucleus	SRD = subnucleus reticularis dorsalis
IC = inferior colliculus	VL = ventrolateral thalamic nucleus
ic = internal capsule	VLM = ventrolateral medulla
InSC = intermediate gray layer of the superior colliculus	VM = ventromedial thalamic nucleus
IO = inferior olive	VMH = ventromedial hypothalamic nucleus
La = lateral amygdaloid nucleus	VPL = ventral posterolateral thalamic nucleus
LC = locus ceruleus	VPM = ventral posteromedial thalamic nucleus
LPGi = lateral paragigantocellular nucleus	
LRt = lateral reticular nucleus	
Me = medial amygdaloid nucleus	
MG = medial geniculate nucleus	
ml = medial lemniscus	
mt = mammillothalamic tract	

noxious stimuli are depressed by intravenous morphine in a dose-dependent and naloxone-reversible fashion (Huang et al. 1993). Receptive fields of PBl neurons are large (generally extending to several parts of the body), whereas the receptive fields of PB-projecting lamina I spinal neurons are generally small (extending, for example, to one or two toes), indicating a large convergence of lamina I input onto PB neurons.

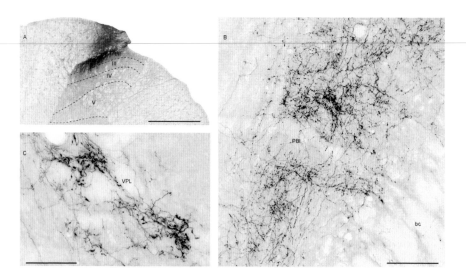

Fig. 2. The two primary projections arising from the spinal lamina I neurons. (A) PHA-L injection site in laminae I–II of the cervical enlargement. (B) Extensive terminal labeling with small varicosities in the PBl area resulting from the injection in A. (C) Terminal labeling with large varicosities in the VPL thalamic nucleus resulting from the injection in A. For abbreviations, see Table I. Scale bars in A = 500 μm, in B and C = 100 μm.

As mentioned above, the second extensive projection of lamina I neuIn summary, the lamina I system is certainly the most specific primary relay for pain, and the brainstem clearly has a complementary function with the thalamus via parallel pathways: (1) the lamina I-(lateral) thalamocortical pathway is probably responsible for pain sensation, as an extention of tactile sensation; (2) the spino-parabrachio-amygdaloid/hypothalamic pathway most likely contributes to the emotional learning and autonomic homeostatic components of pain.

PROJECTIONS ORIGINATING FROM THE DEEP LAMINAE IN THE BRAINSTEM

We studied the ascending projections of laminae IV–VII neurons in the rat by using larger injections of PHA-L or RHO-D that avoided laminae I and II. As shown in Fig. 4 from caudal to rostral, lamina IV–VII neurons terminate chiefly in four brainstem sites as follows: the lateral reticular nucleus (LRt), the SRD (Raboisson et al. 1996), the gigantocellular ventral/paragigantocellular reticular nuclei (Gi), and the parabrachial internal lateral subnucleus (PBil) (Bernard et al. 1995). However, projections to the

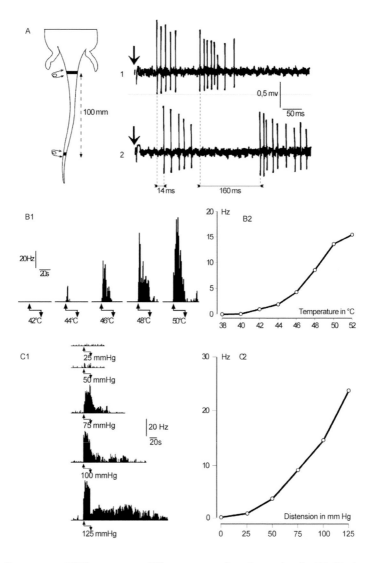

Fig. 3. Responses of PBl neurons to different types of noxious stimuli. (A) Single-sweep recording of the early and late peaks of activation evoked by high-intensity (2 ms, 30 mA) transcutaneous electrical stimulation of the base (1) and the tip (2) of the tail. The increase in latencies of the early (14 ms) and late peak of activation (160 ms), when the stimulus moves from the base to the tip of the tail, indicates peripheral conduction velocities of 100/14 = 7 m/s and 100/160 = 0.6 m/s, i.e., in the range of Aδ- and C-fiber conduction velocities. (B1) Firing of a PBl neuron in response to increasing noxious thermal stimuli applied to the contralateral forepaw (during 20-second periods). (B2) Mean stimulus-response curve of parabrachio-hypothalamic neurons to heat. (C1) Firing of a PBl neuron in response to increasing colorectal distension (20-second periods). (C2) Mean stimulus-response curve of parabrachio-hypothalamic neurons to colorectal distension. Modified from Bernard and Besson (1990), Bernard et al. (1994), and Bester et al. (1995).

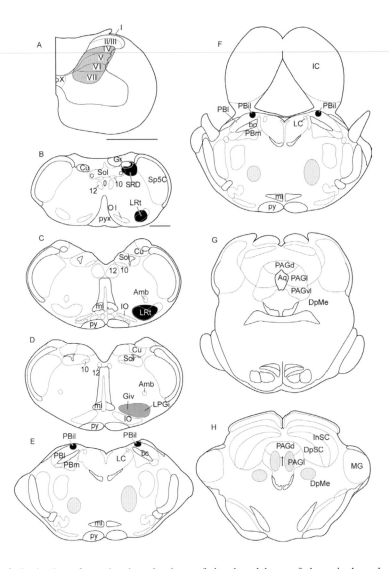

Fig. 4. Projections from the deep laminae of the dorsal horn of the spinal cord. (A) Cervical enlargement of the spinal cord; hatched area, laminae IV–VII projection area; (B–D) medulla; (E) pons; (F–H) mesencephalon. Black, medium, and light gray; high, medium, and low density of projections, respectively. For abbreviations, see Table I. Scale bars in A and B (applies to B–H) = 1 mm.

thalamus appeared consistent only upon the central lateral nucleus (CL) (Gauriau and Bernard 2004).

The LRt is a motor reticular area closely linked to the cerebellum that may be directly involved in motor reactions in response to noxious and proprioceptive stimuli.

The Gi has been considered the most likely candidate to convey nociceptive messages from deep laminae toward the intralaminar thalamus. Indeed, numerous Gi neurons respond to noxious stimuli, and stimulation of this area evokes escape behavior (Casey 1971a,b; Bowsher 1976). However, our PHA-L study demonstrates that the deep laminar projection chiefly targets the caudal portion of Gi, which in turn projects only weakly to the medial thalamus. Thus, it is unlikely that the Gi has an important role in conveying nociceptive messages from the deep laminae of the spinal cord to the medial thalamus. However, Gi neurons project densely to the locus ceruleus, the nucleus of the solitary tract, the motor nuclei of the medulla, and the ventral horn of the spinal cord (Martin et al. 1985; Ohtake 1992; Luppi et al. 1995). Thus, it might be possible that the Gi has an important role in motor, autonomic, and alertness components of pain.

The subnucleus reticularis dorsalis is another reticular area, located caudally in the medulla, just ventral to the cuneate nucleus. Electrophysiological studies demonstrate the involvement of this reticular region in nociceptive processing. Most SRD neurons are strongly excited by noxious stimuli from a low level of spontaneous activity and do not respond to multisensory (visual and auditory) stimuli. SRD neurons encode the intensity of thermal, mechanical, and visceral noxious stimuli. They respond exclusively to the activation of peripheral Aδ and C fibers. Intravenous morphine depresses such responses in a dose-dependent and naloxone-reversible fashion (Villanueva et al. 1996). The receptive fields of SRD neurons are very large and often include the whole body. The main thalamic target of the SRD is the lateral portion of the ventromedial (VM) nucleus, and to a lesser extent, the parafascicular nucleus (Villanueva et al. 1998). Neurons in the lateral portion of the VM, which have recently been reported to be involved in nociceptive processing, project chiefly to layer I of the dorsolateral frontal/prefrontal cortex (Monconduit et al. 1999; Desbois and Villanueva 2001). Given these cortical projections, the spino-SRD-VM link probably has an important role in emotional arousal and in the motor component of pain. Importantly, the SRD also sends substantial projections to the motor nuclei of the brainstem, the inferior olive, the Gi, and the deep laminae (IV–VII) of the spinal cord (Bernard et al. 1990; Villanueva et al. 1995).

The internal lateral parabrachial nucleus (PBil) is a medial subnucleus of the PB area. It does not receive projections from lamina I (contrary to the PBl), but specifically receives a dense projection from deep laminae of the spinal cord and especially from the reticular portion of laminae IV and V (Bernard et al. 1995). PBil neurons project primarily to the paracentral intralaminar thalamic nucleus (Fulwiler and Saper 1984; Bester et al. 1999), a region that in turn projects chiefly to the dorsomedial and lateral orbital prefrontal cortex and to the corresponding striatal compartment (Berendse and Groenewegen 1991). Electrophysiological studies demonstrate the involvement of PBil-thalamic neurons in nociceptive processing. Indeed, most PBil neurons respond to thermal and noxious stimuli, but with a maximal response in the mid-nociceptive scale (48°C and 16 N/cm^2). The PBil neurons exhibit strong wind-up and long-lasting after-discharge in response to noxious stimuli. Intravenous morphine depresses such responses in a dose-dependent and naloxone-reversible fashion (Bourgeais et al. 2001b). The PBil-paracentral-prefrontal link might be involved in emotional and alerting components of pain. As mentioned above, the only substantial thalamic projection of neurons from deep laminae reaches the intralaminar CL nucleus. Interestingly, cortical projections of the CL nucleus are similar to those of the PC nucleus (Berendse and Groenewegen 1991; see also Glenn and Steriade 1982). Thus, the CL-prefrontal link might complement the function of the PC-prefrontal link in nociceptive processing.

In summary, the brainstem clearly has a complementary role with the spinothalamic tract in the functioning of the deep laminar system, which is also an important relay for nociceptive information. Indeed, SRD and PBil neurons and the spinothalamic tract convey nociceptive messages from the deep laminae to the medial (intralaminar and paralaminar) thalamus. As such, this system could deal with alertness, emotional, and motor aspects of pain through a general arousal of the prefrontal and frontal (motor) cortices. Importantly, this conclusion dismisses the Gi as a direct and important link between the spinal cord and the thalamus, but not as an important contributor to motor and alertness reactions to noxious stimuli via other connections, as mentioned above.

FURTHER CONSIDERATIONS ON THE BRAINSTEM AND PAIN

Another nociceptive system, centered on the gracile nucleus, deserves mention. The Willis group proposed the following pathway: the visceral (colorectal) nociceptive messages that reach laminae X and VII of the lumbosacral spinal cord would be conveyed via the medial portion of the dorsal column and the gracile nucleus to the VPL thalamic nucleus. Key evidence of this pathway is the strong effect of a medial commissurotomy (in the middle of the dorsal column fasciculus) upon the response of VPL neurons to visceral noxious stimuli and visceral pain (Al-Chaer et al. 1996; Willis et al. 1999). However, such a pathway remains difficult to reconcile with previous clinical and experimental data. Furthermore, anterograde anatomical study in the rat demonstrated only a moderate projection from the laminae X and VII upon the gracile nucleus (Wang et al. 1999).

Although descending controls of nociception are not within the scope of this chapter, an important point is that ascending pain pathways contact several brainstem areas involved in descending controls. As already mentioned, the Gi, which receives deep laminae projections, is involved in motor and descending control of pain, via major projections to motor nuclei and to the locus coeruleus. The SRD, which receives projections from deep laminae, is involved, at least in part, in diffuse noxious inhibitory control (Bouhassira et al. 1992; see however Almeida et al. 1999), probably via direct projections to laminae IV–VII of the spinal cord (Villanueva et al. 1995). The PAG, which receives projections from lamina I and to a lesser extent from deep laminae and the PB, is an important center for processing motor, autonomic, and antinociceptive integrated responses (Bandler and Shipley 1994) via several reticular projections, notably the rostral ventromedial medulla (the area that controls the transmission of nociceptive information at the level of dorsal horn) and the VLM (the area that controls cardiorespiratory functions).

DUAL ASCENDING NOCICEPTIVE PATHWAYS

Our anatomical and electrophysiological studies described in the rat strongly suggest the existence of two systems that convey nociceptive messages from the dorsal horn to the upper brain centers. In these two systems, the brainstem appears to have a predominant complementary role with regard to the spinothalamic tract (from an anatomical perspective). These nociceptive pain pathways are summarized in Fig. 5 and below.

The first system is centered on lamina I neurons. It includes two parallel subsystems: (1) The lamina I-PB system would be a major contributor to emotional and autonomic features of the pain experience. Indeed, after processing in the PB area, this information is distributed directly to the extended central amygdala, which triggers emotional learning, and to the hypothalamus, which processes autonomic/motivational homeostasis. (2) The lamina I (lateral) thalamic system would be chiefly responsible for sensory discrimination of nociceptive stimuli as an extension of the tactile sensation via thalamic projections to somatosensory cortices (S1, S2, and insular cortex).

The second system is centered on neurons of the deep laminae. It includes two convergent subsystems: (1) the deep laminae-SRD/PBil-medial thalamic system, and (2) the deep laminae-medial thalamic system. Both

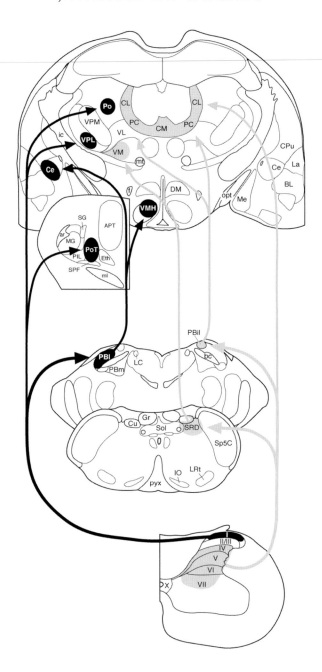

Fig. 5. The main pain pathways in the rat. In black: pathways originating from lamina I of the spinal cord and brain areas driven by lamina I input. In light gray: pathways originating from the deep laminae of the spinal cord and brainstem areas driven by input from deep laminae. For abbreviations, see Table I.

these subsystems could be involved in motor and alertness/arousal emotional features of pain via thalamic projections to frontal motor cortices and prefrontal medial/cingulate cortices.

The spinal ascending axons of all these systems are located around the same spinal lateral/ventrolateral quadrant in the rat. This fasciculus is more ventral in the primate because of the greater volume of the pyramidal tract (in the dorsolateral quadrant). Thus, the striking acute effectiveness of ventrolateral cordotomy is due not only to the interruption of the spinothalamic tract, but also to the interruption of the extensive spino-brainstem pathways described above.

The lamina I-PBl system (Price and Amaral 1981; Wiberg et al. 1987; Craig 1995a) and the lamina I-(lateral) thalamic system we propose in the rat certainly apply to the primate, although the main thalamic target of lamina I in the primate might not be the VPL but rather the VPI, the Po/SG, or VMpo nuclei (Apkarian et al. 1989; Gingold et al. 1991; Ralston and Ralston 1992; Craig et al. 1994; Craig 1995a). However, the projections from deep laminae appear less similar in rats and monkeys. For example, retrograde tracer injections recently showed a substantial projection from deep laminae to the VPL thalamic nucleus in the monkey (Willis et al. 2001, 2002), whereas our recent anterograde tracer anatomical study revealed that such a projection is very weak in the rat (Gauriau and Bernard 2004). It may be a species difference; however, it appears to us that few, if any, anterograde anatomical studies have specifically examined the projection from the deep laminae to the thalamus. An anterograde study focused on the deep laminae is required in primates to settle this point. The projections of deep laminae to the brainstem in the primate also deserve further anterograde tracer investigations.

It is clear that precise knowledge of nociceptive pathways is critically important to understanding the physiology of pain. Nonetheless, powerful descending brainstem controls that may be triggered by noxious messages indicate that pain sensation is the result of a complex and dynamic processing system that cannot be summarized only by knowledge of ascending pain pathways. Furthermore, integrated motor responses that can be processed at the brainstem level, in addition to nociceptive reflexes arising at the spinal level, show the difficulty of interpreting, in terms of sensation, the motor and the behavioral aversive responses to pain in animals.

ACKNOWLEDGMENTS

This chapter primarily addresses experiments conducted in Unit 161 of INSERM (Paris, France), directed for 24 years by Jean-Marie Besson. We warmly thank Jean-Marie for providing the atmosphere of freedom in his laboratory that created an invaluable scientific environment, and for his kindness, support, and advice, which permitted us to complete the studies summarized in this chapter.

REFERENCES

Al-Chaer ED, Lawand NB, Westlund KN, Willis WD. Visceral nociceptive input into the ventral posterolateral nucleus of the thalamus: a new function for the dorsal column pathway. *J Neurophysiol* 1996; 76:2661–2274.

Almeida A, Storkson R, Lima D, Hole K, Tjolsen A. The medullary dorsal reticular nucleus facilitates pain behaviour induced by formalin in the rat. *Eur J Neurosci* 1999; 11:110–122.

Apkarian AV, Hodge CJ. Primate spinothalamic pathways: III. Thalamic terminations of the dorsolateral and ventral spinothalamic pathways. *J Comp Neurol* 1989; 288:493–511.

Bandler R, Shipley MT. Columnar organization in the midbrain periaqueductal gray: modules for emotional expression? *Trends Neurosci* 1994; 17:379–389.

Berendse HW, Groenewegen HJ. Restricted cortical termination fields of the midline and intralaminar thalamic nuclei in the rat. *Neuroscience* 1991; 42:73–102.

Bernard JF, Besson JM. The spino(trigemino)pontoamygdaloid pathway: electrophysiological evidence for an involvement in pain processes. *J Neurophysiol* 1990; 63:473–490.

Bernard JF, Villanueva L, Carroue J, Le Bars D. Efferent projections from the subnucleus reticularis dorsalis (SRD): a *Phaseolus vulgaris* leucoagglutinin study in the rat. *Neurosci Lett* 1990; 122:257–262.

Bernard JF, Alden M, Besson JM. The organization of the efferent projections from the pontine parabrachial area to the amygdaloid complex: a *Phaseolus vulgaris* leucoagglutinin (PHA-L) study in the rat. *J Comp Neurol* 1993; 329:201–229.

Bernard JF, Huang GF, Besson JM. The parabrachial area: electrophysiological evidence for an involvement in visceral nociceptive processes. *J Neurophysiol* 1994; 71:1646–1660.

Bernard JF, Dallel R, Raboisson P, Villanueva L, Le Bars D. Organization of the efferent projections from the spinal cervical enlargement to the parabrachial area and periaqueductal gray: a PHA-L study in the rat. *J Comp Neurol* 1995; 353:480–505.

Bernard JF, Bester H, Besson JM. Involvement of the spino-parabrachio-amygdaloid and hypothalamic pathways in the autonomic and affective emotional aspects of pain. In: Holstege G, Bandler R, Saper CB (Eds). *The Emotional Motor System*. Amsterdam: Elsevier, 1996, pp 243–255.

Besson JM, Chaouch A. Peripheral and spinal mechanisms of nociception. *Physiol Rev* 1987; 67:67–186.

Bester H, Menendez L, Besson JM, Bernard JF. Spino(trigemino)parabrachiohypothalamic pathway: electrophysiological evidence for an involvement in pain processes. *J Neurophysiol* 1995; 73:568–585.

Bester H, Besson JM, Bernard JF. Organization of efferent projections from the parabrachial area to the hypothalamus: a *Phaseolus vulgaris* leucoagglutinin study in the rat. *J Comp Neurol* 1997; 383:245–281.

Bester H, Bourgeais L, Villanueva L, Besson JM, Bernard JF. Differential projections to the intralaminar and gustatory thalamus from the parabrachial area: a PHA-L study in the rat. *J Comp Neurol* 1999; 405:421–449.

Bester H, Chapman V, Besson JM, Bernard JF. Physiological properties of the lamina I spinoparabrachial neurons in the rat. *J Neurophysiol* 2000; 83:2239–2259.

Bouhassira D, Villanueva L, Bing Z, Le Bars D. Involvement of the subnucleus-reticularis-dorsalis in diffuse noxious inhibitory controls in the rat. *Brain Res* 1992; 595:353–357.

Bourgeais L, Gauriau C, Bernard JF. Projections from the nociceptive area of the central nucleus of the amygdala to the forebrain: a PHA-L study in the rat. *Eur J Neurosci* 2001a; 14:229–255.

Bourgeais L, Monconduit L, Villanueva L, Bernard JF. Parabrachial internal lateral neurons convey nociceptive messages from the deep laminas of the dorsal horn to the intralaminar thalamus. *J Neurosci* 2001b; 21:2159–2165.

Bowsher D. Role of the reticular formation in responses to noxious stimulation. *Pain* 1976; 2:361–378.

Casey KL. Somatosensory responses of bulboreticular units in awake cat: relation to escape-producing stimuli. *Science* 1971a; 173:77–80.

Casey KL. Escape elicited by bulboreticular stimulation in the cat. *Int J Neurosci* 1971b; 2:29–34.

Christensen BN, Perl ER. Spinal neurons specifically excited by noxious or thermal stimuli: marginal zone of the dorsal horn. *J Neurophysiol* 1970; 33:293–307.

Craig AD. Spinal distribution of ascending lamina I axons anterogradely labeled with *Phaseolus vulgaris* leucoagglutinin (PHA-L) in the cat. *J Comp Neurol* 1991; 313:377–393.

Craig AD. Distribution of brainstem projections from spinal lamina I neurons in the cat and the monkey. *J Comp Neurol* 1995a; 361:225–248.

Craig AD. Supraspinal projections of lamina I neurons. In: Besson JM, Guilbaud G, Ollat H (Eds). *Forebrain Areas Involved in Pain Processing*. Paris: John Libbey Eurotext, 1995b, pp 13–25.

Craig AD, Bushnell MC, Zhang ET, Blomqvist A. A thalamic nucleus specific for pain and temperature sensation. *Nature* 1994; 372:770–773.

Craig AD, Krout K, Andrew D. Quantitative response characteristics of thermoreceptive and nociceptive lamina I spinothalamic neurons in the cat. *J Neurophysiol* 2001; 86:1459–1480.

Desbois C, Villanueva L. The organization of lateral ventromedial thalamic connections in the rat: a link for the distribution of nociceptive signals to widespread cortical regions. *Neuroscience* 2001; 102:885–898.

Fulwiler CE, Saper CB. Subnuclear organization of the efferent connections of the parabrachial nucleus in the rat. *Brain Res* 1984; 319:229–259.

Gauriau C, Bernard JF. A comparative reappraisal of projections from the superficial laminae of the dorsal horn in the rat: the forebrain. *J Comp Neurol* 2004; 468(1):24–56.

Giesler GJ Jr, Menetrey D, Basbaum AI. Differential origins of spinothalamic tract projections to medial and lateral thalamus in the rat. *J Comp Neurol* 1979; 184:107–126.

Gingold SI, Greenspan JD, Apkarian AV. Anatomic evidence of nociceptive inputs to primary somatosensory cortex: relationship between spinothalamic terminals and thalamocortical cells in squirrel monkeys. *J Comp Neurol* 1991; 308:467–490.

Glenn LL, Steriade M. Discharge rate and excitability of cortically projecting intralaminar thalamic neurons during waking and sleep states. *J Neurosci* 1982; 2:1387–1404.

Huang GF, Besson JM, Bernard JF. Morphine depresses the transmission of noxious messages in the spino(trigemino)-ponto-amygdaloid pathway. *Eur J Pharmacol* 1993; 230:279–284.

Jasmin L, Burkey AR, Card JP, Basbaum AI. Transneuronal labeling of a nociceptive pathway, the spino-(trigemino-) parabrachio-amygdaloid, in the rat. *J Neurosci* 1997; 17:3751–3765.

Light AR, Sedivec MJ, Casale EJ, Jones SL. Physiological and morphological characteristics of spinal neurons projecting to the parabrachial region of the cat. *Somatosens Mot Res* 1993; 10:309–325.

Luppi PH, Aston-Jones G, Akaoka H, Chouvet G, Jouvet M. Afferent projections to the rat locus coeruleus demonstrated by retrograde and anterograde tracing with cholera-toxin B subunit and *Phaseolus vulgaris* leucoagglutinin. *Neuroscience* 1995; 65:119–160.

Malick A, Jakubowski M, Elmquist JK, Saper CB, Burstein R. A neurohistochemical blueprint for pain-induced loss of appetite. *Proc Natl Acad Sci USA* 2001; 98:9930–9935.

Martin GF, Vertes RP, Waltzer R. Spinal projections of the gigantocellular reticular formation in the rat. Evidence for projections from different areas to laminae I and II and lamina IX. *Exp Brain Res* 1985; 58:154–162.

Menendez L, Bester H, Besson JM, Bernard JF. Parabrachial area: electrophysiological evidence for an involvement in cold nociception. *J Neurophysiol* 1996; 75:2099–2116.

Monconduit L, Bourgeais L, Bernard JF, Le Bars D, Villanueva L. Ventromedial thalamic neurons convey nociceptive signals from the whole body surface to the dorsolateral neocortex. *J Neurosci* 1999; 19:9063–9072.

Ohtake T. Ascending projections from the gigantocellular reticular and dorsal paragigantocellular nuclei of the medulla oblongata in the rat: an anterograde PHA-L tracing study. *Neurosci Res* 1992; 14:96–116.

Price JL, Amaral DG. An autoradiographic study of the projections of the central nucleus of the monkey amygdala. *J Neurosci* 1981; 1:1242–1259.

Raboisson P, Dallel R, Bernard JF, Le Bars D, Villanueva L. Organization of efferent projections from the spinal cervical enlargement to the medullary subnucleus reticularis dorsalis and the adjacent cuneate nucleus: a PHA-L study in the rat. *J Comp Neurol* 1996; 367:503–517.

Ralston HJ III, Ralston DD. The primate dorsal spinothalamic tract: evidence for a specific termination in the posterior nuclei (Po/SG) of the thalamus. *Pain* 1992; 48:107–118.

Villanueva L, Bernard JF, Le Bars D. Distribution of spinal cord projections from the medullary subnucleus reticularis dorsalis and the adjacent cuneate nucleus: a *Phaseolus vulgaris*-leucoagglutinin study in the rat. *J Comp Neurol* 1995; 352:11–32.

Villanueva L, Bouhassira D, Le Bars D. The medullary subnucleus reticularis dorsalis (SRD) as a key link in both the transmission and modulation of pain signals. *Pain* 1996; 67:231–240.

Villanueva L, Desbois C, Le Bars D, Bernard JF. Organization of diencephalic projections from the medullary subnucleus reticularis dorsalis and the adjacent cuneate nucleus: a retrograde and anterograde tracer study in the rat. *J Comp Neurol* 1998; 390:133–160.

Wang CC, Willis WD, Westlund KN. Ascending projections from the area around the spinal cord central canal: a *Phaseolus vulgaris* leucoagglutinin study in rats. *J Comp Neurol* 1999; 415:341–367.

Wiberg M, Westman J, Blomqvist A. Somatosensory projection to the mesencephalon: an anatomical study in the monkey. *J Comp Neurol* 1987; 264:92–117.

Willis WD, Al-Chaer ED, Quast MJ, Westlund KN. A visceral pain pathway in the dorsal column of the spinal cord. *Proc Natl Acad Sci USA* 1999; 96:7675–7679.

Willis WD, Coggeshall RE. *Sensory Mechanisms of the Spinal Cord*, 2nd ed. New York: Plenum Press, 1991.

Willis WD Jr, Zhang X, Honda CN, Giesler GJ Jr. Projections from the marginal zone and deep dorsal horn to the ventrobasal nuclei of the primate thalamus. *Pain* 2001; 92:267–276.

Willis WD Jr, Zhang X, Honda CN, Giesler GJ Jr. A critical review of the role of the proposed VMpo nucleus in pain. *J Pain* 2002; 3:79–94.

Zhang X, Honda CN, Giesler GJ. Position of spinothalamic tract axons in upper cervical spinal cord of monkeys. *J Neurophysiol* 2000; 84:1180–1185.

Correspondence to: Dr. Jean-François Bernard, INSERM U-288, Faculté de Médecine Pitié-Salpêtrière, 91 Boulevard de l'Hôpital, 75634 Paris cedex 13, France. Tel: 33-1-4077-9714; Fax: 33-1-4077-9790; email: jfbernar@ext.jussieu.fr.

The Pain System in Normal and Pathological States:
A Primer for Clinicians, Progress in Pain Research
and Management, Vol. 31, edited by Luis Villanueva,
Anthony Dickenson, and Hélène Ollat, IASP Press,
Seattle, © 2004.

9

Spinothalamocortical Processing of Pain

William D. Willis, Jr.

*Department of Neuroscience and Cell Biology, University of Texas
Medical Branch, Galveston, Texas, USA*

A number of ascending pathways convey nociceptive information from the spinal cord to the brain. These include the spinothalamic, spinocervical, postsynaptic dorsal column, spinoreticular, spinomesencephalic, spino-parabrachial, spinohypothalamic, and other spinolimbic pathways (Willis and Coggeshall 2004). All of these are likely to influence the activity of thalamic and cortical neurons that are important for the perception of pain. However, the most direct access from the spinal cord to the thalamus and cortex is by way of the spinothalamic tract (STT). Clinical studies have shown that interruption of ascending spinal cord pathways by anterolateral cordotomy or of their crossing axons by commissural myelotomy can relieve pain for a period of months to years (Gybels and Sweet 1989). Complete pain relief requires interruption of nearly all the anterolateral quadrant at a level rostral and contralateral to the source of the pain (Fig. 1A; Nathan et al. 2001). In monkeys, this area contains the axons of several populations of STT cells, including those whose cell bodies are located in lamina I and those that originate from neurons in the deep layers of the dorsal horn (Fig. 1B; Zhang et al. 2000a). The pain relief is generally attributed to the interruption of the STT, but presumably at least part of the effectiveness of anterolateral cordotomies is due to interruption of other ascending nociceptive tracts, as well. The return of pain some time after an initially successful cordotomy may be due in some cases to enhanced effectiveness of nociceptive pathways in other parts of the spinal cord that were not interrupted. Other reasons are the spread of the disease that caused the pain or the development of central neuropathic pain as a result of the surgical lesion.

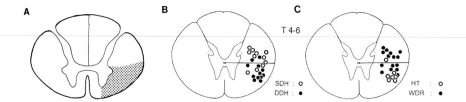

Fig. 1. Location of the ascending nociceptive pathways in the anterolateral quadrant of the spinal cord. (A) Area of the human spinal cord that must be interrupted to result in complete pain relief. (From Nathan et al. 2001.) (B) Locations of the axons of spinotha-lamic tract (STT) cells that were identified by antidromic activation from the ventral posterior lateral nucleus of the monkey thalamus. The positions of the axons were deter-mined by antidromic micromapping at the T4–T6 levels of the spinal cord. Axons from STT cells in the superficial dorsal horn (SDH) are shown by the open circles, and those from STT cells in the deep dorsal horn (DDH) by filled circles. (C) The same axons are identified by the response properties of the STT cells. The axons of high-threshold (HT) STT cells are indicated by the open circles and of wide-dynamic-range (WDR) STT cells by the filled circles. (From Zhang et al. 2000a, with permission.)

THE SPINOTHALAMIC TRACT

There are at least three major subpopulations of nociceptive STT cells in primates, based on the locations of their cell bodies, the course followed by their axons as they ascend rostrally in the spinal cord white matter, their terminations in different parts of the thalamus, and their response properties. There is some overlap between these populations, because some STT cells project to more than one thalamic nucleus. There is also a population of STT cells that are proprioceptive (Milne et al. 1982); this group of cells will not be discussed here.

STT CELLS IN THE SUPERFICIAL DORSAL HORN

The cell bodies of one population of STT cells are located in the super-ficial dorsal horn, mostly in lamina I (Trevino et al. 1973; Willis et al. 1979, 2001; Giesler et al. 1981; Apkarian and Hodge 1989a,b,c; Zhang et al. 2000b). The dendritic trees of these neurons are generally oriented rostro-caudally (Zhang and Craig 1997), and they receive a somatotopically orga-nized input from primary afferent fibers (Willis et al. 1974). The axons of STT cells in the superficial dorsal horn cross to the opposite side of the spinal cord and ascend in the middle of the lateral funiculus (Figs. 1B and 2). The location of these axons shifts to a somewhat more ventral position as the axons ascend into the cervical spinal cord (Zhang et al. 2000a,b).

Many of the axons of the STT cells in the superficial dorsal horn termi-nate in the ventral posterior lateral (VPL) nucleus of the thalamus, as shown

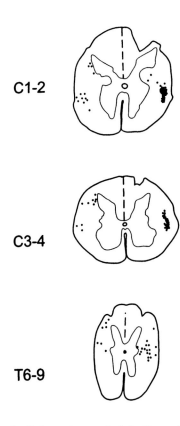

C1-2

C3-4

T6-9

Fig. 2. Positions of axons at thoracic and cervical levels that were labeled by injection of the anterograde tracer, *Phaseolus vulgaris* leuko-agglutinin, into lamina I in the lumbosacral enlargement of a monkey. The largest group of axons were located in the middle of the lateral funiculus contralateral to the injection. Many of these presumably belong to the part of the STT that originates in lamina I. A few labeled axons are observed on the same side as the injection. It was suggested that some of these may belong to the spinocervical tract and others to the STT or to spinoreticular projections. (From Craig 2000, with permission.)

both by retrograde labeling of these neurons from the VPL nucleus (Fig. 3; Willis et al. 1979, 2001) and by antidromic mapping using microstimulation (Fig. 4; Zhang et al. 2000a,b). Other thalamic endings of lamina I STT cells are in the ventral posterior inferior nucleus, the posterior complex, and the central lateral nucleus, which is part of the intralaminar complex (Mehler et al. 1960; Willis et al. 1979; Apkarian and Hodge 1989c; Apkarian and Shi 1994). Craig et al. (1994) have traced the axons of lamina I STT cells to a newly demarcated thalamic nucleus that they have termed VMpo (posterior part of the ventral medial nucleus). However, their claim that few, if any, lamina I STT cells end in the VPL nucleus appears to be erroneous, given evidence such as that shown in Figs. 3 and 4 (see also Willis et al. 2002).

Many of the superficially located STT cells in the monkey spinal cord have a high threshold for activation by mechanical stimuli applied to their cutaneous receptive fields (Willis et al. 1974; Ferrington et al. 1987). These are often called "nociceptive-specific" STT cells (Price and Dubner 1977), although "high-threshold" may be a better term, because other types of STT cells may also signal just pain, even though under the usual experimental conditions they may respond to innocuous as well as to noxious stimuli.

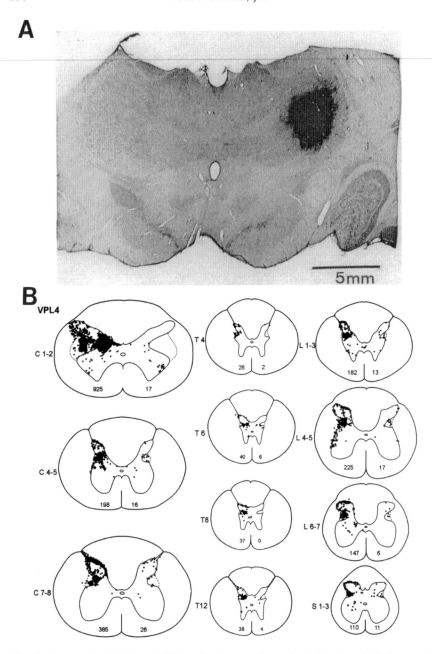

Fig. 3. Retrograde labeling of STT cells in a monkey after injection of cholera toxin subunit B into the ventral posterior lateral nucleus. The injection spread into some adjacent nuclei that do not receive spinal projections, but not into the posterior nuclear complex or the central lateral or dorsal medial nuclei. (A) The injection site at the level of maximal spread of the tracer. (B) The positions of retrogradely labeled STT cells at various segmental levels. The numbers of the neuronal profiles that were counted at each level are indicated. (From Willis et al. 2001, with permission.)

However, over half of the STT cells in the superficial dorsal horn are of the "wide-dynamic-range" (WDR) type, because they respond both to innocuous and noxious mechanical stimuli, but their largest responses are to noxious intensities (Owens et al. 1992). Many lamina I STT cells also respond to noxious heat stimuli (Kenshalo et al. 1979; Surmeier et al. 1986a,b; Ferrington et al. 1987). Others respond to innocuous cooling stimuli (Dostrovsky and Craig 1996). Thus, the lamina I STT cell population is likely to contribute to pain and also to thermal sensations. These STT cells tend to have small receptive fields (Willis 1989), and so they can contribute to the spatial localization of painful or thermal stimuli.

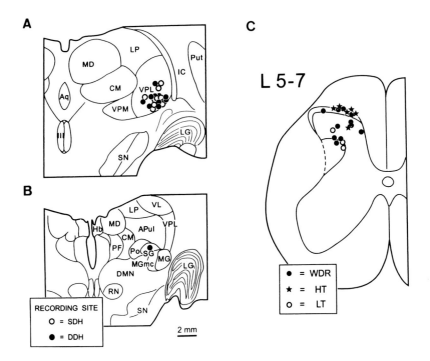

Fig. 4. The locations of sites for antidromic activation of STT cells of the superficial and deep dorsal horn in the ventral posterior lateral (VPL) nucleus and the suprageniculate nucleus of the posterior complex of the monkey thalamus. (A) Sites of microstimulation in the VPL nucleus that were successful in activating STT cells antidromically. Sites that activated STT cells that were in the superficial dorsal horn (SDH) are indicated by the open circles, and those that activated STT cells that were in the deep dorsal horn (DDH) by the filled circles. (B) A site in the suprageniculate nucleus (SG) from which an STT cell in the DDH was activated antidromically. (C) Locations of STT cells that were antidromically activated. Wide-dynamic-range (WDR) neurons are indicated by the filled circles, high-threshold (HT) cells by the stars and several low-threshold (LT) cells by the open circles. (From Zhang et al. 2000b, with permission.)

STT CELLS IN THE DEEP DORSAL HORN

Many primate STT cells are located in the deep dorsal horn (laminae IV–VII), but some are in the intermediate region and even in the ventral horn (laminae VII and VIII), as shown by retrograde tracing and by antidromic mapping (Figs. 3 and 4; Trevino et al. 1973; Willis et al. 1979, 2001; Giesler et al. 1981; Apkarian and Hodge 1989a,b,c; Zhang et al. 2000b). The dendritic trees of these STT cells are often very large, sometimes extending dorsally as far as lamina I (Fig. 5A,B; Surmeier et al. 1988; Westlund et al. 1992). By contrast, the dendrites of some STT cells in the deep dorsal horn are distributed chiefly ventrally (Fig. 5C). There is no obvious somatotopic organization of the primary afferent inputs to these neurons. The axons are often large and can be followed for a distance from the cell body after they are retrogradely or anterogradely labeled. The axons can sometimes be observed to cross the midline very close to the level of the cell body (Fig. 5A–C; see also Willis et al. 1979). The axons ascend on the contralateral side in a position in the lateral funiculus that is generally somewhat ventral to the location of the axons of the STT cells of lamina I (Fig. 1B).

Terminations of the STT cells in the deep dorsal horn are found in the VPL nucleus, as shown by retrograde labeling and by antidromic mapping (Figs. 3 and 4; Willis et al. 1979, 2001; Giesler et al. 1981; Zhang et al. 2000a,b). Some of these cells project to both the VPL and the central lateral nuclei (Giesler et al. 1981). Collaterals may also be given off to structures in the brainstem, such as the reticular formation and the periaqueductal gray (Giesler et al. 1981; Zhang et al. 1990).

This population of STT cells generally responds best to noxious stimuli, including noxious mechanical and thermal stimuli (Willis et al. 1974; Kenshalo et al. 1979; Surmeier et al. 1986a,b; Owens et al. 1992). Most are of the WDR type. However, a substantial proportion of these neurons are of the high-threshold class, and a few of these cells are of the low-threshold variety (Fig. 4), responding only to innocuous mechanical stimuli (Owens et al. 1992; Zhang et al. 2000b). They do not appear to respond to innocuous

Fig. 5. Intracellularly labeled STT cells and immunolabeled synaptic contacts on such labeled STT cells. (A–C) Drawings of primate STT cells that were labeled by intracellular injection of horseradish peroxidase. The neurons were identified by antidromic activation from the thalamic VPL nucleus, and their response properties were noted. After label was injected, the spinal cord tissue containing an STT neuron was prepared for light and electron microscopy. The dendritic trees and the course of the axon (neurite crossing the midline in panel A; those indicated by arrowheads in panels B, C) were reconstructed at the light microscopic level. Below are electron micrographs of sections of such labeled STT cells after immunostaining for glutamate (D) and substance P (E). (Panels A and D are from Westlund et al. 1992; B and C are from Surmeier et al. 1988; E is from Carlton that was published in Willis 2002; reprinted with permission.) ⟶

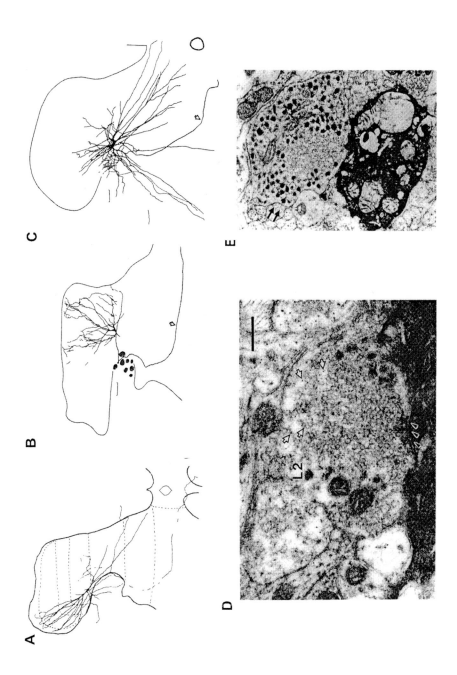

thermal stimuli. Their cutaneous receptive fields tend to be intermediate to large in size (Fig. 6A,B, Giesler et al. 1981; Willis 1989), and so they would not be as capable of signaling the location of noxious stimuli as are lamina I STT cells. STT cells in the deep dorsal horn often receive a convergent input from sensory receptors in muscles (Foreman et al. 1979a,b), joints (Dougherty et al. 1992a), and viscera (Milne et al. 1981; Al-Chaer et al. 1999; see review by Foreman 1989). This population of STT neurons is likely to contribute to referred pain.

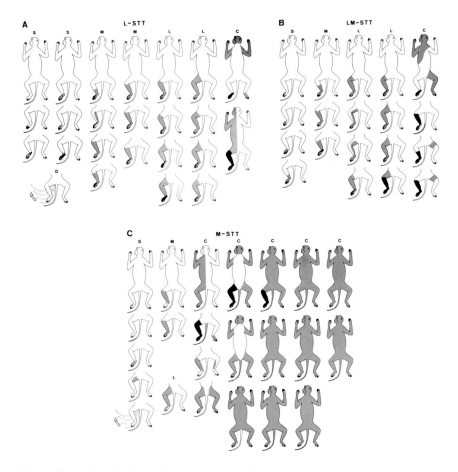

Fig. 6. Receptive fields of STT cells that projected to the lateral thalamus (ventral posterior lateral nucleus), medial thalamus (central lateral nucleus), or both, in the monkey. (A) Receptive fields of STT cells that projected just to the lateral thalamus (L-STT cells). (B) Receptive fields of STT cells that projected to both lateral and medial thalamus (LM-STT cells). (C) Receptive fields of STT cells that projected just to the medial thalamus (M-STT cells). S, M, L = small, medium-sized, and large receptive fields; C = complex and D = deep receptive fields. (From Giesler et al. 1981, with permission.)

STT CELLS THAT PROJECT TO THE CENTRAL LATERAL NUCLEUS

Most of the third population of STT cells is located in the deep dorsal horn and in the ventral horn (Giesler et al. 1981). The axons of these neurons decussate and then ascend to the thalamus through the white matter in the contralateral anterolateral quadrant. Their terminals are in the central lateral nucleus (Giesler et al. 1981).

This population of STT cells that projects to the central lateral nucleus and not to the VPL nucleus is generally of the high-threshold class. These neurons respond best when strong noxious mechanical stimuli are applied to the skin and underlying subcutaneous structures. The receptive fields are large, often extending over the entire surface of the body and face (Fig. 6C; Giesler et al. 1981). These STT cells are not suited to signal stimulus location. Instead, they are likely to contribute to attention, arousal, and motivational affective responses.

SYNAPTIC TRANSMITTERS THAT AFFECT
THE ACTIVITY OF STT CELLS

Morphological studies have demonstrated that primate STT cells labeled by the intracellular injection of horseradish peroxidase are contacted by synaptic endings that contain glutamate (Fig. 5C; Westlund et al. 1992), γ-aminobutyric acid (GABA; Carlton et al. 1992), substance P (Fig. 5E; see illustration by Carlton in Willis 2002), calcitonin gene-related peptide (CGRP; Carlton et al. 1990), serotonin (LaMotte et al. 1988), epinephrine (Carlton et al. 1991), or norepinephrine (Westlund et al. 1990). Glutamate and substance P could have been in either primary afferent or interneuronal terminals. CGRP was presumably in primary afferent terminals, given that all of the CGRP in the dorsal horn is thought to be of primary afferent origin (Chung et al. 1988). Terminals containing serotonin or norepinephrine must have originated, respectively, from neurons in the medullary raphe and dorsolateral pons that give rise to descending control systems (Besson and Chaouch 1987). The GABAergic terminals were most likely derived from interneurons of the dorsal horn, although the terminals of some projections that descend from the brainstem contain GABA colocalized with serotonin (Millhorn et al. 1987).

Pharmacological experiments employing the microiontophoresis technique have demonstrated the actions of a number of transmitter candidates or their agonists or antagonists on the responses of primate STT cells (Jordan et al. 1978; Willcockson et al. 1984a,b, 1986; Dougherty and Willis 1991a,b; Lin et al. 1996). Excitatory effects were produced by iontophoretic release of excitatory amino acids (glutamate, *N*-methyl-D-aspartate [NMDA], α-amino-3-hydroxy-5-methyl-4-isoxazole propionate [AMPA], quisqualic acid) or substance P. Inhibitory actions resulted from iontophoretically released inhibitory amino acids (GABA, glycine), amines (serotonin, norepinephrine, epinephrine), and opioids (morphine, dynorphin, enkephalin, phencyclidine). Sometimes mixed effects were observed. Fig. 7 illustrates the

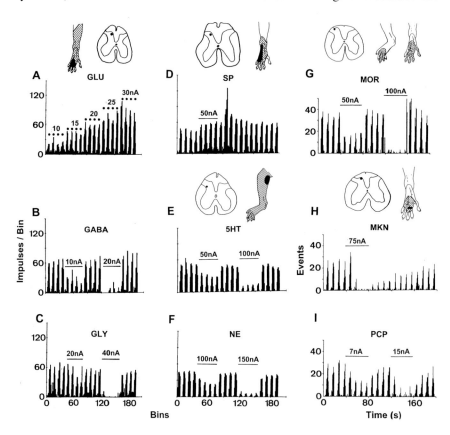

Fig. 7. Responses of STT cells to agents released by iontophoresis. (A) Excitatory effects of graded current doses of glutamate (GLU) on an STT cell in the superficial dorsal horn. The GLU was released by 5-second current pulses at 10-second intervals. (B and C) Reduction in the responses of the same STT cell to GLU by release of two current doses of GABA or of glycine during the times indicated by the horizontal bars. (D) Excitatory effects on the responses of a different STT in the superficial dorsal horn to GLU by co-release of substance P during the time indicated. (E and F) Reduction in the responses of an STT cell in the deep dorsal horn to GLU pulses during release of two current doses of serotonin (5HT) or norepinephrine (NE). (G) Inhibition of responses of an STT cell in the superficial dorsal horn to GLU pulses by release of two doses of morphine (MOR). (H and I) Inhibition of the responses of another STT cell in the superficial dorsal horn by release of methionine enkephalinamide (MKN) and two doses of phencyclidine (PCP). (Panels A, B, C, E, F are from Willcockson et al. 1984a; D is from Willcockson et al. 1984b; G–I are from Willcockson et al. 1986; reprinted with permission.)

actions of several candidate neurotransmitters (glutamate, GABA, glycine, serotonin, norepinephrine) and exogenous opioids (morphine, methionine enkephalinamide, phencyclidine) on primate STT cells. In some instances, it has been possible to block the effects of a transmitter agonist by administration of an antagonist by microdialysis or by iontophoresis. For example, Fig. 8 shows the antagonist action of AP7 infused into the dorsal horn by microdialysis in reducing or blocking the responses of an STT cell to NMDA and aspartate, but not its responses to AMPA or glutamate (Dougherty et al. 1992b).

CHANGES IN RESPONSES OF STT CELLS
AFTER ACUTE INFLAMMATION

The responses of STT cells (and other nociceptive dorsal horn neurons) can undergo substantial changes following inflammation or injury in the area of their receptive fields. For example, the responses of primate STT cells to tactile stimuli are increased following a burn injury of the skin, and

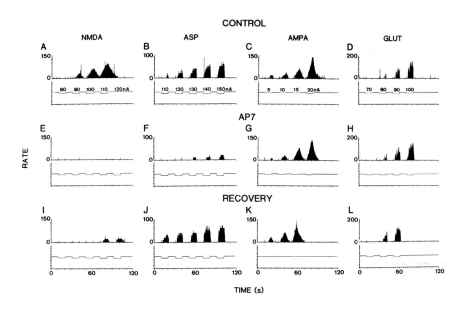

Fig. 8. Antagonist action of AP7 (DL-2-amino-7-phosphonoheptanoic acid) on the responses of a wide-dynamic-range STT cell to iontophoretic release of excitatory amino acids. (A–D) Responses to graded current doses of NMDA, aspartate (ASP), AMPA, and glutamate (GLUT) before microdialysis administration of AP7 into the dorsal horn. (E–H) Responses to the same doses of excitatory amino acids during AP7 administration. (I-L) Partial recovery of the responses 2 hours after termination of the AP7 infusion. (From Dougherty et al. 1992b, with permission.)

responses to innocuous mechanical stimuli applied either inside or outside the burned area are heightened (Kenshalo et al. 1982). It was suggested that such increased responses could help account for the development of secondary mechanical allodynia in the skin surrounding an injury. Repeated strong noxious mechanical stimulation can produce a similar effect (Owens et al. 1992), as can an intradermal injection of capsaicin (Simone et al. 1991; Dougherty and Willis 1992). Recordings from STT cells in anesthetized monkeys given an intradermal capsaicin injection provide a reproducible model of the pain, primary mechanical and heat hyperalgesia, and secondary mechanical allodynia and hyperalgesia seen in human subjects given a similar injection (Simone et al. 1989; LaMotte et al. 1991, 1992). A number of investigations have been conducted to determine what neurotransmitters and signal transduction mechanisms underlie the sensory changes; these studies have been reviewed recently (Willis 2002, 2004; Willis and Coggeshall 2003).

CHANGES IN RESPONSES OF PRIMATE STT CELLS AFTER NERVE INJURY

The responses of primate STT cells have also been used as a model of the changes that underlie neuropathic pain. Tight ligation of the L7 spinal nerve in monkeys (the Chung model of peripheral neuropathic pain adapted to primates; Kim and Chung 1992) results in behavioral changes that can be presumed to reflect the development of mechanical allodynia (Carlton et al. 1994). Recordings from STT cells in monkeys with this model of peripheral neuropathy have shown that the responses of these cells to mechanical stimuli are greatly enhanced compared to those of STT cells on the contralateral side of the spinal cord in the same animals or to those of STT cells in normal monkeys (Fig. 9; Palecek et al. 1992). Responses of the neurons to thermal stimuli are also increased.

RESPONSES OF THALAMIC NEURONS TO NOXIOUS STIMULI

VENTRAL POSTERIOR LATERAL NUCLEUS

Recordings from the primate VPL thalamic nucleus have demonstrated neurons that respond to noxious stimuli (Gaze and Gordon 1954; Perl and Whitlock 1961; Pollin and Albe-Fessard 1979; Kenshalo et al. 1980; Casey and Morrow 1983; Chung et al. 1986a,b; Chandler et al. 1992; Apkarian and Shi 1994; Brüggemann et al. 1994; Apkarian et al. 2000). The search technique in the study by Chung et al. (1986b) involved electrical stimulation of the sciatic nerve at a strength that would activate Aδ fibers. Of 110 neurons

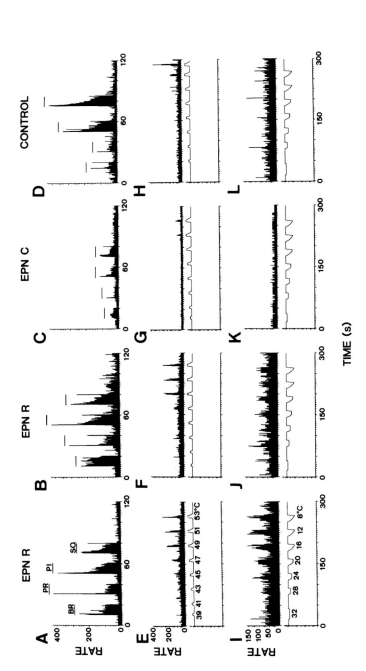

Fig. 9. Responses of STT cells to mechanical and thermal stimuli in a monkey model of experimental peripheral neuropathy (EPN) following tight ligation of the L7 spinal nerve. (A, E, I) Responses of an STT cell in the segment just rostral to the level of spinal nerve ligation (EPN R, rostral to L6/L7 border) to graded mechanical stimuli, graded heat pulses and graded cooling pulses. (B, F, J) Responses of another STT cell in a neuropathic monkey to similar graded mechanical and thermal stimuli. (C, G, K) Responses of an STT cell located at the level of the spinal nerve ligation (EPN C, caudal to L6/L7 border) to graded mechanical and thermal stimuli. (D, H, L) Responses of an STT cell in a control monkey to comparable stimuli. (From Palecek et al. 1992, with permission.)

that were sampled, 56 were classified as low-threshold, as 39 WDR, and 15 as high-threshold neurons. Fig. 10A–F illustrates the responses of a WDR VPL neuron. The locations of the nociceptive neurons correspond to the well-known somatotopic organization of the VPL nucleus. Neurons with receptive fields on the hindlimb are lateral to those with receptive fields on the forelimb (Fig. 10G; Kenshalo et al. 1980). All but one of the nociceptive VPL neurons tested could be activated antidromically when the primary somatosensory (S1) cortex was stimulated electrically (Kenshalo et al. 1980). Electrical stimulation of Aδ or C fibers in a peripheral nerve that supplied the receptive field activated such neurons (Chung et al. 1986b).

VENTRAL POSTERIOR INFERIOR NUCLEUS

Nociceptive neurons have also been recorded in the ventral posterior inferior (VPI) nucleus (Pollin and Albe-Fessard 1979; Apkarian and Shi 1994). As in the VPL nucleus, both WDR and high-threshold neurons were found. The receptive fields were generally larger than those of nociceptive neurons found in the VPL nucleus, and they could include the face. There was a mediolateral somatotopic organization (Apkarian and Shi 1994).

INTRALAMINAR NUCLEI

Nociceptive neurons in the central lateral and parafascicular nuclei have different characteristics than do those in the VPL and VPI nuclei (Casey and Morrow 1983; Bushnell and Duncan 1989; Vogt et al. 1993). Their receptive fields are very large and often bilateral. However, their responses do encode the intensity of noxious heat stimuli (Bushnell and Duncan 1989). In awake, behaving monkeys, the responses can be affected by how attentive the animal is to the stimulus; administration of an anesthetic also alters the responses (Casey and Morrow 1983; Bushnell and Duncan 1989). Presumably these neurons help in the processing of affective responses to painful stimuli.

POSTERIOR PART OF THE VENTRAL MEDIAL NUCLEUS

Craig et al. (1994) recorded from 87 neurons in the region of the proposed VMpo nucleus in monkeys. Almost all of the neurons responded to noxious or to cold stimuli. The receptive fields were often small and were on the tongue or on the hand. The responses were graded with the stimulus intensity. The nucleus had an anteroposterior somatotopic organization.

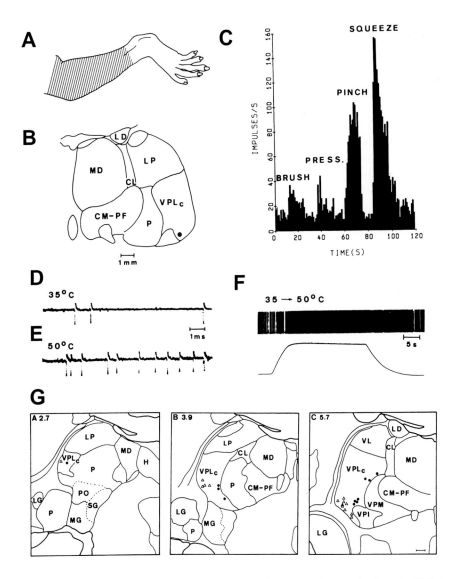

Fig. 10. Nociceptive neurons in the caudal part of the ventral posterior lateral (VPLc) nucleus in the monkey thalamus. (A) Receptive field of a WDR nociceptive VPL neuron. (B) Location of the recording site in the thalamus. (C) Responses of the neuron to graded strengths of mechanical stimulation in the receptive field. (D–F) Responses of the neuron to different temperatures applied to the receptive field. (G) Locations of VPL neurons with receptive fields on the hindlimb (open triangles) or on the forelimb (filled circles). (From Kenshalo et al. 1980, with permission.)

CEREBRAL CORTEX

ROLE OF THE CEREBRAL CORTEX IN PAIN

Clinical studies in the early part of the 20th century led to the conclusion that the cerebral cortex was not responsible for the perception of pain. The evidence came from the examination of patients who had received head wounds that resulted from warfare (Head and Holmes 1911; Head 1920) and from the results of electrical stimulation of the exposed human cerebral cortex during surgery for epilepsy (Penfield and Boldrey 1937). However, recent studies using imaging of the human brain and electrophysiological recordings from the monkey cerebral cortex lead to a different conclusion: the cerebral cortex plays an important role in pain perception and in the motivational-affective component of pain.

IMAGING STUDIES

A number of different regions of the human cerebral cortex have been shown to respond to painful stimuli in imaging studies using either positron emission tomography or functional magnetic resonance imaging (Jones et al. 1991; Talbot et al. 1991; Casey et al. 1994; Coghill et al. 1994, 1999; Rainville et al. 1997; Davis et al. 1998; Iadarola et al. 1998; Bushnell et al. 1999; Gelnar et al. 1999; Ploner et al. 1999; Treede et al. 1999, 2000; see review by Casey and Bushnell 2000). Areas of cortex that are activated by painful stimuli include the primary (S1) and secondary (S2) somatosensory cortices, the insular cortex, and the anterior cingulate cortex. Some areas with motor functions may also respond.

NOCICEPTIVE NEURONS IN THE S1 CORTEX IN MONKEYS

Neurons have been found in area 1 of the S1 cortex in monkeys that respond to noxious stimuli, both in anesthetized animals (Biedenbach et al. 1979; Kenshalo and Isensee 1983; Kenshalo et al. 1988, 2000; Chudler et al. 1990) and in awake, behaving ones (Kenshalo et al. 2000). These include WDR and high-threshold cells (Fig. 11). Nociceptive neurons in the monkey S1 cortex are generally in the middle layers of the cortex; they have relatively small receptive fields and respond to both mechanical and heat stimuli (Fig. 11). The stimulus-response curves of the WDR neurons are steeper than are those of the high-threshold neurons, and the discharge rates of the WDR cells correlate with the ability of the monkeys to recognize noxious heat stimuli, whereas the discharge rates of high-threshold neurons do not

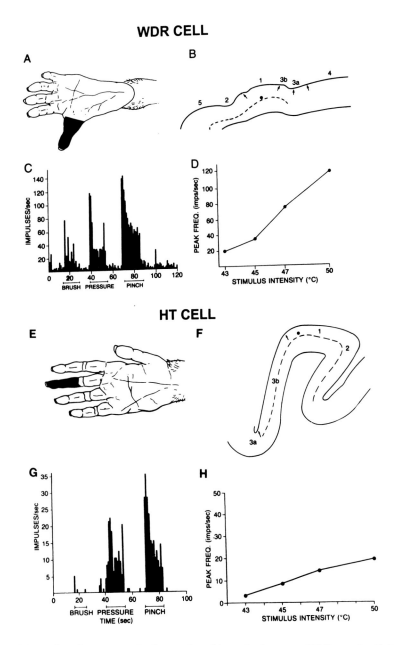

Fig. 11. Nociceptive neurons in the monkey S1 cerebral cortex. (A) Receptive field of a wide-dynamic-range (WDR) S1 neuron; (B) location of the recording site in area 1; (C) responses to graded mechanical stimulation of the receptive field; (D) stimulus-response function for graded noxious heat pulses; (E) receptive field of a high-threshold (HT) neuron in the S1 cortex; (F) location of the recording site in area 1; (G) responses to graded mechanical stimuli; (H) stimulus-response curve for graded noxious heat pulses. (From Kenshalo et al. 2000, with permission.)

(Kenshalo et al. 1988). The properties of the nociceptive neurons in the S1 cortex are appropriate for a role in sensory discrimination of painful stimuli.

NOCICEPTIVE NEURONS IN S2 AND ADJACENT CORTICAL AREAS IN MONKEYS

Nociceptive neurons have also been recorded in the S2 cortex and adjacent parts of the posterior parietal and insular cortex in awake, behaving monkeys (Robinson and Burton 1980a,b; Dong et al. 1989). The response properties of these nociceptive neurons are quite different from those of nociceptive neurons in the S1 cortex. The receptive fields are usually large and often bilateral. They do not encode stimulus intensity well, and they are not somatotopically organized. Therefore, they are not well suited for a role in sensory discrimination. It has been suggested that these cells are concerned with the memory of painful stimuli (Friedman et al. 1986; Dong et al. 1989).

THALAMIC INPUT TO NOCICEPTIVE NEURONS OF THE CEREBRAL CORTEX

S1 AND S2 CORTEX

The main thalamic projections to the S1 and S2 cortex are from the ventral posterior lateral (and ventral posterior medial) nuclei (Jones 1985, 1998). Projections to these cortical areas also come from the ventral posterior inferior nucleus and from the central lateral nucleus (Jones and Leavitt 1974; Jones et al. 1979; Friedman and Murray 1986; Gingold et al. 1991). All of these nuclei receive direct connections from the STT.

ANTERIOR CINGULATE GYRUS

Projections to the anterior cingulate gyrus arise from the anterior thalamic nuclei, the parvicellular part of the medial dorsal nucleus, and the central lateral and parafascicular nuclei (Vogt et al. 1993). The central lateral nucleus receives a direct projection from the STT.

INSULA

The anterior part of the insular cortex receives thalamic input from the parvicellular part of the ventral posterior medial nucleus, the magnocellular part of the medial dorsal nucleus, and several nuclei of the medial thalamus (Mesulam and Mufson 1985; Friedman and Murray 1986). The posterior insula receives input from the VPI nucleus and the pulvinar and the suprageniculate nucleus, as well as from the S1 and S2 cortex and the parietal association cortex (Mesulam and Mufson 1985; Friedman and Murray 1986). There are also reciprocal interconnections between the insula and the amygdala (Mesukam and Mufson 1985). The STT projects directly to the VPI and posterior complex, and the responses of nociceptive neurons in the S1 and S2 cortex would presumably reflect STT input to the VPL nucleus. The input from the amygdala could be influenced by the spino-parabrachio-amygdalar pathway (Bernard and Besson 1990) and the direct spino-amygdalar pathway (Burstein et al. 1987; Burstein and Potrebic 1993).

FUTURE STUDIES

Further experiments are needed to clarify the pharmacology of primate STT cells. For example, the actions of a variety of agents known to have analgesic actions or to depress the activity of nociceptive dorsal horn neurons should be confirmed in recordings from primate STT cells. The pharmacology of neurons in key nuclei of the primate thalamus, including the ventral posterior lateral, the ventral posterior inferior, the posterior, and the central lateral nuclei should be examined more closely than has been accomplished to date. Similarly, the pharmacology of nociceptive cortical neurons needs further investigation. Imaging techniques should be helpful for such studies.

ACKNOWLEDGMENTS

The author thanks Griselda Gonzales for her assistance with the illustrations. The work described that was done in the author's laboratory was supported by National Institutes of Health grants NS 09743 and NS 11255.

REFERENCES

Al-Chaer ED, Feng Y, Willis WD. Comparative study of viscerosomatic input onto postsynaptic dorsal column and spinothalamic tract neurons in the primate. *J Neurophysiol* 1999; 82:1876–1882.

Apkarian AV, Hodge CJ. The primate spinothalamic pathways: I. A quantitative study of the cells of origin of the spinothalamic pathway. *J Comp Neurol* 1989a; 288:447–473.

Apkarian AV, Hodge CJ. The primate spinothalamic pathways: II. The cells of origin of the dorsolateral and ventral spinothalamic pathways. *J Comp Neurol* 1989b; 288:474–492.

Apkarian AV, Hodge CJ. The primate spinothalamic pathways: III. Thalamic terminations of the dorsolateral and ventral spinothalamic pathways. *J Comp Neurol* 1989c; 288:493–511.

Apkarian AV, Shi T. Squirrel monkey lateral thalamus. I. Somatic nociresponsive neurons and their relation to spinothalamic terminals. *J Neurosci* 1994; 14:6779–6795.

Apkarian AV, Shi T, Brüggemann J, Airapetian LR. Segregation of nociceptive and non-nociceptive networks in the squirrel monkey somatosensory thalamus. *J Neurophysiol* 2000; 84:484–494.

Bernard JF, Besson JM. The spino(trigemino)pontoamygdaloid pathway: electrophysiological evidence for an involvement in pain processes. *J Neurophysiol* 1990; 63:473–490.

Besson JM, Chaouch A. Peripheral and spinal mechanisms of nociception. *Physiol Rev* 1987; 67:67–186.

Biedenbach MA, Van Hassel HJ, Brown AC. Tooth pulp-driven neurons in somatosensory cortex of primates: role in pain mechanisms including a review of the literature. *Pain* 1979; 7:31–50.

Brüggemann J, Shi T, Apkarian AV. Squirrel monkey lateral thalamus. II. Viscerosomatic convergent representation of urinary bladder, colon, and esophagus. *J Neurosci* 1994; 14:6796–6814.

Burstein R, Potrebic S. Retrograde labeling of neurons in the spinal cord that project directly to the amygdala or the orbital cortex in the rat. *J Comp Neurol* 1993; 335:469–485.

Burstein R, Cliffer KD, Gieler GJ. Direct somatosensory projections from the spinal cord to the hypothalamus and telencephalon. *J Neurosci* 1987; 7:4159–4164.

Bushnell MC, Duncan GH. Sensory and affective aspects of pain perception: is medial thalamus restricted to emotional issues? *Exp Brain Res* 1989; 78:415–418.

Bushnell MC, Duncan GH, Hofbauer RK, et al. Pain perception: is there a role for primary somatosensory cortex? *Proc Natl Acad Sci USA* 1999; 96:7705–7709.

Carlton SM, Westlund KN, Zhang D, Sorkin LS, Willis WD. Calcitonin gene-related peptide containing primary afferent fibers synapse on primate spinothalamic tract cells. *Neurosci Lett* 1990; 109:76–81.

Carlton SM, Honda CN, Willcockson WS, et al. Descending adrenergic input to the primate spinal cord and its possible role in modulation of spinothalamic cells. *Brain Res* 1991; 543:77–90.

Carlton SM, Westlund KN, Zhang D, Willis WD. GABA-immunoreactive terminals synapse on primate spinothalamic tract cells. *J Comp Neurol* 1992; 322:528–537.

Carlton SM, Lekan HS, Kim SH, Chung JM. Behavioral manifestations of an experimental model for peripheral neuropathy produced by spinal nerve ligation in the primate. *Pain* 1994; 56:155–166.

Casey KL, Bushnell MC (Eds). *Pain Imaging*, Progress in Pain Research and Management, Vol. 18. Seattle: IASP Press, 2000.

Casey KL, Morrow TJ. Ventral posterior thalamic neurons differentially responsive to noxious stimulation of the awake monkey. *Science* 1983; 221:675–677.

Casey KL, Minoshima S, Berger KL, et al. Positron emission tomographic analysis of cerebral structures activated specifically by repetitive noxious heat stimuli. *J Neurophysiol* 1994; 71:802–807.

Chandler MJ, Hobbs SF, Fu QG, et al. Responses of neurons in ventroposterolateral nucleus of primate thalamus to urinary bladder distension. *Brain Res* 1992; 571:26–34.

Chudler EH, Anton F, Dubner R, Kenshalo DR. Responses of nociceptive SI neurons in monkeys and pain sensations in humans elicited by noxious thermal stimulation: effect of interstimulus interval. *J Neurophysiol* 1990; 63:559–569.

Chung JM, Surmeier DJ, Lee KH, et al. Classification of primate spinothalamic and somatosensory thalamic neurons based on cluster analysis. *J Neurophysiol* 1986a; 56:308–327.

Chung JM, Lee KH, Surmeier DJ, et al. Response characteristics of neurons in the ventral posterior lateral nucleus of the monkey thalamus. *J Neurophysiol* 1986b; 56:370–390.

Chung K, Lee WT, Carlton SM. The effects of dorsal rhizotomy and spinal cord isolation on calcitonin gene-related peptide containing terminals in the rat lumbar dorsal horn. *Neurosci Lett* 1988; 90:27–32.

Coghill RD, Talbot JD, Evans AC, et al. Distributed processing of pain and vibration by the human brain. *J Neurosci* 1994; 14:4095–4108.

Coghill RC, Sang CN, Maisog JM, Iadarola MJ. Pain intensity processing within the human brain: a bilateral, distributed mechanism. *J Neurophysiol* 1999; 82:1934–1943.

Craig AD. Spinal location of ascending lamina I axons in the macaque monkey. *J Pain* 2000;1:33–45.

Craig AD, Bushnell MC, Zhang ET, Blomqvist A. A thalamic nucleus specific for pain and temperature sensation. *Nature* 1994; 372:770–773.

Davis KD, Kwan CL, Crawley AP, Mikulis DJ. Functional MRI study of thalamic and cortical activations evoked by cutaneous heat, cold, and tactile stimuli. *J Neurophysiol* 1998; 80:1533–1546.

Dong WK, Salonen LD, Kawakami Y, et al. Nociceptive responses of trigeminal neurons in SII-7b cortex of awake monkeys. *Brain Res* 1989; 484:314–324.

Dostrovsky JO, Craig AD. Cooling-specific spinothalamic neurons in the monkey. *J Neurophysiol* 1996; 76:3656–3665.

Dougherty PM, Willis WD. Modification of the responses of primate spinothalamic neurons to mechanical stimulation by excitatory amino acid agonists and N-methyl-D-aspartate antagonist. *Brain Res* 1991a; 542:15–22.

Dougherty PM, Willis WD. Enhancement of spinothalamic neuron responses to chemical and mechanical stimuli following combined microiontophoretic application of *N*-methyl-D-aspartic acid and substance P. *Pain* 1991b; 47:85–93.

Dougherty PM, Willis WD. Enhanced responses of spinothalamic tract neurons to excitatory amino acids accompany capsaicin-induced sensitization in the monkey. *J Neurosci* 1992; 12:883–894.

Dougherty PM, Sluka KA, Sorkin LS, Westlund KN, Willis WD. Neural changes in acute arthritis in monkeys. I. Parallel enhancement of responses of spinothalamic tract neurons to mechanical stimulation and excitatory amino acids. *Brain Res Rev* 1992a; 17:1–13.

Dougherty PM, Palecek J, Paleckova V, Sorkin LS, Willis WD. The role of NMDA and non-NMDA excitatory amino acid receptors in the excitation of primate spinothalamic tract neurons by mechanical, chemical, thermal and electrical stimuli. *J Neurosci* 1992b; 12:3025–3041.

Ferrington DG, Sorkin LS, Willis WD. Responses of spinothalamic tract cells in the superficial dorsal horn of the primate lumbar spinal cord. *J Physiol* 1987; 388:681–703.

Foreman RD. Organization of the spinothalamic tract as a relay for cardiopulmonary sympathetic afferent fiber activity. In: Ottoson D (Ed). *Progress in Sensory Physiology*, Vol. 9. Heidelberg: Springer-Verlag, 1989, pp 1–51.

Foreman RD, Kenshalo DR, Schmidt RF, Willis WD. Field potentials and excitation of primate spinothalamic neurons in response to volleys in muscle afferents. *J Physiol* 1979a; 286:197–213.

Foreman RD, Schmidt RF, Willis WD. Effects of mechanical and chemical stimulation of fine muscle afferents upon primate spinothalamic tract cells. *J Physiol* 1979b; 286:215–231.

Friedman DP, Murray EA. Thalamic connectivity of the second somatosensory area and neighboring somatosensory fields of the lateral sulcus of the macaque. *J Comp Neurol* 1986; 252:348–373.

Friedman DP, Murray EA, O'Neill JB, Mishkin M. Cortical connections of the somatosensory fields of the lateral sulcus of macaques: evidence for a corticolimbic pathway for touch. *J Comp Neurol* 1986; 252:323–347.

Gaze RM, Gordon G. The representation of cutaneous sense in the thalamus of the cat and monkey. *Q J Exp Physiol* 1954; 39:279–304.

Gelnar PA, Krauss BR, Sheehe PR, Szeverenyi NM, Apkarian AV. A comparative fMRI study of cortical representations for thermal painful, vibrotactile, and motor performance tasks. *Neuroimage* 1999; 10:460–482.

Giesler GJ, Yezierski RP, Gerhart KD, Willis WD. Spinothalamic tract neurons that project to medial and/or lateral thalamic nuclei: evidence for a physiologically novel population of spinal cord neurons. *J Neurophysiol* 1981; 46:1285–1308.

Gingold SI, Greenspan JD, Apkarian AV. Anatomic evidence of nociceptive inputs to primary somatosensory cortex: relationship between spinothalamic terminals and thalamocortical cells in squirrel monkeys. *J Comp Neurol* 1991; 308:467–490.

Gybels JM, Sweet WH. Pain and headache. In: Gildenberg PL (Ed). *Neurosurgical Treatment of Persistent Pain,* Vol. 11. Basel: Karger, 1989.

Head H. *Studies in Neurology,* Vol. 2, Part IV. London: Oxford University Press, 1920, pp 333–862.

Head H, Holmes G. Sensory disturbances from cerebral lesions. *Brain* 1911; 34:102–254.

Iadarola MJ, Berman KF, Zeffiro TA, et al. Neural activation during acute capsaicin-evoked pain and allodynia assessed with PET. *Brain* 1998; 121:931–947.

Jones AKP, Brown WD, Friston KJ, Qi LJ, Frackowiak RSJ. Cortical and subcortical localization of response to pain in man using positron emission tomography. *Proc R Soc Lond B Biol Sci* 1991; 244:39–44.

Jones EG. *The Thalamus.* New York: Plenum Press, 1985.

Jones EG. The primate nervous system, part II. In: Björklund A, Hökfelt T (Eds). *Handbook of Chemical Neuroanatomy,* Vol. 14. Amsterdam: Elsevier, 1998.

Jones EG, Leavitt RY. Retrograde axonal transport and the demonstration of non-specific projections to the cerebral cortex and striatum from thalamic intralaminar nuclei in the rat, cat and monkey. *J Comp Neurol* 1974; 154:349–378.

Jones EG, Wise SP, Coulter JD. Differential thalamic relationships of sensory-motor and parietal cortical fields in monkeys. *J Comp Neurol* 1979; 183:833–882.

Jordan LM, Kenshalo DR, Martin RF, Haber LH, Willis WD. Depression of primate spinothalamic tract neurons by iontophoretic application of 5-hydrotryptamine. *Pain* 1978; 5:135–142.

Kenshalo DR, Isensee O. Responses of primate SI cortical neurons to noxious stimuli. *J Neurophysiol* 1983; 50:1479–1496.

Kenshalo DR, Leonard RB, Chung JM, Willis WD. Responses of primate spinothalamic neurons to graded and to repeated noxious heat stimuli. *J Neurophysiol* 1979; 42:1370–1389.

Kenshalo DR, Giesler GJ, Leonard RB, Willis WD. Responses of neurons in primate ventral posterior lateral nucleus to noxious stimuli. *J Neurophysiol* 1980; 43:1594–1614.

Kenshalo DR, Leonard RB, Chung JM, Willis WD. Facilitation of the responses of primate spinothalamic cells to cold and to tactile stimuli by noxious heating of the skin. *Pain* 1982; 12:141–152.

Kenshalo DR, Chudler EH, Anton F, Dubner R. SI nociceptive neurons participate in the encoding process by which monkeys perceive the intensity of noxious thermal stimulation. *Brain Res* 1988; 454:378–382.

Kenshalo DR, Iwata K, Sholas M, Thomas DS. Response properties and organization of nociceptive neurons in area I of monkey primary somatosensory cortex. *J Neurophysiol* 2000; 84:719–729.

Kim SH, Chung JM. An experimental model for peripheral neuropathy produced by segmental spinal nerve ligation in the rat. *Pain* 1992; 50:355–363.

LaMotte CC, Carlton SM, Honda CN, Surmeier DJ, Willis WD. Innervation of identified primate spinothalamic tract neurons: ultrastructure of serotonergic and other synaptic profiles. *Soc Neurosci Abstr* 1988; 14:852.

LaMotte RH, Shain CN, Simone DA, Tsai EFP. Neurogenic hyperalgesia: psychophysical studies of underlying mechanisms. *J Neurophysiol* 1991; 66:190–211.

LaMotte RH, Lundberg LER, Torebjörk HE. Pain, hyperalgesia and activity in nociceptive C units in humans after intradermal injection of capsaicin. *J Physiol* 1992; 448:749–764.

Lin Q, Peng YB, Willis WD. Role of GABA receptor subtypes in inhibition of primate spino-thalamic tract neurons: difference between spinal and periaqueductal gray inhibition. *J Neurophysiol* 1996; 75:109–123.

Mehler WR, Feferman ME, Nauta WJH. Ascending axon degeneration following anterolateral cordotomy: an experimental study in the monkey. *Brain* 1960; 83:718–751.

Mesulam MM, Mufson EJ. The insula of Reil in man and monkey; architectonics, connectivity, and function. In: Peters A, Jones EG (Eds). *Association and Auditory Cortices,* Cerebral Cortex, Vol. 4. New York: Plenum Press, 1985, pp 179–226.

Millhorn DE, Hökfelt T, Seroogy K, et al. Immunohistochemical evidence for colocalization of γ-aminobutyric acid and serotonin in neurons of the ventral medulla oblongata projecting to the spinal cord. *Brain Res* 1987; 410:179–185.

Milne RJ, Foreman RD, Giesler GJ, Willis WD. Convergence of cutaneous and pelvic visceral nociceptive inputs onto primate spinothalamic neurons. *Pain* 1981; 11:163–183.

Milne RJ, Foreman RD, Wills WD. Responses of primate spinothalamic neurons located in the sacral intermediomedial gray (Stilling's nucleus) to proprioceptive input from the tail. *Brain Res* 1982; 234:227–236.

Nathan PW, Smith M, Deacon P. The crossing of the spinothalamic tract. *Brain* 2001; 124:793–803.

Owens CM, Zhang D, Willis WD. Changes in the response states of primate spinothalamic tract cells caused by mechanical damage of the skin or activation of descending controls. *J Neurophysiol* 1992; 67:1509–1527.

Palecek J, Dougherty PM, Kim SH, et al. Responses of spinothalamic tract neurons to mechani-cal and thermal stimuli in an experimental model of peripheral neuropathy in primates. *J Neurophysiol* 1992; 68:1951–1966.

Penfield W, Boldrey E. Somatic motor and sensory representation in the cerebral cortex of man as studied by electrical stimulation. *Brain* 1937; 60:389–443.

Perl ER, Whitlock DG. Somatic stimuli exciting spinothalamic projections to thalamic neurons in cat and monkey. *Exp Neurol* 1961; 3:256–296.

Ploner M, Schmitz F, Freund HJ, Schnitzler A. Parallel activation of primary and secondary somatosensory cortices in human pain processing. *J Neurophysiol* 1999; 81:3100–3104.

Pollin B, Albe-Fessard D. Organization of somatic thalamus in monkeys with and without section of dorsal spinal tracts. *Brain Res* 1979; 173:431–449.

Price DD, Dubner R. Neurons that subserve the sensory-discriminative aspects of pain. *Pain* 1977; 3:307–338.

Rainville P, Duncan GH, Price DD, Carrier B, Bushnell MC. Pain affect encoded in human anterior cingulate but not somatosensory cortex. *Science* 1997; 277:968–971.

Robinson CJ, Burton H. Organization of somatosensory receptive fields in cortical areas 7b, retroinsula, postauditory and granular insula of *M. fascicularis. J Comp Neurol* 1980a; 192:69–92.

Robinson CJ, Burton H. Somatic submodality distribution within the second somatosensory (SII), 7b, retroinsular, postauditory, and granular insular cortical areas in *M. fascicularis. J Comp Neurol* 1980b; 192:93–108.

Simone DA, Baumann TK, LaMotte RH. Dose-dependent pain and mechanical hyperalgesia in humans after intradermal injection of capsaicin. *Pain* 1989; 38:99–107.

Simone DA, Sorkin LS, Oh U, et al. Neurogenic hyperalgesia: central neural correlates in responses of spinothalamic tract neurons. *J Neurophysiol* 1991; 66:228–246.

Surmeier DJ, Honda CN, Willis WD. Responses of primate spinothalamic neurons to noxious thermal stimulation of glabrous and hairy skin. *J Neurophysiol* 1986a; 56:328–350.

Surmeier DJ, Honda CN, Willis WD. Temporal features of the response of primate spinotha-lamic neurons to noxious thermal stimulation of hairy and glabrous skin. *J Neurophysiol* 1986b; 56:351–369.

Surmeier DJ, Honda CN, Willis WD. Natural groupings of primate spinothalamic neurons based upon cutaneous stimulation. Physiological and anatomical features. *J Neurophysiol* 1988; 59:833–860.

Talbot JD, Marrett S, Evans AC, et al. Multiple representations of pain in human cerebral cortex. *Science* 1991; 251:1355–1358.

Treede RD, Kenshalo DR, Gracely RH, Jones AKP. The cortical representation of pain. *Pain* 1999; 79:105–111.

Treede RD, Apkarian AV, Bromm B, Greenspan JD, Lenz FA. Cortical representation of pain: functional characterization of nociceptive areas near the lateral sulcus. *Pain* 2000; 87:113–119.

Trevino DL, Coulter JD, Willis WD. Location of cells of origin of spinothalamic tract in lumbar enlargement of the monkey. *J Neurophysiol* 1973; 36:750–761.

Vogt BA, Sikes RW, Vogt LJ. Anterior cingulate cortex and the medial pain system. In: Vogt BA, Gabriel M (Eds). *Neurobiology of Cingulate Cortex and Limbic Thalamus: A Comprehensive Handbook.* Boston: Birkhäuser, 1993, pp 313–344.

Westlund KN, Carlton SM, Zhang D, Willis WD. Direct catecholaminergic innervation of primate spinothalamic tract neurons. *J Comp Neurol* 1990; 1299:178–186.

Westlund KN, Carlton SM, Zhang D, Willis WD. Glutamate-immunoreactive terminals synapse on primate spinothalamic tract cells. *J Comp Neurol* 1992; 322:519–527.

Willcockson WS, Chung JM, Hori Y, Lee KH, Willis WD. Effects of iontophoretically released amino acids and amines on primate spinothalamic tract cells. *J Neurosci* 1984a; 4:732–740.

Willcockson WS, Chung JM, Hori Y, Lee KH, Willis WD. Effects of iontophoretically released peptides on primate spinothalamic tract cells. *J Neurosci* 1984b; 4:741–750.

Willcockson WS, Kim J, Shin HK, Chung JM, Willis WD. Actions of opioids on primate spinothalamic tract neurons. *J Neurosci* 1986; 6:2509–2520.

Willis WD. Neural mechanisms of pain discrimination. In: *Sensory Processing in the Mammalian Brain.* Lund JS (Ed). New York: Oxford University Press, 1989, pp 130–143.

Willis WD. Long-term potentiation in spinothalamic neurons. *Brain Res Rev* 2002; 40:2202–2214.

Willis WD. Central sensitization of spinothalamic tract cells is a spinal cord form of long-term potentiation. In: Brune K, Handwerker H (Eds). *Hyperalgesia: Molecular Mechanisms and Clinical Implications,* Progress in Pain Research and Management, Vol. 30. Seattle: IASP Press, 2004, pp 181–199.

Willis WD, Coggeshall RE. *Sensory Mechanisms of the Spinal Cord,* 3rd ed. New York: Kluwer, 2004.

Willis WD, Trevino DL, Coulter JD, Maunz RA. Responses of primate spinothalamic tract neurons to natural stimulation of hindlimb. *J Neurophysiol* 1974; 37:358–372.

Willis WD, Kenshalo DR, Leonard RB. The cells of origin of the primate spinothalamic tract. *J Comp Neurol* 1979; 188:543–574.

Willis WD, Zhang X, Honda CN, Giesler GJ. Projections from the marginal zone and deep dorsal horn to the ventrobasal nuclei of the primate thalamus. *Pain* 2001; 92:267–276.

Willis WD, Zhang X, Honda CN, Giesler GJ. A critical review of the role of the proposed VMpo nucleus in pain. *J Pain* 2002; 3:79–94.

Zhang ET, Craig AD. Morphology and distribution of spinothalamic lamina I neurons in the monkey. *J Neurosci* 1997; 17:3274–3284.

Zhang D, Carlton SM, Sorkin LS, Willis WD. Collaterals of primate spinothalamic tract neurons to the periaqueductal gray. *J Comp Neurol* 1990; 296:277–290.

Zhang X, Wenk HN, Honda CN, Giesler GJ. Locations of spinothalamic tract axons in cervical and thoracic spinal cord white matter in monkeys. *J Neurophysiol* 2000a; 83:2869–2880.

Zhang X, Honda CN, Giesler GJ. Position of spinothalamic tract axons in upper cervical spinal cord of monkeys. *J Neurophysiol* 2000b; 84:1180–1185.

Correspondence to: William D. Willis, Jr., MD, PhD, Department of Neuroscience and Cell Biology, University of Texas Medical Branch, 301 University Boulevard, Galveston, TX 77555-1069, USA. Tel: 409-772-2103; Fax: 409-772-4687; email: wdwillis@utmb.edu.

The Pain System in Normal and Pathological States:
A Primer for Clinicians, Progress in Pain Research
and Management, Vol. 31, edited by Luis Villanueva,
Anthony Dickenson, and Hélène Ollat, IASP Press,
Seattle, © 2004.

10

Forebrain Responses in Normal and Pathological Pain States: Implications for Therapy

Kenneth L. Casey,[a,b,c] Thomas J. Morrow,[a,b,c]
and Jürgen Lorenz[d]

Department of [a]Neurology and [b]Molecular and Integrative Physiology,
University of Michigan, Ann Arbor, Michigan, USA; [c]Neurology Service,
Veterans Affairs Medical Center, Ann Arbor, Michigan, USA; [d]Center for
Experimental Medicine, Institute of Neurophysiology and Pathophysiology,
University Clinic Hamburg-Eppendorf, Hamburg, Germany

Normally, if a noxious stimulus produces tissue damage, there follows a period of inflammation and wound healing that leads to the elimination of pain. In pathological pain states, however, the noxious stimulus produces damage to non-neural or nervous tissue, and pain persists regardless of the state of wound healing. Extreme examples of this clinical condition include complex regional pain syndrome (CRPS) type II (formerly causalgia) and CRPS type I (formerly reflex sympathetic dystrophy) (Allen et al. 1999). Injury of central nervous tissue may also lead to persistent pain in the absence of damage to extraneural tissue (Boivie and Osterberg 1995; Bowsher 1996). In the fibromyalgia syndrome, research has yet to reveal a pathological process that causes the pain experienced by these patients; however, sensitivity to somatic stimuli is abnormally increased so that normally innocuous pressure or heat is perceived as painful (Wolfe et al. 1990; Geisser et al. 2003). A neurophysiological study has shown an abnormally increased response to brief, noxious stimulation with an infrared laser (Lorenz et al. 1996). A recent functional brain-imaging study revealed evidence for abnormal central processing of somatic pressure stimuli, but the cause of this abnormality is not known (Gracely et al. 2002). Indeed, we do not know why some patients are afflicted by these various pathological pain conditions while others are not. Evidence indicates that genetic factors are important determinants of susceptibility to these conditions, but the critical genes have not been identified and the link between the gene, the proteins, and the critical neuronal circuitry is far from being established (Mogil 1999).

Much research has focused on the pathological processes in the tissue, the peripheral nervous system, and the spinal cord dorsal horn that may be responsible for these persistent pain states. The underlying assumption is that treatment directed specifically at the early stages of nociceptive processing will reestablish the normal flow of ascending neuronal activity and that this input, in turn, will act upon a normally functioning forebrain that is the passive recipient of this information. However, ample evidence now shows that peripheral damage, neuronal or non-neuronal, leads to changes in the forebrain that may not only affect ascending processing, but also impair the initiation of descending sensory control mechanisms that modulate nociceptive activity. Because effective analgesic drugs act on both processes, pharmacotherapy may require a significant modification from what would be expected if forebrain mechanisms were fully intact and functioning normally.

These pathological pain states continue to present both a diagnostic and therapeutic challenge to clinicians. Throughout his long career, Professor Jean-Marie Besson and the group he has assembled over the years answered this challenge by conducting seminal neurophysiological and neuropharmacological research at all levels of the nervous system, from the peripheral nerve to the cerebral cortex (for an introduction to the scope of these investigations, see Besson et al. 1987, 1995; Besson and Chaouch 1987a,b,c). These investigations have opened lines of research that have revealed some of the basic mechanisms of nociception, endogenous modulation, and analgesic action that will continue to guide the further development of more effective treatments for pathological pain states.

ANIMAL STUDIES OF PAIN-RELATED FOREBRAIN PLASTICITY

Substantial evidence from animal studies shows that the forebrain undergoes major functional changes following injury to extraneural and to peripheral and central neural tissue (Kaas 1991; Jones and Pons 1998; Woods et al. 2000). However, these studies have focused on a limited set of thalamic and cortical structures that are known to mediate somatic sensation. To obtain a more comprehensive view of the forebrain changes associated with tissue injury, and to relate these changes to quantitative indices of pain in standard behavioral paradigms, we developed a method for functional imaging of the rat brain. The details of the method are described elsewhere and are shown diagrammatically in Fig. 1 (Morrow et al. 1998). We

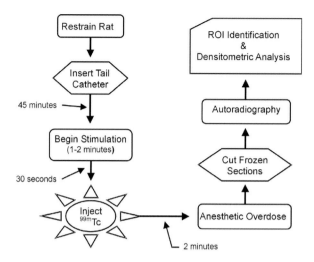

Fig. 1. Diagram of the regional cerebral blood flow (rCBF) functional brain-imaging method in the rat. Briefly, each rat is placed in a soft towel restraint, and a flexible intravenous catheter is inserted into the tail vein. The animals then rest quietly in the restraint for approximately 40 minutes to recover from the stress of catheterization. The radiotracer (10–15 mCi) is injected into the tail vein as a bolus over 10–15 seconds. Approximately 2 minutes after tracer injection, the rat is deeply anesthetized, removed from the restraint, and decapitated. The brain is removed from the skull and quick frozen using powered dry ice. Standard 20-μm coronal frozen sections are then cut at -18°C. Four consecutive coronal brain sections are taken at approximately 250-μm intervals and mounted on glass slides. Standard autoradiograms are generated by direct apposition of the mounted sections to the emulsion side of imaging film. When the radioactivity level of the slides returns to background, the slides are stained with cresyl violet. Precise structural identifications are made by comparing the autoradiograms and stained sections to coronal plates from a stereotactic atlas of the rat brain (Paxinos and Watson 1982). Densitometric analysis of autoradiograms is performed using a microcomputer-assisted video imaging densitometer. Each brain section on film is digitized to produce a high-resolution, 256-level grayscale image. Anatomical location of selected regions of interest (ROIs) is determined by overlaying transparent stereotactic atlas templates on digitized brain images displayed on the video monitor and by comparison with the cresyl violet-stained sections. The densitometer system converts sampled film optical densities to apparent tissue radioactivity concentrations (nCi/mg) by comparison with the optical densities of standards also imaged on each film. The average total brain activity is estimated by sampling all pixels in each brain section and averaging the activity across all sections for each animal. Activation index (AI) values are calculated for each sampled ROI as a percentage difference from the average total activity of the entire brain using the following formula: AI = (sampled ROI activity – [total brain activity])/(total brain activity) × 100%. Finally, the within-subject mean AIs for each sampled region are averaged across all subjects in an experimental group to compute within-group means for each ROI (Morrow et al. 1998).

measured normalized changes in regional cerebral blood flow (rCBF) by an autoradiographic method using the radiotracer ^{99m}Tc-exametazime. The method is analogous to human positron emission tomography (PET), except that the spatial resolution is at the histological level. In the first study using this method, we investigated neural mechanisms involved in the early and late phases of the formalin test. The results revealed the cortical, thalamic, and brainstem structures activated differentially during each phase of the test (Morrow et al. 1998). Specifically, noxious formalin consistently produced detectable, well-localized, and typically bilateral increases in rCBF within multiple forebrain structures and the midbrain periaqueductal gray. Structures showing pain-induced changes in rCBF included limbic and somatosensory forebrain regions. In addition, the spatial pattern and intensity of activation varied as a function of the time following the noxious formalin stimulus. These results highlighted the important role of the limbic forebrain in the neural mechanisms of prolonged pain in this rodent model (Morrow et al. 1998).

In subsequent investigations, we analyzed rat forebrain activity during more prolonged, ongoing neuropathic pain at various times following the chronic constriction injury (CCI) rodent model of this condition (Bennett and Xie 1988). Fig. 2 shows an example of the ongoing (resting) forebrain activity in the early stages of this condition in a sample from one rat (Paulson et al. 2000). Fig. 3 shows examples of the long-term changes in resting forebrain activity that follow a prolonged period of neuropathic injury and coincide with dynamic changes in pain behavior (Paulson et al. 2002). The long-term changes in basal forebrain activation following CCI were region-specific and could be divided into forebrain structures that showed either (1) no change, (2) an increase, or (3) a decrease in activity with respect to the changes that occur within the first two weeks. All rats showed spontaneous pain behaviors that persisted throughout the 12-week observation period, resembling the pattern of change found in the anterior dorsal thalamus, the habenular complex, and the cingulate and retrosplenial cortices. In contrast, heat hyperalgesia was delayed in onset until 4 weeks following CCI, but then persisted, showing a nearly constant level of increased responsiveness. This behavior coincides with increased activity in the somatosensory cortex, the hypothalamic paraventricular nucleus, and the basolateral amygdala (Fig. 3). The time course of mechanical allodynia, however, uniquely matches that of changes in ventrolateral and ventroposterolateral thalamic activity (Fig. 3).

These results show that peripheral nerve damage results in persistent changes in behavior and in resting forebrain systems that modulate pain perception. In particular, the persistent abnormalities in the somatosensory cortex and thalamus suggest that the sensory thalamocortical axis is functionally deranged in certain chronic pain states. These long-term alterations in forebrain activity almost certainly modify ascending nociceptive processing and the descending modulation that emanates from the forebrain. The effects of both centrally and peripherally acting analgesics are likely to be modified accordingly. Although these observations were made in a rodent model of chronic neuropathic pain, the evidence presented below suggests that similar changes in forebrain activity and response occur in humans.

HUMAN STUDIES OF PATHOLOGICAL PAIN STATES

Functional imaging and electrophysiological studies of humans have consistently revealed a group of interconnected brain and brainstem structures that are active following the application of acute experimental pain in healthy subjects (Casey 1999; Derbyshire 2000; Hudson 2000). Depending to some degree on the type of noxious stimulus applied and the gender of the subjects (Casey et al. 1996; Svensson et al. 1997; Paulson et al. 1998), these investigations have shown subcortical activation of the medial midbrain, cerebellum, thalamus, and putamen, with cortical responses seen in the insular, anterior cingulate, prefrontal, premotor, posterior parietal, and primary and secondary somatosensory cortices. Although the neurovascular

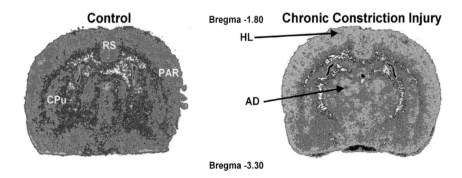

Fig. 2. Color-enhanced digitized brain images showing the pattern of regional cerebral blood flow (rCBF) in a control rat and a rat subjected to chronic constriction injury (CCI). Although each image represents only a single histological section from the brain of one rat, white and gray matter are clearly delineated and multiple brain regions are easily identified due to differences in rCBF. CCI produces bilateral increases in forebrain rCBF as compared to the control, even in the absence of stimulation. AD = anterior dorsal nucleus (thalamus); HL = hindlimb area of primary somatosensory cortex; PAR = secondary somatosensory region of parietal cortex; RS = retrosplenial cortex; CPu = caudate/putamen. Modified from Figs. 1 and 2 of Coghill and Morrow (2000), with permission.

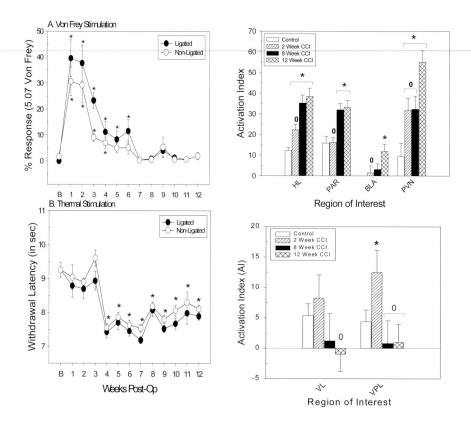

Fig. 3. *Left column*: The mean behavioral response made by animals to (A) mechanical and (B) thermal stimulation when tested before and after chronic constriction injury (CCI). The top panel (A) shows the average percentage of responses made by CCI animals to application of a 5.07-g von Frey hair. The percentage was calculated by dividing the number of foot withdrawals elicited by the von Frey hair by the maximum number of responses possible in that trial. The bottom panel (B) shows the average withdrawal latency to a radiant heat source. CCI produced mechanical allodynia and thermal hyperalgesia in both hindpaws. The asterisk (*) indicates a significant difference in the behavioral response compared to baseline values. *Right column, top*: The average bilateral level of activation in four ROIs (hindlimb [HL], parietal cortex [PAR], basolateral amygdala [BLA], and paraventricular nucleus [PVN]) for unstimulated control and unstimulated CCI groups, 2, 8, and 12 weeks after surgery. The relative levels of activation are expressed as activation index (AI, see Fig. 1 legend), the mean percentage difference from total brain activity. The asterisk (*) indicates a significant increase in activation compared to the control value. The zero (0) indicates a significant difference between the 2-week and the long-term CCI (8- or 12-week) animals. This progressive decrease in activation matches the progressive loss of tactile allodynia shown on the left. *Right column, bottom*: The average bilateral level of activation in the ventral lateral (VL) and ventral posterior lateral (VPL) thalamic nuclei for unstimulated control and unstimulated CCI groups, 2, 8, and 12 weeks after surgery (presentation as in top right panel). This delayed and increasing activation matches the onset and persistence of the heat allodynia shown on the left. Modified from Figs. 2, 4, and 5 (Paulson et al. 2002).

response that underlies these activations does not distinguish between excitatory and inhibitory activity, it is likely that the net effect of excitation dominates the cortical responses and that the "deactivation" detected in some investigations reflects a removal of excitatory inputs (Hudson 2000; Heeger et al. 2000). Functional imaging has moved rapidly beyond the descriptive stage to include investigations that link specific aspects of the forebrain response to critically important components of pain perception such as intensity discrimination (Coghill et al. 1999; Hofbauer et al. 2001) and the cognitive states that accompany pain (Rainville et al. 1997; Peyron et al. 2000b; Rainville 2002). Recent studies have begun to reveal the connectivity and dynamics of forebrain responses to painful stimuli (Casey et al. 2001; Coghill et al. 2001) and their modulation by both exogenous and endogenous analgesia. Both pharmacologically induced (Casey et al. 2000; Petrovic et al. 2002) and endogenous analgesia (Zubieta et al. 2001), including the placebo effect, initiate forebrain pain control mechanisms that act at subcortical, brainstem, and spinal levels (Tracey et al. 2002).

It is now apparent that the forebrain responses to noxious stimuli are altered in various ways during clinically pathological pain states (Peyron et al. 2000a,b; Derbyshire et al. 1994, 1999; Flor et al. 1995; Jones and Derbyshire 1997; Karl et al. 2001; Gracely et al 2002). It is not even necessary to inflict tissue damage to alter forebrain responses; the experimental induction of heat allodynia is sufficient. For example, we have recently shown that, during heat stimuli that are perceived as equally intense, heat allodynia produces a markedly different response pattern that engages the medial thalamus and the orbitofrontal cortex (Fig. 4) (Lorenz et al. 2002). During heat allodynia, there is a unique activation of the medial thalamus, the contralateral right ventral putamen, the dorsal midbrain, and limbic brain structures of both hemispheres such as the right anterior insula, the perigenual cingulate cortex, and the prefrontal and orbitofrontal cortices. These differences between heat allodynia and normal heat pain could not be attributed to differences in perceived intensity because much greater and more sustained differences in the perceived intensities of heat applied to either normal or sensitized skin did not produce significant differences in brain response (Lorenz et al. 2002).

By applying regression and principal components analysis to these results, we showed that heat allodynia is associated with the activation of a prefrontal cortical mechanism that appears to reduce pain affect by uncoupling functional connections between the medial midbrain and medial thalamus (Lorenz et al. 2003). Within a network of 17 distinct anatomical areas specifically activated during heat allodynia, only the bilateral dorsolateral prefrontal cortices (DLPFCs) were negatively correlated with perceived

L. LATERAL   **R. MEDIAL**   **HORIZ.**

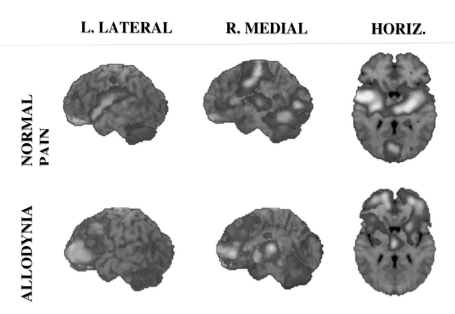

Fig. 4. *Top row* shows statistical brain maps of significant activations ($P < 0.05$; positron emission tomography) during normal heat pain. *Bottom row* shows the difference between normal heat pain and heat allodynia that is perceived as equally intense, revealing the structures uniquely activated during heat allodynia. These images depict the unique activation of the medial thalamus, prefrontal orbitofrontal cortex, and perigenual anterior cingulate cortex during heat allodynia. Modified from Fig. 5 of Lorenz et al. (2002).

intensity or unpleasantness. Right and left DLPFCs accounted for unique factors of the variance-covariance matrix across the repeated scans after capsaicin treatment. These factors were distinct from those that affected areas such as the medial thalamus, perigenual ACC, right ventral striatum, bilateral insulae, and ventral-orbitofrontal cortex, which correlated positively with pain intensity and unpleasantness. The correlation of activity between the midbrain and medial thalamus was significantly higher during scans with low compared to high activity in the left DLPFC. High correlation is thought to indicate high effective connectivity (Salinas and Sejnowski 2001). Although the direction of the modulating action cannot be determined by the regression analysis, our result may indicate a top-down mode of inhibition of neuronal coupling along the ascending midbrain-thalamic-cingulate pathway through descending fibers from the prefrontal cortex. This hypothesis is consistent with invasive studies in animals. For example, electrical stimulation of the prefrontal cortex in rats depressed the midbrain response to noxious stimuli (foot pinch) (Hardy and Haigler 1985), and in cats, electrical stimulation of the periaqueductal gray matter or the frontal (pericruciate) cortex suppressed the medial thalamic response to noxious stimuli (Andersen 1986).

CONCLUSION

The evidence cited here leaves little doubt that clinically relevant pain states modify central processing in a way that alters both the forebrain responses to ascending nociceptive information and the initiation of central control mechanisms that modulate the perception of pain. It is reasonable to expect that pathologically induced forebrain changes will alter the clinical response to drugs or any other form of treatment. Which of these forebrain changes assist or impede therapeutic efforts remains to be determined and presents another challenge to those who follow the path of research pioneered by Professor Jean-Marie Besson and his colleagues.

ACKNOWLEDGMENTS

Supported by the Department of Veteran's Affairs and U.S. Public Health Service NIH grants P01 HD33986 and R01 AR46045. Dr. Jürgen Lorenz was supported by a grant from the Max Kade Foundation.

REFERENCES

Allen G, Galer BS, Schwartz L. Epidemiology of complex regional pain syndrome: a retrospective chart review of 134 patients. *Pain* 1999; 80:539–544.

Andersen E. Periaqueductal gray and cerebral cortex modulate responses of medial thalamic neurons to noxious stimulation. *Brain Res* 1986; 375:30–36.

Bennett GJ, Xie YK. A peripheral mononeuropathy in rat that produces disorders of pain sensation like those seen in man. *Pain* 1988; 33:87–107.

Besson J-M, Chaouch A. Descending serotoninergic systems. In: Akil H, Lewis JW (Eds). *Neurotransmitters and Pain Control.* Karger: Basel, 1987a, pp 64–100.

Besson J-M, Chaouch A. Peripheral and spinal mechanisms of nociception. *Physiol Rev* 1987b; 67:67–184.

Besson J-M, Chaouch A. Descending Serotoninergic Systems. In: Akil H, Lewis JW (Eds). *Neurotransmitters and Pain Control.* Karger: Basel, 1987c, pp 64–100.

Besson J-M, Guilbaud G, Peschanski M. *Thalamus and Pain.* Amsterdam: Excerpta Medica, 1987.

Besson J-M, Guilbaud G, Ollat H. *Forebrain Areas Involved in Pain Processing.* Paris: John Libbey Eurotext, 1995, p 276.

Boivie J, Osterberg A. Central pain syndromes. In: Besson J-M, Guilbaud G, Ollat H (Eds). *Forebrain Areas Involved in Pain Processing.* Paris: John Libbey Eurotext, 1995, pp 239–251.

Bowsher D. Central pain: clinical and physiological characteristics. *J Neurol Neurosurg Psychiatry* 1996; 61:62–69.

Casey KL. Forebrain mechanisms of nociception and pain: analysis through imaging. *Proc Natl Acad Sci USA* 1999; 96:7668–7674.

Casey KL, Minoshima S, Morrow TJ, Koeppe RA. Comparison of human cerebral activation patterns during cutaneous warmth, heat pain, and deep cold pain. *J Neurophysiol* 1996; 76:571–581.

Casey KL, Svensson P, Morrow TJ, et al. Selective opiate modulation of nociceptive processing in the human brain. *J Neurophysiol* 2000; 84:525–533.

Casey KL, Morrow TJ, Lorenz J, Minoshima S. Temporal and spatial dynamics of human forebrain activity during heat pain: analysis by positron emission tomography. *J Neurophysiol* 2001; 85:951–959.

Coghill RC, Morrow TJ. Functional imaging of animal models of pain: high-resolution insights into nociceptive processing. In: Casey KL, Bushnell MC (Eds). *Pain Imaging,* Progress in Pain Research and Management, Vol. 18. Seattle: IASP Press, 2000, pp 211–239.

Coghill RC, Sang CN, Maisog JH, Iadarola MJ. Pain intensity processing within the human brain: a bilateral, distributed mechanism. *J Neurophysiol* 1999; 82:1934–1943.

Coghill RC, Gilron I, Iadarola MJ. Hemispheric lateralization of somatosensory processing. *J Neurophysiol* 2001; 85:2602–2612.

Derbyshire SW. Exploring the pain "neuromatrix." *Curr Rev Pain* 2000; 4:467–477.

Derbyshire SW, Jones AK, Devani P, et al. Cerebral responses to pain in patients with atypical facial pain measured by positron emission tomography. *J Neurol Neurosurg Psychiatry* 1994; 57:1166–1172.

Derbyshire SWG, Jones AKP, Collins M Feinmann C, Harris M. Cerebral responses to pain in patients suffering acute post-dental extraction pain measured by positron emission tomography (PET). *Eur J Pain* 1999; 3:103–113.

Flor H, Elbert T, Knecht S, et al. Phantom-limb pain as a perceptual correlate of cortical reorganization following arm amputation. *Nature* 1995; 375:482–484.

Geisser ME, Casey KL, Brucksch CB, et al. Perception of noxious and innocuous heat stimulation among healthy women and women with fibromyalgia: association with mood, somatic focus, and catastrophizing. *Pain* 2003; 102:243–250.

Gracely RH, Petzke F, Wolf JM, Clauw DJ. Functional magnetic resonance imaging evidence of augmented pain processing in fibromyalgia. *Arthritis Rheum* 2002; 46:1333–1343.

Hardy SGP, Haigler HJ. Prefrontal influences upon the midbrain: a possible route for pain modulation. *Brain Res* 1985; 339:285–294.

Heeger DJ, Huk AC, Geisler WS, Albrecht DG. Spikes versus BOLD: What does neuroimaging tell us about neuronal activity? *Nat Neurosci* 2000; 3:631–633.

Hofbauer RK, Rainville P, Duncan GH, Bushnell MC. Cortical representation of the sensory dimension of pain. *J Neurophysiol* 2001; 86:402–411.

Hudson AJ. Pain perception and response: central nervous system mechanisms. *Can J Neurol Sci* 2000; 27:2–16.

Jones AK, Derbyshire SW. Reduced cortical responses to noxious heat in patients with rheumatoid arthritis. *Ann Rheum Dis* 1997; 56:601–607.

Jones EG, Pons TP. Thalamic and brainstem contributions to large-scale plasticity of primate somatosensory cortex. *Science* 1998; 282:1121–1125.

Kaas JH. Plasticity of sensory and motor maps in adult mammals. *Annu Rev Neurosci* 1991; 14:137–167.

Karl A, Birbaumer N, Lutzenberger W, Cohen LG, Flor H. Reorganization of motor and somatosensory cortex in upper extremity amputees with phantom limb pain. *J Neurosci* 2001; 21:3609–3618.

Lorenz J, Grasedyck K, Bromm B. Middle and long latency somatosensory evoked potentials after painful laser stimulation in patients with fibromyalgia syndrome. *EEG Clin Neurophysiol* 1996; 100:65–168.

Lorenz J, Cross D, Minoshima S, et al. A unique representation of heat allodynia in the human brain. *Neuron* 2002; 35:383–393.

Lorenz J, Minoshima S, Casey KL. Keeping pain out of mind: the role of the dorsolateral prefrontal cortex in pain modulation. *Brain* 2003; 126:1079–1091.

Mogil JS. The genetic mediation of individual differences in sensitivity to pain and its inhibition. *Proc Natl Acad Sci USA* 1999; 96:7744–7751.

Morrow TJ, Paulson PE, Danneman PJ, Casey KL. Regional changes in forebrain activation during the early and late phase of formalin nociception: analysis using cerebral blood flow in the rat. *Pain* 1998; 75:355–365.

Paulson PE, Minoshima S, Morrow TJ, Casey KL. Gender differences in pain perception and patterns of cerebral activation during noxious heat stimulation in humans. *Pain* 1998; 76:223–229.

Paulson PE, Morrow TJ, Casey KL. Bilateral behavioral and regional cerebral blood flow changes during painful peripheral mononeuropathy in the rat. *Pain* 2000; 84:233–245.

Paulson PE, Casey KL, Morrow TJ. Long-term changes in behavior and regional cerebral blood flow associated with painful peripheral mononeuropathy in the rat. *Pain* 2002; 95:31–40.

Paxinos G, Watson C. *The Rat Brain in Stereotaxic Coordinates.* New York: Academic Press, 1982.

Petrovic P, Kalso E, Petersson KM, Ingvar M. Placebo and opioid analgesia—imaging a shared neuronal network. *Science* 2002; 295:1737–1740.

Peyron R, García-Larrea L, Grégoire MC, et al. Parietal and cingulate processes in central pain: a combined positron emission tomography (PET) and functional magnetic resonance imaging (fMRI) study of an unusual case. *Pain* 2000a; 84:77–87.

Peyron R, Laurent B, Garcia-Larrea L. Functional imaging of brain responses to pain: a review and meta-analysis. *Neurophysiol Clin* 2000b; 30:263–288.

Rainville P. Brain mechanisms of pain affect and pain modulation. *Curr Opin Neurobiol* 2002; 12:195–204.

Rainville P, Duncan GH, Price DD, Carrier M, Bushnell MC. Pain affect encoded in human anterior cingulate but not somatosensory cortex. *Science* 1997; 277:968–971.

Salinas E, Sejnowski TJ. Correlated neuronal activity and the flow of neural information. *Nat Rev Neurosci* 2001; 2:539–550.

Svensson P, Minoshima S, Beydoun A, Morrow TJ, Casey KL. Cerebral processing of acute skin and muscle pain in humans. *J Neurophysiol* 1997; 78:450–460.

Tracey I, Ploghaus A, Gati JS, et al. Imaging attentional modulation of pain in the periaqueductal gray in humans. *J Neurosci* 2002; 22:2748–2752.

Wolfe F, Smythe HA, Yunus MB, et al. The American College of Rheumatology 1990 Criteria for the Classification of Fibromyalgia. Report of the Multicenter Criteria Committee. *Arthritis Rheum* 1990; 33:160–172.

Woods TM, Cusick CG, Pons TP, Taub E, Jones EG. Progressive transneuronal changes in the brainstem and thalamus after long-term dorsal rhizotomies in adult macaque monkeys. *J Neurosci* 2000; 20:3884–3899.

Zubieta JK, Smith YR, Bueller JA, et al. Regional mu opioid receptor regulation of sensory and affective dimensions of pain. *Science* 2001; 293:311–315.

Correspondence to: Kenneth L. Casey, MD, Neurology Service, V.A. Medical Center, 2215 Fuller Road, Ann Arbor, MI 48105, USA. Voice mail: 734-769-7100 x5870; Fax: 734-769-7035; email: kencasey@umich.edu.

Part IV

Endogenous Modulatory Systems: Their Role in Analgesia and Pain

The Pain System in Normal and Pathological States: A Primer for Clinicians, Progress in Pain Research and Management, Vol. 31, edited by Luis Villanueva, Anthony Dickenson, and Hélène Ollat, IASP Press, Seattle, © 2004.

11

The Role of the Sympathetic Nervous System in Pain Processing

Ralf Baron[a] and Wilfrid Jänig[b]

[a]Neurological Clinic and [b]Department of Physiology, Christian Albrechts University, Kiel, Germany

Leriche (1916) was the first to report that sympathectomy dramatically relieves causalgia. Several large clinical series, primarily in wounded soldiers, supported this approach. Richards (1967) described the clinical features of causalgia and the effect of sympatholytic interventions in hundreds of cases and was emphatic about the dramatic response of causalgia to sympathetic blockade. He stated: "One of the outstanding surgical lessons that was learned during World War II was that interruption of the appropriate sympathetic nerve fibers is almost invariably effective in the treatment of causalgia. When the sympathetic chain is blocked by a local anesthetic, complete relief occurs almost immediately if the injection has been correctly placed, and the dramatic change in the patient's appearance and attitude is remarkable." The finding that sympatholysis relieves causalgic pain gave rise to the concept of sympathetically maintained pain (SMP).

Despite extensive clinical experience, controversy persists as to whether the sympathetic nervous system plays a role in generating pain (Schott 1994; Verdugo et al. 1994; Verdugo and Ochoa 1994). The pathophysiology of SMP has generated extensive speculation, but well-controlled clinical studies are lacking. This chapter summarizes both animal experiments and clinical observations that address the role of the sympathetic nervous system in neuropathic pain.

EVIDENCE FROM ANIMAL MODELS

BEHAVIORAL ANIMAL MODELS

Studies have used several rat behavioral models involving controlled nerve lesions to determine the contribution of the sympathetic nervous system to neuropathic pain. The interventions performed were surgical or chemical sympathectomy, systemic or local application of adrenoceptor blockers (e.g., phentolamine [α_1, α_2], prazosin [α_1], yohimbine [α_2]) or of adrenoceptor agonists (e.g., clonidine [α_2]), or intraperitoneal application of guanethidine (which is taken up by the noradrenergic terminals and depletes norepinephrine).

Partial lesion of the sciatic nerve. Partial ligation of one-third to one-half of the sciatic nerve leads to signs of spontaneous pain, thermal hyperalgesia, and mechanical allodynia and hyperalgesia (Seltzer et al. 1990). Chemical sympatholysis with intraperitoneal guanethidine prevented thermal hyperalgesia but had little effect on mechanical hyperalgesia (Shir and Seltzer 1991). When performed months after nerve lesion, sympatholysis by guanethidine alleviated all sensory disorders. Similarly, norepinephrine injected locally into the affected paw exacerbated mechanical and thermal hyperalgesic behavior, while the α_2-adrenoceptor antagonist yohimbine and chemical sympathectomy significantly relieved it (Tracey et al. 1995). However, surgical sympathectomy performed 1 week after partial sciatic nerve lesion did not have a significant effect on mechanical or cold allodynia or ongoing pain (Kim et al. 1997). The interpretation of these results depends heavily on the interpretation of the pharmacological interventions.

Chronic constriction injury of the sciatic nerve. Chronic constriction injury of the sciatic nerve generates mechanical and thermal hyperalgesic behavior (Bennett and Xie 1988). Both surgical sympathectomy and depletion of sympathetic transmitters by guanethidine reduce thermal hyperalgesia, but have little effect on mechanical hyperalgesia (Desmeules et al. 1995). Self-mutilating behavior and spontaneous pain behavior did not change after guanethidine injection or surgical sympathectomy, respectively. However, others (Kim et al. 1997) found only a slight (statistically nonsignificant) reduction of mechanical and cold allodynia after surgical sympathectomy.

Spinal nerve lesion. Ligation and transection of the L5 and L6 spinal nerves or only the L5 spinal nerve produces mechanical hyperalgesia and allodynia and thermal hyperalgesia (Kim and Chung 1992; Choi et al. 1994). These pain behaviors were permanently reversed by surgical lumbar sympathectomy, were prevented by surgical sympathectomy prior to spinal nerve lesion, and were temporarily reversed by intraperitoneal injection of phentolamine or guanethidine (Kim et al. 1993). These findings suggest that in this model a coupling between the somatic and sympathetic nervous system is critical not only for the development but also for the maintenance of the behavioral changes. However, rat strains and substrains seem to differ considerably in the development of signs of mechanical allodynia and heat hyperalgesia and in the dependence of mechanical allodynic behavior on adrenoceptors in animals with spinal nerve lesion (Yoon et al. 1999). For example, phentolamine injected intraperitoneally (≤ 2 mg/kg) temporarily abolished mechanical allodynic behavior developing after spinal nerve lesion in Lewis rats but had little or no effect in Fischer, Sprague-Dawley, and Wistar rats. Surgical sympathectomy abolished the mechanical allodynic behavior entirely in Sprague-Dawley rats with spinal nerve lesion (Kim et al. 1993). Another study could not be reproduce this latter result in Sprague-Dawley and Wistar rats despite testing with von Frey hairs of different strengths to measure frequency and threshold of paw withdrawal (Ringkamp et al. 1999).

REDUCED ANIMAL MODELS IN VIVO AND IN VITRO

After *complete nerve injury* in experimental animals, surviving cutaneous afferents may develop noradrenergic sensitivity (Fig. 1A). Myelinated and unmyelinated afferents innervating the stump neuroma can be excited by epinephrine or by stimulation of sympathetic efferents that have regenerated into the neuroma (Devor and Jänig 1981; Scadding 1981; Blumberg and Jänig 1984; Burchiel 1984). In mature neuromas, catecholamine sensitivity is much less pronounced (Blumberg and Jänig 1984; Jänig 1990). However, as late as 1 year after complete section and re-anastomosis of peripheral nerves, electrical stimulation of the sympathetic trunk remains capable of activating regenerated C fibers, probably with nociceptive function (Häbler et al. 1987).

Within 2 weeks of a *partial nerve lesion*, electrical stimulation of the sympathetic trunk and injections of catecholamines can activate or sensitize C nociceptors in the partially injured nerve, including those in continuity with their peripheral targets (Shyu et al. 1990; Sato and Perl 1991; O'Halloran and Perl 1997) (Fig. 1B). More recent in vitro neurophysiological studies, using a primate skin-nerve preparation, have demonstrated that uninjured cutaneous C-fiber nociceptors that innervate skin partially denervated by a spinal nerve ligation have a higher incidence of adrenergic sensitivity than do nociceptive afferents from normal skin (Ali et al. 1999). A recent study reported the development of a novel pattern of sympathetic fiber innervation of the skin after a peripheral nerve injury in the rat (Ruocco et al. 2000). Within a week after bilateral lesions of the mental nerve, fibers positive for

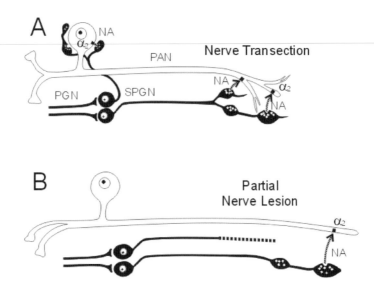

Fig. 1. Influence of sympathetic activity and catecholamines on primary afferent neurons (PAN). (A) Nerve transection. The sympathetic-afferent interaction is located in the neuroma and in the dorsal root ganglion. It is mediated by norepinephrine (NA) released from sympathetic postganglionic neurons (SPGN) and by α_2-adrenoreceptors expressed at the plasma membrane of afferent neurons. PGN, preganglionic neuron. (B) Partial nerve lesion. Partial nerve injury is followed by a decrease of the sympathetic innervation density (stippled sympathetic postganglionic neuron), which induces an upregulation of functional α_2-adrenoceptors at the membrane of intact afferent fibers.

dopamine-β-hydroxylase sprout into the upper dermis, a region usually devoid of such fibers. The migration and branching of these fibers occurred gradually, reaching a peak 4 weeks after the nerve lesion. Ectopic innervation of the superficial dermis by sympathetic fibers may play an important role in the interactions between the sympathetic and regenerating sensory fibers containing substance P.

In addition to the peripheral interaction, coupling of sympathetic and afferent neurons may also occur within the dorsal root ganglion (DRG, Fig. 1A). After a complete nerve lesion, some DRG somata with Aβ fibers and a few with C fibers develop ectopic activity. Electrical stimulation of sympathetic efferents innervating the DRG may lead to an α_2-adrenoceptor-mediated increase of this spontaneous activity (Devor et al. 1994; Chen et al. 1996; Michaelis et al. 1996). Morphological changes within the DRG parallel this increased adrenergic sensitivity (Fig. 1A). After the nerve lesion, sympathetic postganglionic fibers that normally innervate blood vessels within the DRG sprout to form basket-like terminals around large primary afferent somata that project into the injured nerve (McLachlan et al. 1993; Chung et al. 1996, 1997). However, the relationship of this DRG sprouting to pain is uncertain. Sprouting of sympathetic postganglionic terminals largely occurs around the somata of larger, presumably non-nociceptive primary afferents (McLachlan et al. 1993). In the first 20 days after sciatic nerve lesion in the rat, sympathetic stimulation preferentially activates afferent neurons; later, depression of afferent activity predominates. Nevertheless, in the same nerve lesion model, catecholaminergic baskets form around DRG cells after 30 days (Jänig et al. 1996).

Norepinephrine-induced Ca^{2+} influx increased after acute infection of cultured DRG neurons with human varicella-zoster virus, indicating adrenergic sensitivity of these neurons. Interestingly, only infected somata demonstrated these pathological responses. These results may explain that not only mechanical lesion, but also viral infection, may lead to phenotypic changes of afferent neurons (Kress and Fickenscher 2001).

ADRENOCEPTORS INVOLVED IN SYMPATHETIC-AFFERENT COUPLING

The excitation and depression of axotomized DRG cells and the excitation of afferent terminals in neuromas generated by activation of the sympathetic innervation may be mediated by α-adrenoceptors. Any hypothesis about this chemical norepinephrine-mediated coupling between sympathetic and afferent neurons needs to explain how functional adrenoceptors appear on the surface of nociceptive and other afferent neurons as a consequence of a nerve lesion or infection. The cellular mechanisms underlying the increased sensitivity are unknown. An obvious explanation is the novel expression or upregulation of adrenoceptors. Alternatively, the receptors may normally be present on primary nociceptive afferents but not be functional; they may become uncovered and effective during the response to damage or infection. This explanation is consistent with the finding that adrenoceptor mRNA is a normal constituent of DRG cells (Nicholas et al. 1993; Pieribone et al. 1994). The affinity for ligands or the effectiveness of the subsequent cellular transduction may change in injured nociceptive and non-nociceptive afferent neurons. These possibilities are not mutually exclusive, and it is possible that several mechanisms contribute simultaneously to the expression of sympathetically mediated afferent excitation.

Perl and coworkers (Sato and Perl 1991; Perl 1994) suggest, based on their experiments on polymodal nociceptors following partial nerve lesion, that the expression or upregulation of adrenoceptors in primary afferent neurons is related to the sympathetic denervation of the target tissue, analogous to the development of the denervation supersensitivity that is observed in effector tissues following their denervation (Fleming and Westfall 1988). This idea is supported by the observation that cutaneous nociceptive C fibers in the rabbit ear may develop adrenoceptor sensitivity following surgical sympathectomy (Bossut et al. 1996). However, close-arterial injection of norepinephrine excites only a small percentage of afferents, generating few impulses.

Knowledge about the subtypes of α-adrenoreceptor involved in the sympathetic-afferent coupling following nerve trauma is important for understanding the underlying neural mechanisms and may be useful in the design of more specific treatment modalities for neuropathic pain conditions involving sympathetic efferent activity. Excitation and sensitization of polymodal nociceptors in the rabbit ear skin generated by electrical stimulation of the sympathetic supply, or by norepinephrine after partial lesion of the auricular nerve, are largely mediated by α_2-adrenoceptors (Sato and Perl 1991). Investigation of sympathetic-sensory coupling at the site of experimental nerve injury in neuromas and at the cell bodies of axotomized afferent neurons using type-selective agonists and antagonists has shown that this transmission is also largely mediated by α_2-adrenoreceptors (Chen et al. 1996). Recordings from primate cutaneous C-fiber nociceptors after an L6 spinal nerve ligation, however, showed a significantly higher incidence of response to both the selective α_1- and α_2-adrenergic agonists, phenylephrine and brimonidine, respectively (Ali et al. 1999). Normal (uninjured) DRG neurons have mRNAs for α_{2A}- and particularly α_{2B}-adrenoceptors, whereas mRNA for α_1-adrenoceptors is either absent or scarce (Pieribone et al. 1994). mRNA for α_{2A}-adrenoceptors is clearly upregulated in DRG neurons after nerve lesion (Shi et al. 2000). Furthermore, immunohistochemistry with polyclonal antibodies supports the upregulation of α_{2A}-receptors after partial nerve lesion in 15–20% of mainly large afferent neurons. Importantly, both injured and uninjured neurons showed this phenotypic switch (Birder and Perl 1999).

However, caution is required in generalizing from these results. These changes only lasted for up to 72 days, an indication that this noradrenergic sensitivity is unlikely to be relevant for chronic changes occurring in patients. Moreover, these results were obtained in rats. Species may differ in the expression of adrenoceptors following trauma.

In conclusion, the behavioral and reduced animal models, in vivo and in vitro, show that sympathetic-afferent coupling can occur under pathophysiological conditions, involving expression of functional adrenoceptors by the lesioned or infected afferent neurons and plastic changes of both sympathetic and afferent neurons. However, the data from these models are inconsistent with observations of SMP in patients. The experimental interventions used in the animal models to date (e.g., frequency of stimulation of sympathetic neurons, concentrations of applied adrenoceptor agonists) seem out of proportion to what occurs under normal conditions. Therefore, the experimental data must be considered with utmost care.

CLINICAL DATA FROM SYMPATHOLYTIC INTERVENTIONS

The important question for clinical practice is whether findings in the animal models are also valid in patients. As mentioned above, long-standing but nonquantitative clinical observations indicate that interruption of the efferent sympathetic nerve supply can relieve pain in several neuropathic pain states including complex regional pain syndromes (CRPS types I and II), acute herpetic neuralgia, and phantom limb pain. However, this effect only occurs in a subgroup of patients. Neuropathic pain patients with similar clinical signs and symptoms can be divided into two groups based on their response to selective sympathetic blockade or antagonism of α-adrenoceptor mechanisms (Arnér 1991; Raja et al. 1991). The pain component that is relieved by specific sympatholytic procedures is considered sympathetically maintained pain. SMP is a general term that includes spontaneous pain and evoked pains (by mechanical and thermal stimuli). Thus, SMP is now defined as a symptom and not a clinical entity. The positive effect of a sympathetic blockade is not essential for the diagnosis of the clinical entity, e.g., CRPS. However, the only way to differentiate between SMP and sympathetically independent pain (SIP) is the efficacy of a correctly applied sympatholytic intervention (Stanton-Hicks et al. 1995).

Two therapeutic techniques are used to block sympathetic activity: (1) injections of a local anesthetic around sympathetic paravertebral ganglia that project to the affected body part (sympathetic ganglion blocks), and (2) regional intravenous (i.v.) application of guanethidine, bretylium, or reserpine (which all deplete norepinephrine in the postganglionic axon) to an isolated extremity blocked with a tourniquet (intravenous regional sympatholysis, IVRS).

Many uncontrolled surveys in the literature review the effect of sympathetic interventions in CRPS. About 70% of patients with CRPS types I and II report a full or partial response (Cepeda et al. 2002). The efficacy of these procedures is, however, a topic of continuing controversy (Schott 1989, 1994, 1998; Verdugo et al. 1994; Verdugo and Ochoa 1994; Kingery 1997; Ochoa 1999). In fact, the specificity, the long-term results, and the techniques used have rarely been adequately evaluated.

One controlled study in patients with CRPS-I has shown that sympathetic ganglion blocks with local anesthetic have the same immediate effect on pain as a control injection with saline (Price et al. 1998). However, after 24 hours patients in the local anesthetic group were much better, indicating that nonspecific effects are important initially and that evaluating the efficacy of sympatholytic interventions is best done after 24 hours. We must keep these data in mind and cautiously interpret the uncontrolled studies mentioned above. Only few studies assessed long-term effects. The results of studies using IVRS with reserpine, guanethidine, or bretylium are still inconsistent. Most studies, however, show negative results (Hord and Oaklander 2003).

A problem inherent in the evaluation of sympatholytic procedures is the high potential for false-negative results. Several factors could contribute to this problem: (1) A technically inadequate blockade of sympathetic activity may be due either to anatomical maldistribution or inadequate concentration of drug at the site of action. (2) The sympathetic chain may have anatomical variability. (3) Neurons as far caudal as T2 that contribute to the upper limb innervation may escape the stellate ganglion block. (4) A proximal sympathetic-afferent interaction (e.g., in the DRG) may escape IVRS.

It is not possible to completely rule out false-negative results, and thus the percentage of patients that could benefit from sympatholytic interventions may be underestimated. Even the careful monitoring of Horner's syndrome and cutaneous vasodilatation during a sympathetic block does not ensure the block of sympathetic innervation of deep tissues, the DRG, or both.

In conclusion, we urgently need controlled studies that assess both the acute and long-term effects of sympathetic blockade and IVRS on pain and other CRPS symptoms, in particular motor function. Studies should use well-performed sympathetic ganglion blocks rather than IVRS (Hord and Oaklander 2003).

EXPERIMENTAL DATA FROM HUMAN PAIN MODELS AND NEUROPATHIC PAIN PATIENTS

INFLUENCE OF SYMPATHETIC ACTIVITY AND CATECHOLAMINES ON INTACT PRIMARY AFFERENTS AFTER TISSUE INFLAMMATION

Cutaneous application of the algogenic agent capsaicin causes neurogenic inflammation by activating and sensitizing nociceptors. Use of this model in human subjects revealed an adrenergic effect on sensitized cutaneous nociceptors. Iontophoresis of norepinephrine enhanced the heat hyperalgesia that develops after topical application of capsaicin to the skin of human volunteers (Drummond 1995). Phentolamine, a mixed α_1- and α_2-antagonist, inhibited the norepinephrine-induced pain and mechanical hyperalgesia in capsaicin-sensitized skin (Liu et al. 1996; Kinnman et al. 1997). However, iontophoresis of the nonadrenergic vasoconstrictors, angiotensin II and vasopressin (Drummond 1998), and occlusion of blood flow (Drummond et al. 1996) mildly enhanced hyperalgesia in capsaicin-treated skin. This response suggests that changes in blood flow may account for some aspects of the enhanced cutaneous sensibility seen in capsaicin-induced hyperalgesia.

When sympathetic cutaneous vasoconstrictor activity was modulated in physiological ranges by thermoregulatory stress, it did not measurably influence capsaicin-induced pain (Baron et al. 1999). Accordingly, activation of sympathetic vasoconstrictor neurons in the skin does not change the irritant-induced discharge of single cutaneous C nociceptors recorded by microneurography (Elam et al. 1996).

One controlled study has evaluated the effect of sympathetic blockade on pain after experimental tissue inflammation. Pedersen et al. (1997) used a cutaneous heat injury pain model to show that sympathetic blocks with bupivacaine did not alter spontaneous pain or heat hyperalgesia (Raja 1995). In patients with rheumatoid arthritis, however, regional i.v. guanethidine decreased pain and increased pinch strength (Levine et al. 1986).

INFLUENCE OF SYMPATHETIC ACTIVITY AND CATECHOLAMINES ON PRIMARY AFFERENTS IN NEUROPATHIC PAIN STATES

Amputation pain. Long after limb amputation, patients report that injection of epinephrine around a stump neuroma is intensely painful (Chabal et al. 1992). Recent studies also demonstrate that the perineuromal administration of physiological doses of norepinephrine induces more pain than do saline injections (Raja et al. 1998).

Postherpetic neuralgia. In some patients with postherpetic neuralgia, injection of epinephrine or phenylephrine enhances spontaneous pain and mechanical hyperalgesia (Choi and Rowbotham 1997).

Polyneuropathy. In patients with painful and nonpainful polyneuropathy of different origins, we quantified spontaneous pain and measured warm and heat pain thresholds on the dorsum of the foot before and after iontophoresis of norepinephrine and saline. The groups with polyneuropathy and the controls showed no differences in the decrease in heat-pain thresholds. Pain perception did not change. Thus, in human polyneuropathy, adrenergic mechanisms are obviously not involved in the generation of pain (Schattschneider and Baron, unpublished data).

Post-traumatic neuralgia and complex regional pain syndrome type II. CRPS-II (causalgia) is characterized by a demonstrable lesion of a peripheral nerve. It is thus by definition a neuropathic disorder. Intraoperative stimulation of the sympathetic chain induces an increase of spontaneous pain in patients with CRPS-II but not in patients with hyperhidrosis (White and Sweet 1969). In addition, i.v. phentolamine, but not propranolol, relieves pain in CRPS-II patients (Arnér 1991; Raja et al. 1991). In these patients, pain relief following a local anesthetic sympathetic ganglion block and pain relief following a phentolamine infusion were correlated.

In CRPS-II and post-traumatic neuralgias, intracutaneous application of norepinephrine into a symptomatic area rekindles spontaneous pain and dynamic mechanical hyperalgesia that had been relieved by sympathetic blockade, supporting the idea that noradrenergic sensitivity of human nociceptors occurs after partial nerve lesion (Torebjörk et al. 1995).

A potential criticism of the above-mentioned studies is that they rekindled plain by using much higher doses of norepinephrine than are likely to occur physiologically. Another study thus compared the algesic effects of peripheral administration of physiologically relevant doses of norepinephrine in patients with SMP and normal subjects (Ali et al. 2000). Pain evoked by intradermal norepinephrine was greater in the affected limbs of patients with SMP than in the contralateral unaffected limb, and greater than in control subjects. Moreover, most patients who had increased pain in the affected extremity after injection of norepinephrine also reported decreased pain after systemic administration of phentolamine.

Topical application of the α_2-adrenoceptor agonist clonidine relieves hyperalgesia at the site of application in patients with SMP but not in those with SIP (Davis et al. 1991). This effect was considered secondary to a reduction in the release of norepinephrine via activation of the α_2-adrenergic autoreceptor on the sympathetic terminal. Injection of norepinephrine and the α_1-adrenoceptor agonist phenylephrine into the clonidine-treated area produced marked pain and hyperalgesia.

In further support of this concept, quantitative autoradiographic studies indicate that the number of α_1-adrenoceptors in hyperalgesic skin of patients with SMP is significantly greater than in the skin of normal subjects (Drummond et al. 1996). Finally, an increase in venous α-adrenoceptor responsiveness has been observed in patients with CRPS-I (Arnold et al. 1993).

Complex regional pain syndrome type I. Per definition, no CRPS-I patients have a demonstrable nerve lesion. It is questionable whether CRPS-I is a neuropathic disorder and, especially in the acute stage, whether its mechanisms differ from those operating in syndromes associated with nerve lesions.

In patients with CRPS-I with identified SMP, spontaneous pain and mechanical hyperalgesia are augmented when sympathetic cutaneous vaso-constrictor neurons are activated physiologically by cold stress (Baron et al. 2002) (Fig. 2). In these patients, sympathetic blocks with a local anesthetic (leading to an increase of the skin temperature of the hand to ≥ 35°C) significantly decreased spontaneous pain and mechanical allodynia; thus, pain relief during sympathetic blocks and augmentation of pain during ther-moregulatory cold stress showed a high correlation. Patients with CRPS-I who had SIP served as controls. In these patients, thermoregulatory cold stress did not augment spontaneous pain or mechanical allodynia, nor was either symptom relieved after sympathetic blocks. This experiment in CRPS patients does not indicate whether direct or indirect coupling between sym-pathetic and afferent fibers evokes the SMP.

The experimental setup used in the above study selectively alters sym-pathetic cutaneous vasoconstrictor activity without influencing other sympa-thetic systems innervating the extremities, i.e., piloerector, sudomotor, and muscle vasoconstrictor neurons. The interaction of sympathetic and afferent neurons measured here is thus likely to be located within the skin, as pre-dicted by the pain-enhancing effect of intracutaneous norepinephrine injec-tions (Torebjörk et al. 1995; Ali et al. 2000). Interestingly, the relief of spontaneous pain after sympathetic blockade was more pronounced than changes in spontaneous pain that could be induced experimentally by sym-pathetic activation. One explanation for this discrepancy might be that a complete sympathetic block affects all sympathetic outflow channels pro-jecting to the affected extremity. It is likely that in addition to a coupling in the skin, a sympathetic-afferent interaction may also occur in other tissues, in particular in the deep somatic domain such as bone, muscle, or joints. These structures are extremely painful in some patients with CRPS (Baron and Wasner 2001). Furthermore, some patients may have a selective or predominant sympathetic-afferent interaction in deep somatic tissues with sparing of the skin (Wasner et al. 1999).

As mentioned above, CRPS-I patients have no overt nerve lesion. It is thus likely that different mechanisms may be involved in SMP in these patients. One possible explanation is that sympathetic activity influences the acute inflammatory component of this disorder. Studies have repeatedly suggested an inflammatory processes in the affected extremity, in particular in the deep somatic tissues, including bones (Birklein et al. 2000). Fig. 3 illustrates the possible interactions between sympathetic fibers, afferent fi-bers, blood vessels, and non-neural cells related to the immune system (e.g., macrophages) leading theoretically to the inflammatory changes observed in CRPS-I patients (Jänig and Baron 2003).

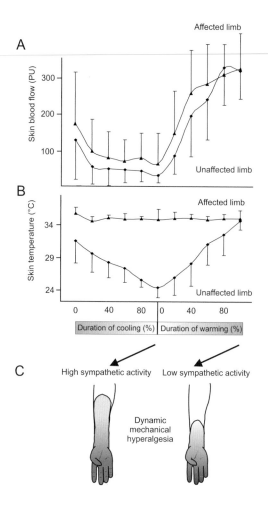

Fig. 2. Experimental modulation of cutaneous sympathetic vasoconstrictor neurons by the physiological thermoregulatory reflex stimuli in 13 CRPS patients. Whole-body cooling and warming altered sympathetic skin nerve activity. The subjects lay in a thermal suit supplied by tubes that delivered running water of 12°C and 50°C (inflow temperature) to cool or warm the whole body so as to switch sympathetic activity on and off. (A) High sympathetic vasoconstrictor activity during cooling induces a considerable drop in skin blood flow in both the affected and unaffected extremity (laser-Doppler flowmetry). Measurements were taken at 5-minute intervals (mean + SD). (B) A secondary decrease of skin temperature was documented on the unaffected side. On the affected side the forearm temperature was clamped at 35°C by a feedback-controlled heat lamp to exclude temperature effects on the sensory receptor level. Measurements were taken at 5-minute intervals (mean + SD). (C). Effect of cutaneous sympathetic vasoconstrictor activity on dynamic mechanical hyperalgesia in one CRPS patient with sympathetically maintained pain (SMP). Activation of sympathetic neurons (during cooling) leads to a considerable increase of the area of dynamic mechanical hyperalgesia. From Baron et al. (2002), with permission.

INTERPRETATION OF THE CLINICAL AND EXPERIMENTAL DATA OBTAINED IN HUMANS

Although these studies of human patients are the basis for the belief that the sympathetic nervous system is involved in the generation of pain, they do not reveal which mechanisms are involved. Several conclusions can be drawn from these clinical observation. (1) Primary afferent nociceptors are excited and possibly sensitized by norepinephrine released by the sympathetic fibers. (2) Either the primary afferent nociceptive neurons have expressed adrenoceptors, or their increased excitability is generated indirectly, via the vascular bed (e.g., change of blood flow) or other components. For example, inflammatory cells in the environment of the nociceptive neurons may have a permissive effect on sympathetic to nociceptor coupling or are modulated directly by molecules released from sympathetic postganglionic neurons. (3) Sympathetically maintained spontaneous and evoked activity in

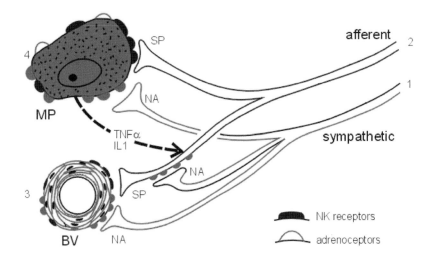

Fig. 3. Hypothetical interaction of sympathetic noradrenergic nerve fibers (1), peptidergic afferent nerve fibers (2), blood vessels (BV, 3), and macrophages (MP, 4). The activated and sensitized afferent nerve fibers activate macrophages (via substance P release). The immune cells start to release cytokines, such as tumor necrosis factor α (TNF-α) and interleukin 1 (IL1), which further activate afferent fibers by enhancing sodium influx into the cells. Substance P (SP) (and CGRP) released from the afferent nerve fibers reacts with neurokinin 1 (NK1) receptors in the blood vessels (arteriolar vasodilation, venular plasma extravasation; neurogenic inflammation). The sympathetic nerve fibers interact with this system on three levels: (1) via adrenoceptors (mainly alpha) on the blood vessels (vasoconstriction); (2) via adrenoceptors (mainly beta) on macrophages (further release of cytokines), and (3) via adrenoceptors (mainly alpha) on afferents (further sensitization of these fibers). From Jänig and Baron (2003), with permission.

nociceptive neurons may generate a state of central sensitization/hyperexcitability, e.g., of dorsal horn neurons. (4) Central sensitization leads to spontaneous pain and pain evoked by stimulation of mechanoreceptors, thermoreceptors, or nociceptors (mechanical and thermal allodynias and hyperalgesias). The most important question, however, is still unsolved: Which factors determine adrenergic sensitivity in different human neuropathies?

As shown above, human peripheral painful neuropathies differ considerably in the development of adrenergic sensitivity, although all peripheral neuropathies involve lesions of peripheral nerves. Furthermore, only a subgroup of patients with an identical disorder (e.g., CRPS-I) develop noradrenergic sensitivity. Some disorders involve a peripheral nerve lesion that never develops adrenergic sensitivity (e.g., polyneuropathies). Thus, additional factors other than nerve damage per se must be responsible for adrenergic sensitivity and SMP.

First, the etiology of the lesion might determine the expression of adrenergic receptors on afferent neurons. For example, evidence is sufficient that virus infection triggers adrenoreceptor expression on afferent neurons. This particular mechanism might be responsible for the catecholamine response in patients with zoster-associated pain (Choi and Rowbotham 1997).

Second, the type and severity of nerve lesion might be important. Phantom limb pain is characterized by an entire severance of all nerves supplying one extremity, whereas no major nerve lesion is demonstrable in CRPS-I. These differences may be responsible for the different mechanisms of adrenergic sensitivity.

One feature of most polyneuropathies that is distinct from the aforementioned norepinephrine-sensitive syndromes is a chronic underlying disease, such as diabetes mellitus or alcoholism. This chronic process leads to neuronal degeneration and regeneration occurring in parallel, a phenomenon that might account for a decline of norepinephrine sensitivity.

Third, evidence suggests that acute CRPS and acute mechanical nerve lesions are associated with a profound inflammatory reaction (Birklein et al. 2001). Acute inflammation leads to nociceptor sensitization with an enhanced response to adrenergic substances (Nakamura and Ferreira 1987; Hu and Zhu 1989). This adrenergic component induced by inflammatory reactions is thought to be time dependent. Accordingly, clinical data show that a subgroup of patients with acute CRPS (SMP patients) responds well to sympathetic blocks, but the effect diminishes over time (Torebjörk et al. 1995). A decline of the inflammatory component over the course of the disease (Birklein et al. 2001) may be followed by a reduction of the SMP component. Thus, it is possible that patients with long-standing painful neuropathy lose the SMP component over time.

Finally, we have learned from animal models that different rat strains with spinal nerve lesions appear to differ considerably in the occurrence of sympathetically maintained allodynic behavior. These results point to genetic differences and predispositions that might determine the expression of adrenoreceptors on afferent neurons in human neuropathies.

In summary, it seems obvious from animal and human research that afferent neurons may develop adrenergic sensitivity after trauma, infection, or inflammation. The efferent sympathetic nervous system is thus involved in pain processing. Further research is needed to establish the exact mechanisms of afferent adrenergic sensitivity in human neuropathies of different etiologies and in particular the time course during the disease process and the genetic predisposition for the development of adrenergic sensitivity.

ACKNOWLEDGMENT

The work was supported by the German Research Foundation (Deutsche Forschungsgemeinschaft) (Ba 1921/1-3) and by the Bundesministerium für Bildung und Forschung (German Research Network on Neuropathic Pain [BMBF, 01EM01/04]). There is no financial or other relationship that might lead to a conflict of interest.

REFERENCES

Ali Z, Ringkamp M, Hartke TV, et al. Uninjured C-fiber nociceptors develop spontaneous activity and alpha-adrenergic sensitivity following L6 spinal nerve ligation in monkey. *J Neurophysiol* 1999; 81:455–466.

Ali Z, Raja SN, Wesselmann U, et al. Intradermal injection of norepinephrine evokes pain in patients with sympathetically maintained pain. *Pain* 2000; 88:161–168.

Arnér S. Intravenous phentolamine test: diagnostic and prognostic use in reflex sympathetic dystrophy. *Pain* 1991; 46:17–22.

Arnold JM, Teasell RW, MacLeod AP, et al. Increased venous alpha-adrenoceptor responsiveness in patients with reflex sympathetic dystrophy. *Ann Intern Med* 1993; 118:619–621.

Baron R, Wasner G. Complex regional pain syndromes. *Curr Pain Headache Rep* 2001; 5:114–123.

Baron R, Wasner GL, Borgstedt R, et al. Effect of sympathetic activity on capsaicin evoked spontaneous pain, hyperalgesia and vasodilatation. *Neurology* 1999; 52:923–932.

Baron R, Schattschneider J, Binder A, et al. Relation between sympathetic vasoconstrictor activity and pain and hyperalgesia in complex regional pain syndromes: a case-control study. *Lancet* 2002; 359:1655–1660.

Bennett GJ, Xie YK. A peripheral mononeuropathy in rat that produces disorders of pain sensation like those seen in man. *Pain* 1988; 33:87–107.

Birklein F, Weber M, Neundorfer B. Increased skin lactate in complex regional pain syndrome: evidence for tissue hypoxia? *Neurology* 2000; 55:1213–1215.

Birklein F, Schmelz M, Schifter S, Weber M. The important role of neuropeptides in complex regional pain syndrome. *Neurology* 2001; 57:2179–2184.

Birder LA, Perl ER. Expression of alpha-2-adrenergic receptors in rat primary afferent neurones after peripheral nerve injury or inflammation. *J Physiol* 1999; 515:533–542.

Blumberg H, Jänig W. Discharge pattern of afferent fibers from a neuroma. *Pain* 1984; 20:335–353.

Bossut DF, Shea VK, Perl ER. Sympathectomy induces adrenergic excitability of cutaneous C-fiber nociceptors. *J Neurophysiol* 1996; 75:514–517.

Burchiel KJ. Spontaneous impulse generation in normal and denervated dorsal root ganglia: sensitivity to alpha-adrenergic stimulation and hypoxia. *Exp Neurol* 1984; 85:257–272.

Cepeda MS, Lau J, Carr DB. Defining the therapeutic role of local anesthetic sympathetic blockade in complex regional pain syndrome: a narrative and systematic review. *Clin J Pain* 2002; 18:216–233.

Chabal C, Jacobson L, Russell LC, Burchiel KJ. Pain response to perineuromal injection of normal saline, epinephrine, and lidocaine in humans. *Pain* 1992; 49:9–12.

Chen Y, Michaelis M, Jänig W, Devor M. Adrenoreceptor subtype mediating sympathetic-sensory coupling in injured sensory neurons. *J Neurophysiol* 1996; 76:3721–3730.

Choi B, Rowbotham MC. Effect of adrenergic receptor activation on post-herpetic neuralgia pain and sensory disturbances. *Pain* 1997; 69:55–63.

Choi Y, Yoon YW, Na HS, et al. Behavioral signs of ongoing pain and cold allodynia in a rat model of neuropathic pain. *Pain* 1994; 59:369–376.

Chung K, Lee BH, Yoon YW, Chung JM. Sympathetic sprouting in the dorsal root ganglia of the injured peripheral nerve in a rat neuropathic pain model. *J Comp Neurol* 1996; 376:241–252.

Chung K, Yoon YW, Chung JM. Sprouting sympathetic fibers form synaptic varicosities in the dorsal root ganglion of the rat with neuropathic injury. *Brain Res* 1997; 751:275–280.

Davis KD, Treede RD, Raja SN, et al. Topical application of clonidine relieves hyperalgesia in patients with sympathetically maintained pain. *Pain* 1991; 47:309–317.

Desmeules JA, Kayser V, Weil-Fuggaza J, et al. Influence of the sympathetic nervous system in the development of abnormal pain-related behaviours in a rat model of neuropathic pain. *Neuroscience* 1995; 67:941–951.

Devor M, Jänig W. Activation of myelinated afferents ending in a neuroma by stimulation of the sympathetic supply in the rat. *Neurosci Lett* 1981; 24:43–47.

Devor M, Jänig W, Michaelis M. Modulation of activity in dorsal root ganglion neurons by sympathetic activation in nerve-injured rats. *J Neurophysiol* 1994; 71:38–47.

Drummond PD. Noradrenaline increases hyperalgesia to heat in skin sensitized by capsaicin. *Pain* 1995; 60:311–315.

Drummond PD. The effect of noradrenaline, angiotensin II and vasopressin on blood flow and sensitivity to heat in capsaicin-treated skin. *Clin Auton Res* 1998; 8:87–93.

Drummond PD, Skipworth S, Finch PM. Alpha 1-adrenoceptors in normal and hyperalgesic human skin. *Clin Sci (Colch)* 1996; 91:73–77.

Elam M, Skarphedinsson JO, Olhausson B, Wallin BG. No apparent sympathetic modulation of single C-fiber afferent transmission in human volunteers. In: *Abstracts: 8th World Congress on Pain.* Seattle: IASP Press, 1996, p 398.

Fleming WW, Westfall DP. Adaptive supersensitivity. In: Trendelenburg U, Weiner N (Eds). *Catecholamines I.* Handbook of Experimental Pharmacology, Vol. 90. New York: Springer Verlag, 1988, pp 509–559.

Häbler HJ, Jänig W, Koltzenburg M. Activation of unmyelinated afferents in chronically lesioned nerves by adrenaline and excitation of sympathetic efferents in the cat. *Neurosci Lett* 1987; 82:35–40.

Hord ED, Oaklander AL. Complex regional pain syndrome: a review of evidence-supported treatment options. *Curr Pain Headache Rep* 2003; 7:188–196.

Hu SJ, Zhu J. Sympathetic facilitation of sustained discharges of polymodal nociceptors. *Pain* 1989; 38:85–90.

Jänig W. Activation of afferent fibers ending in an old neuroma by sympathetic stimulation in the rat. *Neurosci Lett* 1990; 111:309–314.

Jänig W, Baron R. Complex regional pain syndrome: mystery expained? *Lancet Neurol* 2003; 2:687–697.

Jänig W, Levine JD, Michaelis M. Interactions of sympathetic and primary afferent neurons following nerve injury and tissue trauma. *Prog Brain Res* 1996; 113:161–184.

Kim SH, Chung JM. An experimental model for peripheral neuropathy produced by segmental spinal nerve ligation in the rat. *Pain* 1992; 50:355–363.

Kim SH, Na HS, Sheen K, Chung JM. Effects of sympathectomy on a rat model of peripheral neuropathy. *Pain* 1993; 55:85–92.

Kim KJ, Yoon YW, Chung JM. Comparison of three rodent neuropathic pain models. *Exp Brain Res* 1997; 113:200–206.

Kingery WS. A critical review of controlled clinical trials for peripheral neuropathic pain and complex regional pain syndromes. *Pain* 1997; 73:123–139.

Kinnman E, Nygards EB, Hansson P. Peripheral alpha-adrenoreceptors are involved in the development of capsaicin induced ongoing and stimulus evoked pain in humans. *Pain* 1997; 69:79–85.

Kress M, Fickenscher H. Infection by human varicella-zoster virus confers norepinephrine sensitivity to sensory neurons from rat dorsal root ganglia. *FASEB J* 2001; 15:1037–1043.

Leriche R. De la causalgie envisagée comme une névrite du sympathique et de son traitement par la dénudation et l'excision des plexus nerveux péri-artériels. *Presse Med* 1916; 24:178–180.

Levine JD, Fye K, Heller P, et al. Clinical response to regional intravenous guanethidine in patients with rheumatoid arthritis. *J Rheumatol* 1986; 13:1040–1043.

Liu M, Max MB, Parada S, et al. The sympathetic nervous system contributes to capsaicin-evoked mechanical allodynia but not pinprick hyperalgesia in humans. *J Neurosci* 1996; 16:7331–7335.

McLachlan EM, Jänig W, Devor M, Michaelis M. Peripheral nerve injury triggers noradrenergic sprouting within dorsal root ganglia. *Nature* 1993; 363:543–546.

Michaelis M, Devor M, Jänig W. Sympathetic modulation of activity in dorsal root ganglion neurons changes over time following peripheral nerve injury. *J Neurophysiol* 1996; 76:753–763.

Nakamura M, Ferreira SH. A peripheral sympathetic component in inflammatory hyperalgesia. *Eur J Pharmacol* 1987; 135:145–153.

Nicholas AP, Pieribone V, Hökfelt T. Distributions of mRNAs for alpha-2 adrenergic receptor subtypes in rat brain: an in situ hybridization study. *J Comp Neurol* 1993; 328:575–594.

Ochoa JL. Truths, errors, and lies around "reflex sympathetic dystrophy" and "complex regional pain syndrome." *J Neurol* 1999; 246:875–879.

O'Halloran KD, Perl ER. Effects of partial nerve injury on the responses of C-fiber polymodal nociceptors to adrenergic agonists. *Brain Res* 1997; 759:233–240.

Pedersen JL, Rung GW, Kehlet H. Effect of sympathetic nerve block on acute inflammatory pain and hyperalgesia. *Anesthesiology* 1997; 86:293–301.

Perl ER. A reevaluation of mechanisms leading to sympathetically related pain. In: Fields HL, Liebeskind JC (Eds). *Pharmacological Approaches to the Treatment of Chronic Pain: New Concepts and Critical Issues*, Progress in Pain Research and Management, Vol. 1. Seattle: IASP Press, 1994, pp 129–150.

Pieribone VA, Nicholas AP, Dagerlind A, Hökfelt T. Distribution of alpha 1 adrenoceptors in rat brain revealed by in situ hybridization experiments utilizing subtype-specific probes. *J Neurosci* 1994; 14:4252–4268.

Price DD, Long S, Wilsey B, Rafii A. Analysis of peak magnitude and duration of analgesia produced by local anesthetics injected into sympathetic ganglia of complex regional pain syndrome patients. *Clin J Pain* 1998; 14:216–226.

Raja SN. Role of the sympathetic nervous system in acute pain and inflammation. *Ann Med* 1995; 27:241–246.

Raja SN, Treede RD, Davis KD, Campbell JN. Systemic alpha-adrenergic blockade with phentolamine: a diagnostic test for sympathetically maintained pain. *Anesthesiology* 1991; 74:691–698.

Raja SN, Abatzis V, Frank SM. Role of alpha-adrenoceptors in neuroma pain in amputees. *Anesthesiology* 1998; 89:A1083.

Richards RL. Causalgia: a centennial review. *Arch Neurol* 1967; 16:339–350.

Ringkamp M, Eschenfelder S, Grethel EJ, et al. Lumbar sympathectomy failed to reverse mechanical allodynia- and hyperalgesia-like behavior in rats with L5 spinal nerve injury. *Pain* 1999; 79:143–153.

Ruocco I, Cuello AC, Ribeiro-Da-Silva A. Peripheral nerve injury leads to the establishment of a novel pattern of sympathetic fibre innervation in the rat skin. *J Comp Neurol* 2000; 422:287–296.

Sato J, Perl ER. Adrenergic excitation of cutaneous pain receptors induced by peripheral nerve injury. *Science* 1991; 251:1608–1610.

Scadding JW. Development of ongoing activity, mechanosensitivity, and adrenaline sensitivity in severed peripheral nerve axons. *Exp Neurol* 1981; 73:345–364.

Schott G. Clinical features of algodystrophy: is the sympathetic nervous system involved? *Funct Neurol* 1989; 4:131–134.

Schott GD. Visceral afferents: their contribution to 'sympathetic dependent' pain. *Brain* 1994; 117:397–413.

Schott GD. Interrupting the sympathetic outflow in causalgia and reflex sympathetic dystrophy. *BMJ* 1998; 316:792–793.

Seltzer Z, Dubner R, Shir Y. A novel behavioral model of neuropathic pain disorders produced in rats by partial sciatic nerve injury. *Pain* 1990; 43:205–218.

Shi T-JS, Winzer-Serhan U, Leslie F, Hökfeldt T. Distribution and regulation of alpha-2 adrenoceptors in rat dorsal root ganglia. *Pain* 2000; 84:319–330.

Shir Y, Seltzer Z. Effects of sympathectomy in a model of causalgiform pain produced by partial sciatic nerve injury in rats. *Pain* 1991; 45:309–320.

Shyu BC, Danielsen N, Andersson SA, Dahlin LB. Effects of sympathetic stimulation on C-fibre response after peripheral nerve compression: an experimental study in the rabbit common peroneal nerve. *Acta Physiol Scand* 1990; 140:237–243.

Stanton-Hicks M, Jänig W, Hassenbusch S, et al. Reflex sympathetic dystrophy: changing concepts and taxonomy. *Pain* 1995; 63:127–133.

Torebjörk E, Wahren L, Wallin G, et al. Noradrenaline-evoked pain in neuralgia. *Pain* 1995; 63:11–20.

Tracey DJ, Cunningham JE, Romm MA. Peripheral hyperalgesia in experimental neuropathy: mediation by alpha 2-adrenoreceptors on post-ganglionic sympathetic terminals. *Pain* 1995; 60:317–327.

Verdugo RJ, Ochoa JL. 'Sympathetically maintained pain.' I. Phentolamine block questions the concept. *Neurology* 1994; 44:1003–1010.

Verdugo RJ, Campero M, Ochoa JL. Phentolamine sympathetic block in painful polyneuropathies. II. Further questioning of the concept of 'sympathetically maintained pain'. *Neurology* 1994; 44:1010–1014.

Wasner G, Heckmann K, Maier C, Baron R. Vascular abnormalities in acute reflex sympathetic dystrophy (CRPS I)—complete inhibition of sympathetic nerve activity with recovery. *Arch Neurol* 1999; 56:613–620.

White JC, Sweet WH. *Pain and the Neurosurgeon*. Springfield, Illinois: Charles C. Thomas, 1969.

Yoon YW, Lee DH, Lee BH, et al. Different strains and substrains of rats show different levels of neuropathic pain behaviors. *Exp Brain Res* 1999; 129:167–171.

Correspondence to: Prof. Ralf Baron, Dr med, Klinik für Neurologie, Christian-Albrechts-Universität Kiel, Niemannsweg 147, 24105 Kiel, Germany. Tel: 49-431-597-8504; Fax: 49-431-597-8502; email: r.baron@neurologie.uni-kiel.de.

The Pain System in Normal and Pathological States:
A Primer for Clinicians, Progress in Pain Research
and Management, Vol. 31, edited by Luis Villanueva,
Anthony Dickenson, and Hélène Ollat, IASP Press,
Seattle, © 2004.

12

Sensitization of Trigeminovascular Neurons and Migraine Therapy with Triptans

Rami Burstein,[a,b,c] Itay Goor-Aryeh,[a] and Moshe Jakubowski[a]

[a]Departments of Anesthesia and Critical Care, Beth Israel Deaconess Medical Center, Boston, Massachusetts, USA; [b]Department of Neurobiology and [c]Program in Neuroscience, Harvard Medical School, Boston, Massachusetts, USA

Migraine is a neurological disorder of recurring, unilateral, throbbing headache that affects 27 million women and 10 million men in the United States (Stewart et al. 1992). Migraine is associated with variable incidence of aura (visual, sensory and motor function disturbances), nausea and vomiting, photophobia and phonophobia, fatigue, and enhanced irritability (Olesen and Cutrer 2000; Zagami and Rasmussen 2000). We have recently shown that migraine headache is also associated with high incidence of ipsilateral cutaneous allodynia, particularly in periorbital and temporal skin areas. Patients who experience cutaneous allodynia during migraine feel that their skin hurts in response to otherwise innocuous activities such as combing, shaving, taking a shower, or wearing glasses or earrings.

This chapter presents evidence to support the view that the development of throbbing in the initial phase of migraine is mediated by sensitization of *peripheral* trigeminovascular neurons that innervate the meninges (Fig. 1), and that the development and maintenance of cutaneous allodynia later in the attack is propelled by sensitization of *central* trigeminovascular neurons that receive converging sensory input from the meninges as well as from the scalp and facial skin (Fig. 1). We will than present evidence that the development of cutaneous allodynia during migraine is detrimental to termination of acute migraine attacks using triptans ($5HT_{1B/1D}$-receptor agonists).

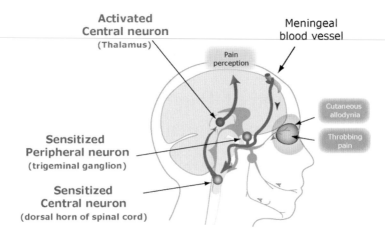

Fig. 1. Peripheral and central sensitization. Sensitization of peripheral trigeminovascular neurons in the trigeminal ganglion mediates the throbbing pain. Sensitization of central trigeminovascular neurons in the nucleus caudalis mediates cutaneous allodynia.

SENSITIZATION OF FIRST-ORDER TRIGEMINOVASCULAR NEURONS DRIVES THE THROBBING PAIN

The induction of headache following electrical stimulation of the dura in awake patients (Penfield and McNaughton 1940; Ray and Wolff 1940) provided the first clue that activated peripheral sensory fibers that innervate the dura may play a critical role in migraine. Since then, a number of theories have emerged regarding the role of peripheral activation during migraine (Goadsby and Edvinsson 1993; Moskowitz and Macfarlane 1993). The most widely acknowledged theories proposed that the release of potassium and hydrogen ions in the vicinity of sensory fibers that innervate the dura following transient disturbances in cortical sensory functions (Csiba et al. 1985; Scheller et al. 1992; Lauritzen 1994; Mayevsky et al. 1996) could activate C-fiber meningeal nociceptors, potassium ions through direct depolarization, and hydrogen ions through the vanilloid receptor (Caterina et al. 1997) or the acid-sensitive ion channel receptor (Waldmann et al. 1997). According to these theories, activation of meningeal nociceptors could cause these sensory fibers to secrete from their peripheral branches calcitonin-gene-related peptide (Ebersberger et al. 1999), a neuropeptide capable of initiating neurogenic inflammation in the dura (Goadsby and Edvinsson 1993; Moskowitz and Macfarlane 1993) and the extracellular release of inflammatory agents such as histamine, serotonin, bradykinin, and prostaglandins.

This theory, together with the anti-migraine action of multiple over-the-counter nonsteroidal anti-inflammatory drugs, has provided a strong rational for the use of "inflammatory soup" (Steen et al. 1992, 1995) in our animal model of intracranial pain.

In the first study with this animal model, we found that mechanically insensitive meningeal nociceptors (i.e., peripheral trigeminovascular neurons) in the trigeminal ganglion became mechanosensitive several minutes after chemical stimulation of their dural receptive fields and as a result, began to respond to dural indentation (Strassman et al. 1996). The slightest mechanical pressure (producing no visible indentation of the dura) was sufficient to induce activity in the sensitized neurons, so we concluded that when meningeal nociceptors become sensitized, they become responsive to otherwise unperceived rhythmic fluctuations in intracranial pressure (i.e., throbbing) produced by normal arterial pulsation (Fig. 1). Based on this conclusion, we proposed that during migraine, such mechanical hypersensitivity could mediate the throbbing of the headache and its worsening during coughing, bending, or other physical activities that increase intracranial pressure (Blau 1981; Anthony 1993).

SENSITIZATION OF SECOND-ORDER TRIGEMINOVASCULAR NEURONS DRIVES THE CUTANEOUS ALLODYNIA

The potential contribution of inflammatory agents to the perception of migraine pain was also assessed by recording their impact on dorsal horn neurons that receive input from meningeal sensory fibers. Response properties of individual brainstem trigeminal neurons that receive convergent input from the dura and the periorbital skin were analyzed before, during, and after the application of the inflammatory agents to the dura. The findings showed that the inflammatory agents not only activate these dorsal horn neurons (Ebersberger et al. 1997; Schepelmann et al. 1999), but also sensitize them for up to 10 hours (Burstein et al. 1998). The sensitized neurons in the medullary dorsal horn showed increased responsiveness to mechanical indentation of dural receptive fields and to mechanical and thermal stimulation of cutaneous receptive fields; their response thresholds decreased and their response magnitudes increased. Based on these findings, we expected migraine to be associated with central sensitization, the clinical manifestation of which should be *extracranial* (periorbital skin) *sensory hypersensitivity* during migraine.

We tested this hypothesis using repeated measurements of mechanical and thermal pain thresholds of periorbital and forearm skin areas in the absence of, and during (4 hours from onset), unilateral migraine attacks (Burstein et al. 2000b). The study showed that in 79% of the patients, migraine was associated with cutaneous allodynia on the facial skin ipsilateral to the migraine pain, and in 21% of the patients cutaneous allodynia was not detected. These findings were consistent with patients' testimonies that they avoid brushing their hair or touching their scalp (Liveing 1873; Selby and Lance 1960); shaving; wearing glasses, contact lenses, earrings, or hats; or resting the affected side of the head on a pillow as it hurts them during migraine attacks. Based on the animal studies, we interpreted the pathophysiology of migraine in the patients as follows: In non-allodynic migraine patients, there is peripheral sensitization of sensory trigeminal ganglion neurons that innervate the dura. In migraine patients who have cutaneous allodynia in the referred pain area, there is peripheral sensitization of meningeal nociceptors and central sensitization of medullary dorsal horn neurons with periorbital receptive fields (Fig. 1).

TEMPORAL ASPECTS OF PERIPHERAL AND CENTRAL SENSITIZATION DURING MIGRAINE

There are remarkable similarities between the temporal changes in the development of peripheral and central sensitization in the rat and their corresponding clinical manifestations during the course of migraine. The induction of peripheral sensitization in the rat occurs rapidly within 5–20 minutes after applying inflammatory soup (IS) onto the dura (Strassman et al. 1996; Levy and Strassman 2002), whereas central sensitization develops over 20–120 minutes and becomes firmly established only 120–240 minutes after application of IS (Burstein et al. 1998). Similarly in patients, throbbing transpires some 5–20 minutes after the onset of headache, whereas cutaneous allodynia starts within 20–120 minutes and becomes firmly established only 120–240 minutes after the onset of headache (Burstein et al. 2000a). According to our scenario, meningeal nociceptors become sensitized a few minutes after their initial activation, resulting in throbbing headache and its exacerbation by bending over. The continued barrage of impulses arriving from sensitized meningeal nociceptors gradually stimulates the development of central sensitization in spinal trigeminovascular neurons, resulting in cutaneous allodynia in the same area as the referred head pain. Eventually, as we observed in the rat (Burstein et al. 1998), central trigeminovascular neurons change their physiological properties and remain inveterately sensitized, independent of incoming impulses from meningeal nociceptors.

DEFEATING MIGRAINE PAIN WITH TRIPTANS IS A RACE AGAINST THE DEVELOPMENT OF CUTANEOUS ALLODYNIA

To test whether central sensitization, as manifested by cutaneous allodynia, presents an obstacle to migraine therapy, we studied migraine patients repeatedly on three visits to the clinic: in the absence of migraine (baseline); before and after *early* triptan treatment (initiated within the first hour of one attack, before the establishment of central sensitization); and before and after *late* triptan treatment (initiated 4 hours from onset of another attack, after the establishment of central sensitization). Triptans, a family of $5HT_{1B/1D}$-receptor agonists originally designed to constrict dilated blood vessels (Friberg et al. 1991; Humphrey and Feniuk 1991), are among the most commonly prescribed migraine drugs.

We found that the success rate of rendering a migraine patient pain-free is tightly associated with the absence or presence of cutaneous allodynia at the time of triptan therapy (Burstein et al. 2004). Patients who developed allodynia during the course of an attack were far more likely to be rendered pain-free when triptan therapy was administered before rather than after the establishment of cutaneous allodynia (Fig. 2), and those who never developed allodynia were highly likely to be rendered pain-free at any time after the onset of pain (Fig. 3). In the presence of allodynia, triptan treatment brought about complete pain relief in only 5/34 attacks (15%). In the other 29 attacks (85%), triptan treatment reduced the pain level by about 40%. Pain thresholds for heat, cold, and mechanical stimuli of the periorbital skin shifted significantly ($P < 0.0001$) from normal values at baseline into the allodynic zone during migraine (before treatment) and remained in the allodynic zone after treatment: pain thresholds dropped from $45.6° \pm 0.6°C$ to $40.1° \pm 0.6°C$ for heat, increased from $12.7° \pm 1.2°C$ to $20.7° \pm 1.5°C$ for cold, and dropped from 112.6 ± 6.6 g to 29.8 ± 6.6 g for mechanical skin stimulation. Notwithstanding the partial pain relief, triptan treatment did terminate the throbbing in 70% of the attacks and reduced throbbing intensity by more than half in an additional 19% of these attacks. In contrast, in the absence of allodynia, triptan treatment effectively eliminated the pain in 25/27 attacks (93%), and abolished throbbing. In these attacks, pain thresholds for heat, cold, and mechanical stimuli of the periorbital skin remained well outside the allodynic zone throughout the attacks and were unchanged from baseline levels (i.e., between attacks): heat pain thresholds remained above 46°C, cold pain thresholds remained below 13°C, and mechanical pain thresholds remained above 100 g.

These results have led us to propose a new guideline for triptan treatment: (1) patients with allodynia should take triptans as early as possible

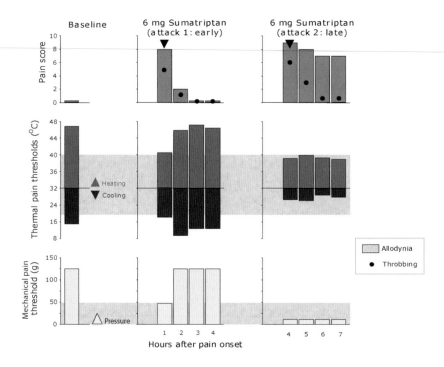

Fig. 2. Sumatriptan relieves the pain of migraine in allodynic patients only when taken before the establishment of allodynia. A representative patient illustrating the effects of sumatriptan on migraine pain intensity and periorbital skin sensitivity in the absence (attack 1) and presence (attack 2) of allodynia at the time of the treatment. Pain scores and pain thresholds to heat, cold, and mechanical stimulation of the referred pain area in the ipsilateral periorbital skin were collected in the absence of migraine (pain free), and during two migraine attacks. Heat, cold, and mechanical pain thresholds falling *outside* the shaded allodynia zone are considered normal (adapted from Burstein et al. 2004).

during the attack before the emergence of any sign of allodynia; (2) after the onset of allodynia, patients may still use triptans if they find significant benefits in partial pain relief; (3) allodynia-free patients can expect excellent results from triptans at any time during the attack.

THE RACE AGAINST THE DEVELOPMENT OF CUTANEOUS ALLODYNIA IS A RACE AGAINST THE ESTABLISHMENT OF CENTRAL SENSITIZATION

Given that cutaneous allodynia of migraine is a manifestation of sensitization of central trigeminovascular neurons, we used our rat model for cutaneous allodynia induced by intracranial pain to examine whether *early* sumatriptan administration can *prevent* the development of central sensitization, and whether *late* sumatriptan administration can *reverse* inveterate central sensitization. The study was based on recording changes in response properties of spinal trigeminal nucleus neurons that received convergent inputs from the dura and facial skin. To mimic the clinical study, sumatriptan (300 µg/kg i.v.) was administered either 2 hours after induction of central sensitization by topical application of IS to the dura (late intervention), or at the same time as IS (early intervention).

We found that the effects of sumatriptan on spinal trigeminovascular neurons depend on whether the drug is given before or after the establishment of central sensitization and cutaneous allodynia (Burstein and Jakubowski 2004). Early sumatriptan intervention effectively prevented the induction of central sensitization, whereas late sumatriptan intervention could not reverse an already established central sensitization.

Late sumatriptan intervention effectively counteracted neuronal measures of central sensitization that depend on peripheral input from the meninges: dural receptive fields, which initially expanded after application

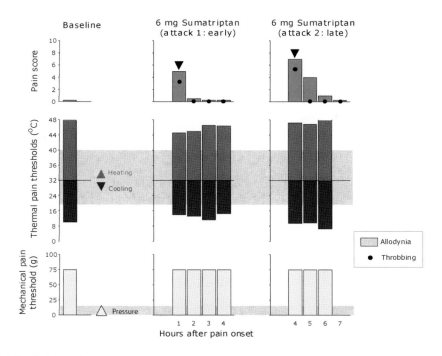

Fig. 3. Sumatriptan relieves migraine pain in non-allodynic patients at any time after the onset of the attack. A representative patient illustrating the effects of sumatriptan on migraine pain intensity and periorbital skin sensitivity in the absence (attacks 1 and 2) of allodynia at the time of treatment. Presentation as in Fig. 2 (adapted from Burstein et al. 2004).

of IS in 78% of the cases, shrank back to their original size after treatment (Fig. 4); neuronal response threshold to dural indentation, which initially decreased from 3.0 ± 0.6 g at baseline to 1.0 ± 0.2 g after IS, increased significantly to 1.9 ± 0.3 g after sumatriptan. On the other hand, late

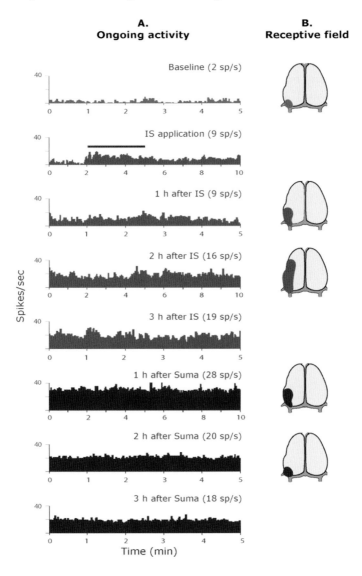

Fig. 4. *Late* sumatriptan treatment cannot reverse inflammatory soup (IS)-induced increase in spontaneous activity (A) but effectively reverses expansion of the dural receptive field (B) of central trigeminovascular neurons in the medullary dorsal horn. Shown in panel B is a dorsal view of the rat's hemispheres and meningeal sinuses (adapted from Burstein and Jakubowski 2004).

sumatriptan intervention did not reverse aspects of central sensitization that reflect intrinsic activity: spontaneous firing rate (spikes/second), which initially increased from 3.4 ± 1.3 at baseline to 20.0 ± 6.0 after IS, remained elevated at 16.4 ± 5.0 after sumatriptan (Fig. 4); neuronal response magnitude to skin brushing (spikes/second), which initially increased from 20.8 ± 3.8 at baseline to 45.1 ± 7.6 after IS, remained elevated at 47.8 ± 6.0 after sumatriptan; and neuronal response threshold to heating of the skin, which initially dropped from 46.7° ± 1.0°C at baseline to 42.2° ± 0.6°C after IS, remained at 43.2° ± 1.1°C after sumatriptan. Early sumatriptan intervention effectively blocked the development of all aspects of central sensitization expected to be induced by IS 2 hours later (Fig. 5): dural receptive fields did not expand; neuronal response threshold to dural indentation did not decrease (1.6 ± 0.2 g vs. 2.5 ± 0.4 g); spontaneous firing rate did not increase (8.5 ± 4.9 vs. 6.2 ± 3.7 spikes/second); and neuronal response thresholds to skin stimuli remained unchanged (brushing: 17.6 ± 6.2 vs. 18.9 ± 5.9 spikes/second; heat: 45.7° ± 1.2°C vs. 46.5° ± 1.5°C).

Both the clinical (Burstein et al. 2004) and preclinical (Burstein and Jakubowski 2004) studies suggest that triptans act peripherally to block transmission of pain signals from the dura, but do not act directly on the central neurons in the spinal trigeminal nucleus. This functional conclusion is further supported by anatomical studies in which $5HT_{1B/1D}$-receptor immunoreactivity appears to be absent from cell bodies of central nociceptive neurons of the spinal and medullary dorsal horn (Longmore et al. 1997; Riad et al. 1998; Potrebic et al. 2003), but present on peripheral terminals of meningeal nociceptors, and also on central terminals of yet unidentified nociceptors in the spinal and medullary dorsal horn (Potrebic et al. 2003).

The peripheral action of triptans that blocks transmission of pain signals from the dura to the central trigeminovascular neurons can explain our observations that these drugs are highly effective, *whether given early or late*, in terminating throbbing in patients, and in reversing hypersensitivity to mechanical stimulation of the dura in central trigeminovascular neurons. This peripheral action also explains why *early* triptan intervention is effective in terminating migraine pain and blocking the development of cutaneous allodynia, as it disrupts the input necessary for the development of central sensitization. The evidence that the peripheral action of triptans cannot counteract the inveterate, ongoing sensitization in the central trigeminovascular neurons can explain the failure of *late* triptan intervention to terminate migraine pain or reverse the exaggerated skin sensitivity in attacks already associated with allodynia, as well as the inability of triptans to abolish the increased spontaneous activity and hypersensitivity to mechanical and thermal stimulation of the skin in central trigeminovascular neurons.

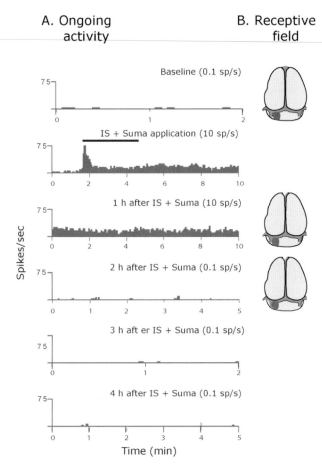

Fig. 5. *Early* sumatriptan treatment effectively prevents IS-induced increase in spontaneous activity (A) and expansion of the dural receptive field (B) of central trigeminovascular neurons in the medullary dorsal horn. Shown in panel B is a dorsal view of the rat's hemispheres and meningeal sinuses (adapted from Burstein and Jakubowski 2004).

Based on the relatively high incidence of cutaneous allodynia during migraine, plus the importance of the timing of triptan therapy to precede the onset of allodynia, we call for adding a new classification to the diagnosis of migraine: migraine with and without allodynia.

ACKNOWLEDGMENTS

Supported by National Institutes of Health grants DE-10904 (National Institutes of Dental and Craniofacial Research) and NS-35611 (National Institutes of Neurological Disorder and Stroke), and by a grant from GlaxoSmith-Kline.

REFERENCES

Burstein R, Jakubowski M. Analgesic triptan action in an animal model of intracranial pain: a race against the development of central sensitization. *Ann Neurol* 2004; 55:27–36.

Burstein R, Yamamura H, Malick A, et al. Chemical stimulation of the intracranial dura induces enhanced responses to facial stimulation in brain stem trigeminal neurons. *J Neurophysiol* 1998; 79:964–982.

Burstein R, Cutrer FM, Yarnitsky D. The development of cutaneous allodynia during a migraine attack: clinical evidence for the sequential recruitment of spinal and supraspinal nociceptive neurons in migraine. *Brain* 2000a; 123:1703–1709.

Burstein R, Yarnitsky D, Goor-Aryeh I, et al. An association between migraine and cutaneous allodynia. *Ann Neurol* 2000b; 47:614–624.

Burstein R, Jakubowski M, Collins B. Defeating migraine pain with triptans: a race against the development of cutaneous allodynia. *Ann Neurol* 2004; 55:19–26.

Csiba L, Paschen W, Mies G. Regional changes in tissue pH and glucose content during cortical spreading depression in rat brain. *Brain Res* 1985; 336:167–170.

Ebersberger A, Ringkamp M, Reeh PW, et al. Recordings from brain stem neurons responding to chemical stimulation of the subarachnoid space. *J Neurophysiol* 1997; 77:3122–3133.

Ebersberger A, Averbeck B, Messlinger K, et al. Release of substance P, calcitonin gene-related peptide and prostaglandin E2 from rat dura mater encephali following electrical and chemical stimulation in vitro. *Neuroscience* 1999; 89:901–907.

Friberg L, Olesen J, Iversen HK, et al. Migraine pain associated with middle cerebral artery dilatation: reversal by sumatriptan. *Lancet* 1991; 338:13–17.

Goadsby PJ, Edvinsson L. The trigeminovascular system and migraine: studies characterizing cerebrovascular and neuropeptide changes seen in humans and cats. *Ann Neurol* 1993; 33:48–56.

Humphrey PP, Feniuk W. Mode of action of the anti-migraine drug sumatriptan. *Trends Pharmacol Sci* 1991; 12:444–446.

Lauritzen M. Pathophysiology of the migraine aura: the spreading depression theory. *Brain* 1994; 117:199–210.

Levy D, Strassman AM. Distinct sensitizing effects of the cAMP-PKA second messenger cascade on rat dural mechanonociceptors. *J Physiol* 2002; 538:483–493.

Liveing E. *On Megrim, Sick Headache*. Nijmegen: Arts & Boeve, 1873.

Longmore J, Shaw D, Smith D, et al. Differential distribution of 5HT1D- and 5HT1B-immunoreactivity within the human trigemino-cerebrovascular system: implications for the discovery of new antimigraine drugs. *Cephalalgia* 1997; 17:833–842.

Mayevsky A, Doron A, Manor T, et al. Cortical spreading depression recorded from the human brain using a multiparametric monitoring system. *Brain Res* 1996; 740:268–274.

Moskowitz MA, Macfarlane R. Neurovascular and molecular mechanisms in migraine headaches. *Cerebrovasc Brain Metab Rev* 1993; 5:159–177.

Olesen J, Cutrer FM. Migraine with aura and its subforms. In: Olesen J, Tfelt-Hansen P, Welch K (Eds). *The Headaches.* New York: Raven Press, 2000, pp 345–357.

Penfield W, McNaughton F. Dural headache and innervation of the dura mater. *Arch Neurol Psychiatry* 1940; 44:43–75.

Potrebic S, Ahn AH, Skinner K, et al. Peptidergic nociceptors of both trigeminal and dorsal root ganglia express serotonin 1D receptors: implications for the selective antimigraine action of triptans. *J Neurosci* 2003; 23:10988–10997.

Ray BS, Wolff HG. Experimental studies on headache: pain-sensitive structures of the head and their significance in headache. *Arch Surg* 1940; 41:813–856.

Riad M, Tong XK, el Mestikawy S, et al. Endothelial expression of the 5-hydroxytryptamine-1B antimigraine drug receptor in rat and human brain microvessels. *Neuroscience* 1998; 86:1031–1035.

Scheller D, Kolb J, Tegtmeier F. Lactate and pH change in close correlation in the extracellular space of the rat brain during cortical spreading depression. *Neurosci Lett* 1992; 135:83–86.

Schepelmann K, Ebersberger A, Pawlak M, et al. Response properties of trigeminal brain stem neurons with input from dura mater encephali in the rat. *Neuroscience* 1999; 90:543–554.

Selby G, Lance JW. Observations on 500 cases of migraine and allied vascular headache. *J Neurol Neurosurg Psychiatry* 1960; 23–32.

Steen KH, Reeh PW, Anton F, et al. Protons selectively induce lasting excitation and sensitization to mechanical stimulation of nociceptors in rat skin, in vitro. *J Neurosci* 1992; 12:86–95.

Steen KH, Steen AE, Reeh PW. A dominant role of acid pH in inflammatory excitation and sensitization of nociceptors in rat skin, in vitro. *J Neurosci* 1995; 15:3982–3989.

Stewart WF, Lipton RB, Celentano DD, et al. Prevalence of migraine headache in the United States: relation to age, income, race, and other sociodemographic factors. *JAMA* 1992; 267:64–69.

Strassman AM, Raymond SA, Burstein R. Sensitization of meningeal sensory neurons and the origin of headaches. *Nature* 1996; 384:560–564.

Zagami AS, Rasmussen BK. Symptomology of migraine without aura. In: Olesen J, Tfelt-Hansen P, Welch MA (Eds). *The Headaches.* New York: Raven Press, 2000, pp 337–343.

Correspondence to: Rami Burstein, PhD, Department of Anesthesia and Critical Care, Harvard Institutes of Medicine, Room 830, 77 Avenue Louis Pasteur, Boston, MA 02115, USA. Tel: 617-667-0806, Fax: 617-975-5329, email: rburstei@caregroup.harvard.edu.

The Pain System in Normal and Pathological States:
A Primer for Clinicians, Progress in Pain Research
and Management, Vol. 31, edited by Luis Villanueva,
Anthony Dickenson, and Hélène Ollat, IASP Press,
Seattle, © 2004.

13

Endogenous Central Mechanisms of Pain Modulation

Luis Villanueva[a] and Howard L. Fields[b]

[a]Faculty of Dental Surgery, INSERM E-216, Clermont-Ferrand, France; [b]Department of Neurology, University of California, San Francisco, California, USA

Les concepts sont des outils: ils s'usent en assurant leur fonction (Claude Bernard)

During the last few decades, most studies of central mechanisms that modulate nociceptive transmission have focused on segmental or brainstem controls triggered by primary afferent inputs and acting at the level of the spinal or medullary dorsal horn. This chapter considers the functional organization of central nervous system (CNS) networks that modulate nociceptive information.

SEGMENTAL MODULATION

The gate control theory proposed that segmental inhibitions are elicited by activity in large-diameter cutaneous afferent fibers and can be activated naturally by innocuous mechanical stimuli (Melzack and Wall 1965). In fact, the activation of fine-diameter fibers not only elicits pain but also triggers both segmental and heterosegmental inhibitory mechanisms that must have a functional basis beyond the dorsal horn scope of the original gate control hypothesis. Although transcutaneous electrical nerve stimulation (TENS) can be effective when applied at frequencies and intensities that activate mainly large afferent fibers, the resulting pain relief is localized and often limited to the stimulated segment (see Andersson 1979). Stronger analgesic effects can be obtained with TENS by using a stimulation intensity that produces an unpleasant, but not quite painful, sensation (Andersson

1979; Melzack 1984). In summary, a substantial amount of data has implicated the activation of fine-diameter fibers in analgesic procedures based on percutaneous electrical stimulation (Woolf et al. 1980; Chung et al. 1984; Bouhassira et al. 1987). This conclusion is supported by a meta-analysis that showed that the intensity of stimulation is a critical parameter for obtaining analgesia using segmental TENS (Delisle and Plaghki 1990).

On the basis of the gate control theory, it was also proposed that antidromic activation of large-diameter afferent fibers underlies the analgesic effects elicited by stimulation of the dorsal columns (usually termed "spinal cord stimulation" in humans). This type of stimulation produces inhibitions of dorsal horn nociceptive neurons. These inhibitions were explained by the activation of collaterals from primary afferent fibers in the dorsal columns, which passed into the spinal gray matter. However, in animal experiments, dorsal column stimulation induced only a brief inhibition of activity in dorsal horn nociceptive neurons, whereas pain relief lasting for hours after spinal cord stimulation was observed in humans. In addition, spinal cord stimulation may relieve ischemic pain and increase peripheral circulation and skin temperature in human subjects (Linderoth and Meyerson 1995). It is possible that central inhibitory mechanisms influencing sympathetic efferent neurons could be conveyed by axons descending from dorsal column cells and terminating in the superficial dorsal horn (Burton and Loewy 1977; Villanueva et al. 1995), given that lamina I dorsal horn neurons provide a direct propriospinal pathway that is responsible for somatosympathetic reflexes elicited by noxious stimuli (Craig 2003).

BULBOSPINAL MODULATION

DIFFUSE NOXIOUS INHIBITORY CONTROLS

In contrast to segmental controls, heterosegmental controls are elicited mainly by noxious stimuli. A painful focus can induce widespread inhibitory phenomena, mainly on deep dorsal horn neurons. These inhibitions are mediated by both propriospinal (Cadden et al. 1983) and supraspinal mechanisms, such as diffuse noxious inhibitory controls (DNICs; Le Bars et al. 1979). These controls have several anatomical and functional analogues in animals and human beings. The supraspinal structures responsible for DNICs include the subnucleus reticularis dorsalis (SRD) in the caudal-dorsal medulla, which contains a homogeneous population of neurons whose properties mirror the functional characteristics of DNICs in that they are activated exclusively by noxious stimuli applied to any region of the body and they precisely encode the intensity of these stimuli (Villanueva et al. 1996).

Moreover, lesions of the caudal medulla reduce DNICs in both animals (Bouhassira et al. 1992) and humans (De Broucker et al. 1990). These caudal medullary networks have been proposed to facilitate the extraction of nociceptive information by increasing the signal-to-noise ratio between a pool of deep dorsal horn neurons activated by a painful focus and the remaining population of such neurons, which are simultaneously inhibited. These studies also suggested that DNIC mediates the "pain inhibits pain" or "counter-stimulation" phenomenon, whereby there is a mutual inhibition between the pathways that mediate sensations elicited concomitantly by two separate painful foci.

Interestingly, more than half the SRD neurons projecting to the thalamus provide monosynaptic connections to the spinal cord (Monconduit et al. 2002b), suggesting that this nucleus simultaneously regulates the flow of sensory information in spinal and thalamic nociceptive pathways. Double-projecting neurons are concentrated in the dorsal-most aspect of the SRD, in a region of "whole body" nociceptive convergence that projects to several areas of the CNS involved in motor processing. These areas include the deep dorsal horn and the more dorsal part of the ventral horn at all levels of the spinal cord (Almeida et al. 1995; Villanueva et al. 1995), as well as brainstem motor nuclei, the giganto- and parvocellular reticular formation (Bernard et al. 1990), and motor-related areas of the forebrain such as the ventromedial, parafascicular thalamic nuclei and the ventral zona incerta (Villanueva et al. 1998). Conversely, various regions of the deep dorsal horn (laminae V–VII), containing neurons that respond to noxious cutaneous or visceral stimuli, provide the main input to the dorsal-most aspect of the SRD (Lima 1990; Villanueva et al. 1991; Raboisson et al. 1996). The SRD, via its reciprocal connections, exerts both inhibitory (Bouhassira et al. 1992) and excitatory (Dugast et al. 2003) influences on deep dorsal horn neurons.

THE ROSTRAL VENTROMEDIAL MEDULLA

Early systematic studies of what was originally termed "stimulation-produced analgesia" in animals (Mayer et al. 1971; Oliveras et al. 1975; Basbaum et al. 1976) showed that the brainstem sites where microstimulation most effectively elicited strong antinociceptive effects were the ventral periaqueductal gray matter (PAG) and the rostral ventromedial medulla (RVM; see references in Oliveras and Besson 1988). The RVM sends dense descending projections to the spinal and trigeminal dorsal horn that modulate the activity of both superficial and deep dorsal horn cells (Basbaum et al. 1978; Fields et al. 1995) at the origin of spinal ascending nociceptive pathways. RVM cells receive spinal inputs indirectly via the PAG and the adjacent medullary nucleus reticularis gigantocellularis, and they constitute a key link for descending modulation because the PAG projects minimally to the dorsal horn. In common with caudal medullary systems, RVM networks are both excitatory and inhibitory, because noxious inputs can modulate spinal outflow, via the RVM, in a bidirectional fashion (Fields et al. 1983a; Morgan et al. 1994).

Electrophysiological studies of RVM neurons have elucidated the mechanism of their bidirectional control. There are three classes of RVM neuron: off cells, which pause just prior to withdrawal reflexes; on cells, which show a burst of activity prior to such reflexes; and neutral cells, which have no reflex-related activity. On and off cells project directly to dorsal horn laminae I, II, and V (Fields et al. 1995). Off cells are activated by local infusions of μ-opioid agonists or bicuculline, and their activity inhibits nociceptive transmission (Heinricher and Tortorici 1994; Heinricher et al. 1994). In contrast, on cells, whose activity facilitates nociceptive transmission, are inhibited by local or systemic opioids and are activated by tonic noxious stimuli and during acute morphine abstinence (Bederson et al. 1990; Kaplan and Fields 1991; Morgan and Fields 1994).

In contrast to the caudal medullary systems that preferentially modulate deep dorsal horn neurons, RVM cells modulate not only deep dorsal horn but also lamina I neurons, a key relay for nociceptive inputs to CNS areas that process signals relevant to homeostasis (Craig 2003). This suggests that a broader modulatory role is exerted by the RVM. It has been proposed that, under appropriate environmental circumstances, RVM neurons integrate activities from the somatomotor and autonomic systems in response to different bodily needs. They could contribute not only to the modulation of pain but also to arousal reactions and homeostatic regulations such as changes in vasomotor, temperature, and sexual function in a manner appropriate to the behavioral status of the body (Lovick 1997; Mason 2001).

Accordingly, in unanesthetized animals, robust antinociceptive effects can be elicited by exposure to stressful and threatening situations, such as inescapable noxious stimuli, the presence of a predator, or contextual cues associated with intense or prolonged noxious stimuli. In many of these situations, the behavioral antinociceptive effect clearly involves the PAG-RVM network (Fields et al. 2004). The PAG-RVM system also contributes to hyperalgesia and allodynia in inflammatory and neuropathic models, including spinal nerve ligation (Gardell et al. 2003).

Electrophysiological studies in unanesthetized rats are also illuminating in this regard because they demonstrate powerful state-dependent changes in RVM neurons. For example, RVM off cells are only intermittently active when the animals are awake but become continuously active when they transition to slow-wave sleep (Leung and Mason 1999) or when they are given barbiturate anesthesia (Oliveras et al. 1991) or morphine (McGaraughty et al. 1993). On cells show a reciprocal pattern, becoming much less active during slow-wave sleep. Interestingly, compared to the anesthetized and sleeping states, in awake rats both on and off cells are more responsive to a variety of innocuous stimuli.

It is important to point out that about 20% of RVM neurons are serotonergic. Although similar to other RVM neurons in that they project to the dorsal horn via the dorsolateral funiculus, serotonergic RVM neurons are neither on nor off cells (Potrebic et al. 1994). Furthermore, the firing of RVM serotonergic neurons is not affected by morphine (Gao et al. 1998) or by electrical stimulation of the PAG (Gao et al. 1997), and their responses to noxious stimulation are either absent or minimal (Gao and Mason 2000). Serotonergic RVM neurons are, however, strongly activated by baroreceptor inputs. Thus, while they probably contribute to the control of nociceptive transmission, serotonergic neurons form a modulatory channel that is parallel to and can be activated independently of the bidirectional control exerted by RVM on and off cells (Yaksh 1979; Le Bars 1988; Mason and Gao 1998).

FUNCTIONAL IMPLICATIONS

The studies described above show that several ascending and bulbospinal descending modulatory "pain pathways" are activated simultaneously when a noxious stimulus occurs. Such networks, which are not somatotopically organized, provide widespread negative and positive spino-bulbo-spinal feedback loops by which nociceptive signals may attenuate or increase their own magnitudes.

Perhaps the main difficulty in attempting to correlate the activity of bulbospinal modulatory systems with behavioral analgesia is that several pain modulation networks operate in parallel, and so the net effect cannot be attributed exclusively to activity in any single network. This complexity is illustrated below by two examples: the counterstimulation phenomenon and morphine analgesia.

Counterstimulation-induced analgesia. DNIC were proposed to underlie the analgesic effects elicited by counterstimulation procedures ("pain inhibits pain") because they both reduce spinal (R-III) and trigeminal reflexes and diminish the perception of experimental, acute pain following heterotopic noxious stimulation in humans (Villanueva and Le Bars 1995). In contrast to animal studies, in chronic pain patients, several mechanisms, sometimes not involving DNICs, are implicated in counterstimulation phenomena. For example, in neuropathic pain patients, counterstimulation produced differential effects, thus showing that DNIC mechanisms are not universal (Bouhassira et al. 2003). Light pressure applied to an allodynic area induced inhibitions of both the R-III reflex and the concomitant painful sensation, whereas stroking within the same neural territory, which elicited a similar level of pain, reduced the painful sensation but did not modify the R-III reflex. One can conclude that in this latter situation, dynamic mechano-allodynia elicited a counterstimulation effect that involved supraspinal rather than spinal circuitry. Furthermore, DNIC effects against experimental pain (Kosek and Hansson 1997) and temporally summated second pain are absent in fibromyalgia patients. Indeed, a lack of DNIC-like effects against temporally summated second pain is also found in normal female subjects (Staud et al. 2003).

Morphine analgesia. The existence of opioidergic links in the medulla led to the proposal that noxious stimuli release opioid peptides and, via descending bulbospinal controls, elicit endogenous analgesia. It was suggested that in addition to its well-known spinal action, morphine analgesia could be mediated by a depression of spinal transmission following the activation of inhibitory controls originating within the rostral-ventral medulla (Fields et al. 1983b). It was also proposed that morphine analgesia may result from a DNIC-mediated blockade of the amplification of nociceptive spinal outputs (Le Bars et al. 1981).

In fact, it is likely that morphine produces analgesia by interacting with several CNS modulatory systems in addition to its direct effects on bulbospinal modulatory systems. The CNS targets for morphine analgesia are multiple and include a number of subcortical and cortical areas. Recent functional imaging studies of metabolic brain activity have shown that the CNS structures activated by the endogenous μ-opioid system following sustained pain in human beings are similar to those observed under equivalent experimental conditions in animals. In addition to the PAG and RVM, these areas include the cingulate, prefrontal, and insular cortices and subcortical areas such as the hypothalamus, amygdala, and ventrolateral thalamus (Zubieta et al. 2001; Petrovic et al. 2002). Also, the activation of μ-opioid receptors reduces the activity of all cortical and subcortical areas activated by pain (Casey et al. 2000). The high sensitivity of forebrain areas to opioids is illustrated by animal studies showing that activity evoked in thalamic neurons is depressed by morphine at doses several times lower that that required to reduce the activity in dorsal horn or ascending axons in the spinal cord under similar experimental conditions (see references in Monconduit et al. 2002a).

THE CORTEX AS A MAJOR SOURCE OF TOP-DOWN MODULATION

Powerful endogenous control of nociception probably originates from the cortex because, as we will see below, almost all nociceptive relays within the CNS are under corticofugal modulation, including the networks involved in segmental and heterosegmental modulation at the dorsal horn level (Fig 1). In contrast to bulbospinal descending controls, corticofugal modulation often occurs in the absence of a painful stimulus. For example, the insular cortex contributes to the processing of paradoxical pain elicited by the concomitant application of innocuous cold and warm stimuli (Craig et al. 1996), whereas frontal cortical areas may selectively alter the unpleasantness of pain perception following manipulation of attentional factors or the anticipation of pain (Rainville 2002). Some of these same cortical areas are involved in the analgesia produced by placebo or hypnotic manipulations (see Rainville 2002; Ploghaus et al. 2003). However, the mechanisms underlying these modulations are still poorly understood.

ATTENTION, EXPECTATION, AND THE ROLE OF THE LIMBIC CORTEX IN TOP-DOWN MODULATION OF PAIN

ATTENTION

Attention as a powerful modulator of perceived pain intensity is well established (see Villemure and Bushnell 2002 for a review). When human subjects are trained to either make a visual or noxious thermal discrimination, attending to the pain increases its perceived intensity and distraction reduces it (Miron et al. 1989; Tracey et al. 2002). While the neural circuits involved in attentional modulation are uncertain, functional imaging studies in humans suggest that the PAG-to-RVM system might be involved. In fact, when normal human subjects rated thermal pain in the presence of a visual distractor, pain intensity ratings were significantly lower and there was a concomitant increase in activity in the PAG (Tracey et al. 2002). In addition, Bantick et al. (2002) found that pain reaction times were increased and intensity ratings were lowered during distraction. Concomitant brain imaging demonstrated an increase in the rostral anterior cingulate cortex (ACC) during distraction but a decrease in pain transmission pathways including the contralateral thalamus, insular cortex, and mid-cingulate. Thus, the imaging results indicate that the ACC and PAG are activated during attentional distraction associated with reduced pain intensity, and they support a mechanism for attentional effects involving reduced activity in afferent pathways.

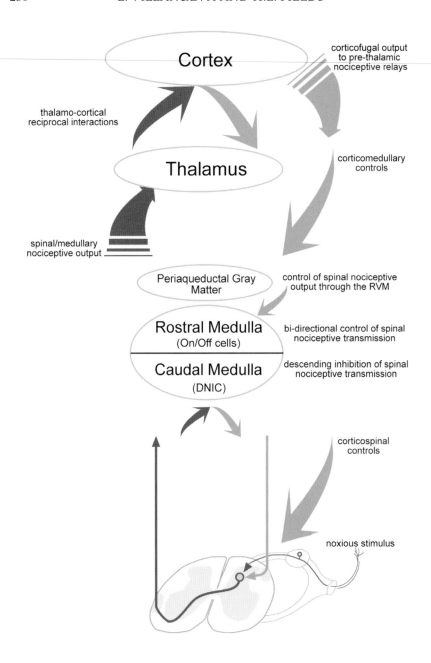

Fig. 1. Diagram of the main central mechanisms of pain modulation. A noxious stimulus activates both segmental and bulbospinal modulatory mechanisms by which nociceptive signals may attenuate or increase their own magnitudes. The most important, and widespread, source of top-down modulation arises from the cortex because both thalamic and prethalamic nociceptive relays are under corticofugal modulation.

EXPECTATION

Initially neutral exteroceptive sensory cues can acquire the power to modulate the activity of nociceptive dorsal horn neurons *in the absence of a noxious stimulus* (see the primate studies described below). When subjects are conditioned with specific cues that predict either painful or neutral stimuli, the cues can exert powerful pain-modulating effects (Sawamoto et al. 2000; Ploghaus et al. 2003). For example, pain-predictive cues presented just prior to nonpainful warm stimuli cause human subjects to report the warm stimuli as painful. In the same subjects, the rostral ACC and anterior insular cortex were activated by cues predicting pain (Ploghaus et al. 1999). Consistent with the human brain-imaging studies, recordings in the ACC of awake primates have demonstrated neurons specifically activated during pain avoidance behaviors (Koyama et al. 2001). Furthermore lesions of the rostral ACC prevent rats from learning to avoid environments associated with tonic noxious stimulation (e.g., Johansen et al. 2001).

Ploghaus and colleagues (2003) suggested that certain and uncertain expectation are mediated by different networks. The former is associated with activity in the rostral ACC and posterior cerebellum, and the latter with activity changes in the ventromedial prefrontal cortex, mid-cingulate cortex, and hippocampus. Certain expectation is related with fear that leads to decreased pain sensitivity and hypoalgesia, whereas uncertain expectation, associated with anxiety rather than fear, has the opposite effect on pain perception, leading to increased pain sensitivity.

How do neurons in the rostral ACC and anterior insula exert modulatory control in expectancy-related situations? There are direct projections from the ACC to the PAG (Marchand and Hagino 1983; An et al. 1998). There is also a dense projection from the rostral ACC to the nucleus accumbens (Kunishio and Haber 1994), which in turn projects to the hypothalamus and basolateral amygdala. There are also direct anterior insular connections to the RVM and dorsolateral pontine tegmentum (Jasmin et al. 2003). Further research is required to determine how expectancy-related cortical activation modulates pain. Some possibilities are described in the following sections.

CORTICOFUGAL MODULATION OF DORSAL HORN ACTIVITIES

Corticofugal controls act as early as the termination areas of nociceptive primary afferents. Anatomical studies have shown direct projections of the primary somatosensory corticospinal tract to the superficial laminae of the dorsal horn in several species (Cheema et al. 1984; Ralston and Ralston 1985; Casale et al. 1988). Some of these axons have collaterals terminating in the deeper laminae of the dorsal horn, thus raising the possibility that this system simultaneously modulates the activity of both superficial and deep dorsal horn nociceptive neurons. Early electrophysiological studies showed that stimulation of the somatosensory and motor cortices elicited mainly inhibitory effects on the responses of dorsal horn neurons following low-threshold cutaneous stimulation (Besson and Rivot 1972; Coulter et al. 1974). Later studies showed that stimulation of the sensorimotor cortex excited or inhibited nociceptive spinothalamic cells in the monkey. Inhibitory actions were obtained mainly from stimulation of the primary somatosensory (S1) cortical area, whereas excitation or mixed effects were elicited from the motor cortex (Yezierski et al. 1983). In addition, local application of morphine in S1 reduced the evoked potentials in the ventrolateral funiculus following percutaneous electrical stimulation of the rat hindpaw (Hernandez and Soto-Moyano 1986).

As demonstrated by the studies of Jasmin's group, similar effects can be elicited from other cortical areas (Burkey et al. 1996, 1999). This group showed that both opioidergic and dopaminergic manipulation of the rostral anterior insular cortex (RAIC) can strongly modulate the activity of dorsal horn neurons. Interestingly, a recent study in freely moving animals showed that GABAergic manipulation of the rostral insula may elicit bidirectional effects on nociceptive processing (Jasmin et al. 2003). This control appears to involve brainstem structures including the RVM and noradrenergic neurons in the dorsolateral pontine tegmentum. Increasing γ-aminobutyric acid (GABA) locally within the RAIC elicits antinociceptive effects by releasing the activity of brainstem noradrenergic descending controls, whereas selectively activating $GABA_B$ receptors produces hyperalgesia by releasing a pronociceptive circuit within the amygdala. Taken together, these studies show that a number of cortical areas may exert direct and indirect influences in the processing of nociceptive inputs at the level of the dorsal horn.

CORTICOFUGAL MODULATION OF TRIGEMINAL MEDULLARY DORSAL HORN ACTIVITIES

Anatomical studies in the trigeminal system have also shown direct projections of the corticomedullary tract to the trigeminal nucleus caudalis (Jacquin et al. 1990; Desbois et al. 1999). Furthermore, as in the spinal dorsal horn, early electrophysiological studies showed that stimulation of the primary somatosensory cortex inhibited the evoked responses of a proportion of trigeminal nucleus caudalis nociceptive neurons (Sessle et al. 1981). A systematic study of corticofugal projections to the trigeminal nucleus caudalis showed that they originate mainly from the primary somatosensory and insular cortices and innervate both superficial and deep layers (Constandil et al. 2003). Corticofugal afferents arise primarily from contralateral structures and are somatotopically organized, as shown by the fact that distinct cortical projections are confined to the area in the trigeminal nucleus caudalis that contains the dura-sensitive neurons reported by Burstein and his colleagues (1998). Considering the experimental data that point to cortical spreading depression as the key event in the activation of the trigemino-vascular system (Bolay et al. 2002), and also taking into account the enhanced cortical excitability commonly found in migraine sufferers (see references and discussion in Pietrobon and Striessnig 2003), it is possible that the somatosensory and insular cortices contribute to central sensitization mechanisms that underlie migraines and other types of headache. These cortical areas could control trigeminal nucleus caudalis neurons via the amygdala or by more direct connections via the descending pain-modulating pathway. Support for this idea comes from functional imaging studies that implicate the midbrain PAG in the pathogenesis of the painful attack in acute migraine (Weiller et al. 1995).

Although the mediating pathways have not been identified, corticofugal controls are likely to be involved in the modulation of neurons in the medullary dorsal horn by behaviorally significant stimuli, as demonstrated in trained monkeys (Bushnell et al. 1984). This type of modulation, termed "task-related," may produce a greater neuronal response than that produced by equivalent stimuli in the absence of the relevant behavioral state. Indeed, the modulated responses were not necessarily occurring to cutaneous stimuli that invariably activated the neuron under passive conditions. Thus, thermally responsive cells may exhibit an additional task-related response to visual or motor cues involved in the behavioral task, but not to similar stimuli presented outside the task (Duncan et al. 1987). Many of these task-related responses demonstrated a consistent preferential association with either the visual stimulus or the motor response (hand movement), which indicates that the mechanism of the behavioral modulation was mediated by distinct modulatory networks involved in either sensory or motor preparation. Interestingly, neither the detection of the visual stimulus nor the movement of the hand were related to the functions normally ascribed to the trigeminal nucleus caudalis. This finding indicates that relevant information regarding the environment is disseminated to parts of the nervous system that may be directly or indirectly involved in the animal's ongoing behavior. Thus, neuronal responsiveness may bear no relationship to the features of stimuli that a sensory nucleus is capable of detecting and may be dependent entirely on the behavioral context within which a sensory signal is received. Given that similar task-related responses have been demonstrated in several cortical areas, the task-related changes in trigeminal neuronal activity could represent a corticofugal reiteration of the paradigm instructions.

CORTICOFUGAL MODULATION OF BULBOSPINAL CONTROLS

Corticofugal modulation of the subnucleus reticularis dorsalis: a substrate for the processing of nociceptive and motor activities? The dorsalmost aspect of the SRD receives strong, direct influences from numerous cortical regions including the motor, somatosensory, and insular cortices (Desbois et al. 1999). Various corticofugal influences could, via SRD collaterals, reach rostral and caudal sites in the CNS almost simultaneously. Perhaps one of the advantages conferred by single SRD cells projecting to both thalamic structures and the dorsal horn is that it allows for more precise temporal synchrony between the two target areas. From a general point of view, it has been suggested that the pyramidal system might implement and refine basic motor patterns generated by brainstem reticulospinal circuits (see Canedo 1997), and this could apply to those relayed at the level of the SRD. Based on findings showing that SRD efferents terminate in several CNS areas that influence motor processing, it is tempting to speculate that the SRD is a medullary link for the processing of nociceptive and motor activities. The cortex might, via pyramidal influences onto SRD neurons, coordinate the nociceptive information that ascends to it. Corticofugal mechanisms could allow the cortex to select its own inputs by suppressing or augmenting transmission of signals through SRD-hindbrain/forebrain pathways or by coordinating activities in spino-SRD-spinal circuits and thus selecting the relevant information caused by the noxious stimulus itself. Consistent with this proposal, behavioral studies in rats (Almeida et al. 1996) have shown modifications of motor responses, such as decreases in the latency of tail-flick withdrawal reactions, following glutamate injections in the SRD. In addition, the same studies showed that lesions that included the dorsal aspect of the SRD increased the latencies of the hot-plate, tail-flick (Almeida et al. 1996), and formalin-elicited withdrawal reactions (Almeida et al. 1999).

Corticofugal modulation of the PAG/RVM network: a common substrate for placebo and morphine analgesia? The first evidence that the opioid-linked PAG-RVM network could be activated by the psychological process of expectancy was pharmacological. Levine et al. (1978), using the dental postoperative pain model, demonstrated that placebo analgesia is reversed by systemic administration of the opioid antagonist naloxone. This observation has been repeatedly confirmed in both clinical and experimental pain models (Amanzio and Benedetti 1999). Furthermore, Lipman et al.

(1990) have reported endogenous opioid-like material in the cerebrospinal fluid of chronic pain patients whose pain level dropped following placebo administration. Evidence consistent with the view that this naloxone effect is through an action on central pain-modulating pathways comes from studies on human subjects by Petrovic and his colleagues (2002). These authors used positron emission tomography to study brain activity in subjects who were given the μ-opioid agonist fentanyl or a saline placebo and then were subjected to a painful thermal stimulus. They found a significant overlap between the areas of the brain activated by fentanyl and the saline placebo. These areas included the ACC and regions within the caudal pons/rostral medulla. Interestingly, they also observed that ACC activity covaried with activity in areas close to the PAG during both opioid and placebo analgesia, but not during the pain-only condition. This finding raises the possibility that a similar modulatory effect is mediated by the ACC, via the PAG, contributing to both placebo and morphine analgesia.

CORTICOTHALAMIC MODULATION

Cortical activity must be highly dependent on reciprocal interactions with thalamic relays, because there are nearly 10 times as many fibers projecting back from the cortex to the thalamus as there are in the forward direction from thalamus to cortex (Deschênes et al. 1998). The function of this massive feedback network in the processing of pain has not been fully elucidated, but attempts to address this question by Casey and his colleagues showed that the primary somatosensory cortex facilitates sensory transmission to ventrobasal thalamic neurons (Yuan et al. 1986). More recently, Krupa et al. (1999) showed that inactivation of the S1 cortex resulted not only in rapid changes in the receptive field properties of ventrobasal thalamic cells but also in a significant reduction in their ability to reorganize their receptive fields following peripheral deafferentation.

Moreover, Ergenzinger et al. (1998) showed that after several months of chronic delivery of an *N*-methyl-D-aspartate antagonist into the monkey primary somatosensory cortex, at the site at which the hand is represented, the tactile receptive fields of ventrobasal thalamic cells dramatically increased, but only in the hand region. As in other sensory systems, corticothalamic controls seem to excite relay cells directly by reducing the strength of the intrinsic inhibitory mechanisms affecting these cells, i.e., by disinhibiting them. Overall, these studies suggest that the primary sensory cortices, via their corticofugal projections, provide positive feedback for the "correct" input while at the same time suppressing irrelevant information (the "egocentric selection"; Rauschecker 1998).

The rat ventrobasal thalamus contains only excitatory neurons that project mainly to layer 4 of the S1 cortex. Descending projections in the thalamo-cortical loop originate primarily in layer 6 of the S1 cortex (Deschênes et al. 1998). The distal dendrites of ventrobasal neurons are densely innervated by these projections, which activate both ionotropic and metabotropic glutamate receptors. On their way to the thalamus, corticothalamic projections also send branches to reticular thalamic neurons, which are exclusively inhibitory and which project locally in the reticular thalamus or to the ventrobasal thalamus. Crick and Koch (1998) suggested, on the basis of the similar organization for the visual system, that the primary sensory cortices and their thalamic targets never form a strong, reciprocal loop. The reason for this "no-strong loop hypothesis" is that a reciprocal excitatory loop would be strong enough to throw the cortex into uncontrolled oscillations, as in epilepsy. Thus, it would be difficult for such a network to constrain its effects, probably because thalamic neurons are near the edge of excitation by the highly specific positive feedback loop circuitry (see Fig. 1 in Rauscheker 1998). However, because epilepsy or phenomena related to cortical spreading depression do occur, it is tempting to propose that disturbances in normal sensory processing within these loops could lead to modifications in perception and thus to the pain produced in absence of an organic lesion.

CONCLUSIONS

Taken together, these studies support the concept that CNS mechanisms that modulate pain do not consist only of a bottom-up process whereby a painful focus modifies the inputs to the next-higher level. The most important, most widespread source of top-down modulation arises from the cortex. Indeed, several cortical regions mediate subtle forms of plasticity by adjusting both thalamic and prethalamic maps and consequently altering all the modulatory mechanisms downstream as a result of sensory experience. Accordingly, functional imaging studies have shown that the activity of distinct cortical areas is closely related to the unpleasantness of the experience of pain and to changes in pain perception following manipulation of environmental factors (Rainville 2002; Ploghaus et al. 2003).

In the field of pain research, P.D. Wall and P.W. Nathan were among the first to propose that the brain has many ways and strategies for modifying the incoming information it receives, and sensations are not merely facsimiles in consciousness of every stimulus to the CNS. Selection is the main mechanism that generates a sensation, and thus, by means of modulation, the brain modifies the efficacy of certain inputs to the nervous system. The sensory pathways that convey nociceptive inputs are simultaneously collecting information from many sources. This basic somesthetic activity is not only relevant for pain, but could have a role in the continual transmission of information relevant to the integrity of the body. This information is constantly being selected and modulated in the context of producing an appropriate response.

As suggested by Wall (1989), such dynamic states may explain the extreme variability of painful stimuli and responses in apparently identical experiments with highly trained subjects performed by different laboratories and in studies on patients admitted to an emergency clinic. The brain's selection process could also explain another mismatch between experimental and clinical studies of pain modulation, such as the brief inhibitions of responses of dorsal horn neurons or spinal reflexes in experimental situations and the pain relief that persists for hours following the clinical manipulation of endogenous modulatory systems (e.g., see Carlsson 2002).

The relevance of corticofugal controls in pathological pain is underlined by their role in phantom limb perception and in the pain that occurs in the absence of detectable organic lesions. As shown by Ramachandran and his colleagues (1998), light touch on an amputee's face referred sensations from the face to a precise area on the phantom hand. The authors suggested that these changes could be due to modifications in cortical topography and that when the region of the somatosensory cortex formerly receiving inputs from the hand becomes silent, synapses from neighboring regions, which had previously been subliminal, now become active—a process that can be reinforced later by sprouting of neurites. This idea is supported by the fact that a facial map of the phantom hand may be present immediately after surgery (Borsook et al. 1998) and by psychophysical studies showing that in healthy subjects, complete local anesthesia of the thumb increased the perception of the size of the lips by approximately 50% without affecting the perception of the adjacent finger or digits on the contralateral side (Gandevia and Phegan 1999).

Harris (1999) proposed that pain without organic lesions such as those that result from phantom limbs and focal hand dystonias in writers, musicians, or keyboard operators could be due to a mismatch between motor intention, awareness of movement, and visual feedback. This situation would elicit plastic changes in the sensorimotor cortex, leading to an inappropriate cortical control of proprioception that produces a false mismatch between intention and movement, which in turn results in pain—in the same way that a mismatch between vestibular and visual sensations results in motion sickness. Support for this hypothesis includes the fact that watching a virtual image of a phantom limb move in synchrony with motor commands may relieve phantom limb pain (Ramachandran et al. 1998). In a similar way, motion sickness induced by optokinetic stimulation increases nausea and headache that persist longer in migraine sufferers compared to non-headache controls. Also, scalp tenderness increased during optokinetic stimulation in nauseated subjects, and pain in the fingertips, increased to a greater extent, and photophobia persisted longer, in migraine sufferers than in controls (Drummond 2002).

As a concluding statement, this chapter invites us to consider modulatory mechanisms in line with psychophysical, behavioral, and clinical evidence that pain perception is an active process. Curiously enough, these ideas bring together two a priori antagonistic views of CNS mechanisms of pain processing: "Pain would join sensations such as hunger and thirst and itch, which are best defined as needs that signify the next probable action. Pain is an attribute assigned by the brain as a quality" (Wall 1999). "Pain is a homeostatic emotion, akin to temperature, itch, hunger and thirst. That is, pain is both an aspect of interoception and a specific behavioral motivation" (Craig 2003).

ACKNOWLEDGMENTS

Luis Villanueva was supported by the CNRS, Institut UPSA de la Douleur, and Fonds Benoît. Howard Fields was supported by the University of California and by grants from the United States Public Health Service.

REFERENCES

Almeida A, Tavares I, Lima D. Projection sites of superficial or deep dorsal horn in the dorsal reticular nucleus. *Neuroreport* 1995; 6:1245–1248.

Almeida A, Tjolsen A, Lima D, Coimbra A, Hole K. The medullary dorsal reticular nucleus facilitates acute nociception in the rat. *Brain Res Bull* 1996; 39:7–15.

Almeida A, Storkson R, Lima D, Hole K, Tjolsen A. The medullary dorsal reticular nucleus facilitates pain behaviour induced by formalin in the rat. *Eur J Neurosci* 1999; 11:110–122.

Amanzio M, Benedetti F. Neuropharmacological dissection of placebo analgesia: expectation-activated opioid systems versus conditioning-activated specific subsystems. *J Neurosci* 1999; 19:484–494.

An X, Bandler R, Ongur D, et al. Prefrontal cortical projections to longitudinal columns in the midbrain periaqueductal gray in macaque monkeys. *J Comp Neurol* 1998; 401:455–479.

Andersson SA. Pain control by sensory stimulation. In: Bonica J, Liebeskind JC, Albe-Fessard D (Eds). *Proceedings of the Second World Congress on Pain,* Advances in Pain Research and Therapy, Vol. 3. New York: Raven Press, 1979, pp 569–585.

Bantick SJ, Wise RG, Ploghaus A, et al. Imaging how attention modulates pain in humans using functional MRI. *Brain* 2002; 125:310–319.

Basbaum AI, Clanton CH, Fields HL. Opiate and stimulus-produced analgesia: functional anatomy of a medullospinal pathway. *Proc Natl Acad Sci USA* 1976; 73:4685–4688.

Basbaum AI, Clanton CH, Fields HL. Three bulbospinal pathways from the rostral medulla of the cat: an autoradiographic study of pain modulating systems. *J Comp Neurol* 1978; 178:209–224.

Bederson JB, Fields HL, Barbaro NM. Hyperalgesia during naloxone-precipitated withdrawal from morphine is associated with increased ON-cell activity in the rostral ventromedial medulla. *Somatosens Motor Res* 1990; 7:185–203.

Bernard JF, Villanueva L, Carroué J, Le Bars D. Efferent projections from the subnucleus reticularis dorsalis (SRD): a *Phaseolus vulgaris* leucoagglutinin study in the rat. *Neurosci Lett* 1990; 116:257–262.

Besson JM, Rivot JP. Heterosegmental, heterosensory and cortical inhibitory effects on dorsal horn interneurones in the cat's spinal cord. *Electroenceph Clin Neurophysiol* 1972; 33:195–206.

Bolay H, Reuter U, Dunn AK, et al. Intrinsic brain activity triggers trigeminal meningeal afferents in a migraine model. *Nat Med* 2002; 8:136–142.

Borsook D, Becerra L, Fishman S, et al. Acute plasticity in the human somatosensory cortex following amputation. *Neuroreport* 1998; 9:1013–1017.

Bouhassira D, Le Bars D, Villanueva L. Heterotopic activation of Aδ and C fibres triggers inhibition of trigeminal and spinal convergent neurones in the rat. *J Physiol (Lond)* 1987; 389:301–317.

Bouhassira D, Villanueva L, Bing Z, Le Bars D. Involvement of the subnucleus reticularis dorsalis in diffuse noxious inhibitory controls in the rat. *Brain Res* 1992; 595:353–357.

Bouhassira D, Danziger N, Attal N, Guirimand F. Comparison of the pain suppressive effects of clinical and experimental painful conditioning stimuli. *Brain* 2003; 126:1068–1078.

Burkey AR, Carstens E, Wenniger JJ, Tang J, Jasmin L. An opioidergic cortical antinociception triggering site in the agranular insular cortex of the rat that contributes to morphine antinociception. *J Neurosci* 1996; 16:6612–6623.

Burkey AR, Carstens E, Jasmin L. Dopamine reuptake inhibition in the rostral agranular insular cortex produces antinociception. *J Neurosci* 1999; 19:4169–4179.

Burstein R, Yamamura H, Malick A, Strassman AM. Chemical stimulation of the intracranial dura induces enhanced responses to facial stimulation in brain stem trigeminal neurons. *J Neurophysiol* 1998; 79:964–982.

Burton H, Loewy D. Projections to the spinal cord from medullary somatosensory relay nuclei. *J Comp Neurol* 1977; 173:773–792.

Bushnell MC, Duncan GH, Dubner R, He LF. Activity of trigeminothalamic neurons in medullary dorsal horn of awake monkeys trained in a thermal discrimination task. *J Neurophysiol* 1984; 52:170–187.

Cadden SW, Villanueva L, Le Bars D. Depression of activities of dorsal horn convergent neurones by propriospinal mechanisms triggered by noxious inputs: comparison with diffuse noxious inhibitory controls (DNIC). *Brain Res* 1983; 275:1–11.

Canedo A. Primary motor cortex influences on the descending and ascending systems. *Prog Neurobiol* 1977; 51:287–335.

Carlsson C. Acupuncture mechanisms for clinically relevant long-term effects—reconsideration and a hypothesis. *Acupunct Med* 2002; 20:56–73.

Casale E, Light AR, Rustioni A. Direct projection of the corticospinal tract to the superficial laminae of the spinal cord in the rat. *J Comp Neurol* 1988; 278:275–286.

Casey KL, Svensson P, Morrow TJ, et al. Selective opiate modulation of nociceptive processing in the human brain. *J Neurophysiol* 2000; 84:525–533.

Cheema SS, Rustioni A, Whitsel BL. Light and electron microscopic evidence for a direct corticospinal projection to superficial laminae of the dorsal horn in cats and monkeys. *J Comp Neurol* 1984; 225:276–290.

Chung JM, Lee KH, Hori Y, Endo K, Willis WD. Factors influencing peripheral nerve stimulation produced inhibition of primate spinothalamic tract cells. *Pain* 1984; 19:277–293.

Constandil L, Monconduit L, Villanueva L. Corticofugal modulation of trigeminal nociception: anatomical studies in the rat. *Soc Neurosci Abstr* 2003.

Coulter JD, Maunz RA, Willis WD. Effects of stimulation of sensorimotor cortex on primate spinothalamic neurons. *Brain Res* 1974; 65:351–356.

Craig AD. A new view of pain as a homeostatic emotion. *Trends Neurosci* 2003; 26:303–307.

Craig AD, Reiman EM, Evans A, Bushnell MC. Functional imaging of an illusion of pain. *Nature* 1996; 384:258–260.

Crick F, Koch C. Constraints on cortical and thalamic projections: the no-strong loops hypothesis. *Nature* 1998; 391:245–250.

De Broucker T, Cesaro P, Willer JC, Le Bars D. Diffuse noxious inhibitory controls (DNIC) in man: involvement of a spino-reticular tract. *Brain* 1990; 113:1223–1234.

Desbois C, Le Bars D, Villanueva L. Organization of cortical projections to the medullary subnucleus reticularis dorsalis: a retrograde and anterograde tracing study in the rat. *J Comp Neurol* 1999; 410:178–196.

Deschênes M, Veinante P, Zhang ZW. The organization of corticothalamic projections: reciprocity versus parity. *Brain Res Rev* 1998; 28:286–308.

Delisle D, Plaghki L. La neurostimulation électrique transcutanée est-elle capable de modifier la perception de la douleur? Une méta-analyse. *Douleur Analgésie* 1990; 3:115–122.

Drummond PD. Motion sickness and migraine: optokinetic stimulation increases scalp tenderness, pain sensitivity in the fingers and photophobia. *Cephalalgia* 2002; 22:117–124.

Dugast C, Almeida A, Lima D. The medullary dorsal reticular nucleus enhances the responsiveness of spinal nociceptive neurons to peripheral stimulation in the rat. *Eur J Neurosci* 2003; 18:580–588.

Duncan GH, Bushnell MC, Dubner R. Task-related responses of monkey medullary dorsal horn neurons. *J Neurophysiol* 1987; 57:289–310.

Ergenzinger ER, Glasier MM, Hahm JO, Pons TP. Cortically induced thalamic plasticity in the primate somatosensory system. *Nat Neurosci* 1998; 1:226–229.

Fields HL, Bry J, Hentall I, Zorman G. The activity of neurons in the rostral medulla of the rat during withdrawal from noxious heat. *J Neurosci* 1983a; 3:2545–2552.

Fields HL, Vanegas H, Hentall ID, Zorman G. Evidence that disinhibition of brainstem neurones contributes to morphine analgesia. *Nature* 1983b; 306:684–686.

Fields HL, Malick A, Burstein R. Dorsal horn projection targets of on and off cells in the rostral ventromedial medulla. *J Neurophysiol* 1995; 74:1742–1759.

Fields HL, Basbaum AI, Heinricher MM. Central nervous system mechanisms of pain modulation. In: McMahon S, Koltzenburg M (Eds). *Textbook of Pain*. Edinburgh: Churchill Livingstone, 2004, in press.

Gandevia SC, Phegan CML. Perceptual distortions of the human body image produced by local anaesthesia, pain and cutaneous stimulation. *J Physiol (Lond)* 1999; 514.2:609–616.

Gao K, Mason P. Serotonergic raphe magnus cells that respond to noxious tail heat are not ON or OFF cells. *J Neurophysiol* 2000; 84(4):1719–1725.

Gao K, Kim YH, Mason P. Serotonergic pontomedullary neurons are not activated by antinociceptive stimulation in the periaqueductal gray. *J Neurosci* 1997; 17:3285–3292.

Gao K, Chen DO, Genzen JR, et al. Activation of serotonergic neurons in the raphe magnus is not necessary for morphine analgesia. *J Neurosci* 1998; 18(5):1860–1868.

Gardell LR, Vanderah TW, Gardell SE, et al. Enhanced evoked excitatory transmitter release in experimental neuropathy requires descending facilitation. *J Neurosci* 2003; 23:8370–8379.

Harris AJ. Cortical origin of pathological pain. *Lancet* 1999; 354:1464–1466.

Heinricher MM, Tortorici V. Interference with GABA transmission in the rostral ventromedial medulla: disinhibition of off-cells as a central mechanism in nociceptive modulation. *Neuroscience* 1994; 63(2):533–546.

Heinricher MM, Morgan MM, Tortorici V, et al. Disinhibition of off-cells and antinociception produced by an opioid action within the rostral ventromedial medulla. *Neuroscience* 1994; 63:279–288.

Hernandez A, Soto-Moyano R. Effect of morphine-induced cortical excitation on spinal sensory transmission. *J Neurosci Res* 1986; 15:217–222.

Jacquin MF, Wiegand MR, Renehan WE. Structure-function relationships in rat brain stem subnucleus interpolaris. VIII. Cortical inputs. *J Neurophysiol* 1990; 64:3–27.

Jasmin L, Rabkin SD, Granato A, Boudah A, Ohara P. Analgesia and hyperalgesia from GABA-mediated modulation of the cerebral cortex. *Nature* 2003; 424:316–320.

Johansen JP, Fields HL, Manning BH. The affective component of pain in rodents: direct evidence for a contribution of the anterior cingulate cortex. *Proc Natl Acad Sci USA* 2001; 98(14):8077–8082.

Kaplan H, Fields HL. Hyperalgesia during acute opioid abstinence: evidence for a nociceptive facilitating function of the rostral ventromedial medulla. *J Neurosci* 1991; 11(5):1433–1439.

Kosek E, Hansson P. Modulatory influence on somatosensory perception from vibration and heterotopic noxious conditioning stimulation (HCNS) in fibromyalgia patients and healthy subjects. *Pain* 1997; 70:41–51.

Koyama T, Kato K, Tanaka YZ, et al. Anterior cingulate activity during pain-avoidance and reward tasks in monkeys. *Neurosci Res* 2001; 39(4):421–30.

Krupa DJ, Ghazanfar AA, Nicolelis MA. Immediate thalamic sensory plasticity depends on corticothalamic feedback. *Proc Natl Acad Sci USA* 1999; 96:8200–8205.

Kunishio K, Haber SN. Primate cingulostriatal projection: limbic striatal versus sensorimotor striatal input. *J Comp Neurol* 1994; 350(3):337–356.

Le Bars D. Neuronal serotonin. In: Osborne NM, Hamon M (Eds). *Serotonin and Pain*. New York: John Wiley, 1988, pp 171–226.

Le Bars D, Dickenson AH, Besson JM. Diffuse noxious inhibitory controls (DNIC): I. Effects on dorsal horn convergent neurones in the rat. *Pain* 1979; 6:283–304.

Le Bars D, Chitour D, Kraus E, et al. The effect of systemic morphine upon diffuse noxious inhibitory controls (DNIC) in the rat: evidence for a lifting of certain descending inhibitory controls of dorsal horn convergent neurones. *Brain Res* 1981; 215:257–274.

Leung CG, Mason P. Physiological properties of raphe magnus neurons during sleep and waking. *J Neurophysiol* 1999; 81:584–595.

Levine JD, Gordon NC, Fields HL. The mechanism of placebo analgesia. *Lancet* 1978; 2:654–657.

Lima D. A spinomedullary projection terminating in the dorsal reticular nucleus of the rat. *Neuroscience* 1990; 34:577–589.

Linderoth B, Meyerson BA. Dorsal column stimulation: modulation of somatosensory and autonomic function. *Semin Neurosci* 1995; 7:263–277.

Lipman JJ, Miller BE, Mays KS, et al. Peak beta endorphin concentration in cerebrospinal fluid: reduced in chronic pain patients and increased during the placebo response. *Psychopharmacology* 1990; 102:112–116.

Lovick TA. The medullary raphe nuclei: a system for integration and gain control in autonomic and somatomotor responsiveness? *Exp Physiol* 1997; 82:31–41.

Marchand JE, Hagino N. Afferents to the periaqueductal gray in the rat: a horseradish peroxidase study. *Neuroscience* 1983; 9:95–106.

Mason P. Contributions of the medullary raphe and ventromedial reticular region to pain modulation and other homeostatic functions. *Annu Rev Neurosci* 2001; 24:737–777.

Mason P, Gao K. Raphe magnus serotonergic neurons tonically modulate nociceptive transmission. *Pain Forum* 1998; 7:143–150.

Mayer DJ, Wolfle TL, Akil H, Carder B, Liebeskind JC. Analgesia from electrical stimulation in the brainstem of the rat. *Science* 1971; 174:1351–1354.

McGaraughty S, Reinis S, Tsoukatos J. Two distinct unit activity responses to morphine in the rostral ventromedial medulla of awake rats. *Brain Res* 1993; 604:331–333.

Melzack R. Acupuncture and related forms of folk medicine. In: Wall PD, Melzack R (Eds). *Textbook of Pain*. Edinburgh: Churchill Livingstone, 1984, pp 691–700.

Melzack R, Wall PD. Pain mechanisms: a new theory. *Science* 1965; 150:971–979.

Miron D, Duncan GH, Bushnell MC. Effects of attention on the intensity and unpleasantness of thermal pain. *Pain* 1989; 39:345–352.

Monconduit L, Bourgeais L, Bernard JF, Villanueva L. Systemic morphine selectively depresses a thalamic link of widespread nociceptive inputs in the rat. *Eur J Pain* 2002a; 6:81–87.

Monconduit L, Desbois C, Villanueva L. The integrative role of the rat medullary subnucleus reticularis dorsalis in nociception. *Eur J Neurosci* 2002b; 16:937–944.

Morgan MM, Fields HL. Pronounced changes in the activity of nociceptive modulatory neurons in the rostral ventromedial medulla in response to prolonged thermal noxious stimuli. *J Neurophysiol* 1994; 72:1161–1170.

Morgan MM, Heinricher MM, Fields HL. Inhibition and facilitation of different nocifensor reflexes by spatially remote noxious thermal stimuli. *J Neurophysiol* 1994; 72(2):1152–1160.

Oliveras JL, Besson JM. Stimulation-produced analgesia in animals: behavioural investigations. *Prog Brain Res* 1988; 77:141–157.

Oliveras JL, Redjemi F, Guilbaud G, Besson JM. Analgesia induced by electrical stimulation of the inferior centralis nucleus of the raphe in the cat. *Pain* 1975; 1:139–145.

Oliveras JL, Montagne-Clavel J, Martin G. Drastic changes of ventromedial medulla neuronal properties induced by barbiturate anesthesia. I. Comparison of the single-unit types in the same awake and pentobarbital-treated rats. *Brain Res* 1991; 563:241–250.

Petrovic P, Kalso E, Petersson KM, Ingvar M. Placebo and opioid analgesia-imaging a shared neuronal network. *Science* 2002; 295:1737–1740.

Pietrobon D, Striessnig J. Neurobiology of migraine. *Nat Rev Neurosci* 2003; 4:386–398.

Ploghaus A, Tracey I, Gati JS, et al. Dissociating pain from its anticipation in the human brain. *Science* 1999; 284(5422):1979–1981.

Ploghaus A, Becerra L, Borras C, Borsook D. Neural circuitry underlying pain modulation: expectation, hypnosis, placebo. *Trends Cogn Sci* 2003; 7:197–200.

Potrebic SB, Fields HL, Mason P. Serotonin immunoreactivity is contained in one physiological cell class in the rat rostral ventromedial medulla. *J Neurosci* 1994; 14:1655–1665.

Raboisson, P, Dallel R, Bernard JF, Le Bars D, Villanueva L. Organization of efferent projections from the spinal cervical enlargement to the medullary subnucleus reticularis dorsalis and the adjacent cuneate nucleus: a PHA-L study in the rat. *J Comp Neurol* 1996; 367:503–517.

Rainville P. Brain mechanisms of pain affect and pain modulation. *Curr Opin Neurobiol* 2002; 12:195–204.

Ralston DD, Ralston HJ. The terminations of corticospinal tract axons in the macaque monkey. *J Comp Neurol* 1985; 242:325–337.

Ramachandran VS. Consciousness and body image: lessons from phantom limbs, Capgras syndrome and pain asymbolia. *Philos Trans R Soc Lond B Biol Sci* 1998; 353:1851–1859.

Rauscheker JP. Cortical control of the thalamus: top-down processing and plasticity. *Nat Neurosci* 1998; 1:179–180.

Sawamoto N, Honda M, Okada T, et al. Expectation of pain enhances responses to nonpainful somatosensory stimulation in the anterior cingulate cortex and parietal operculum/posterior insula: an event-related functional magnetic resonance imaging study. *J Neurosci* 2000; 20(19):7438–7445.

Sessle BJ, Hu JW, Dubner R, Lucier GE. Functional properties of neurons in cat trigeminal subnucleus caudalis (medullary dorsal horn). II. Modulation of responses to noxious and nonnoxious stimuli by periaqueductal gray, nucleus raphe magnus, cerebral cortex, and afferent influences, and effect of naloxone. *J Neurophysiol* 1981; 45:193–207.

Staud R, Robinson ME, Vierck CJ, Price DD. Diffuse noxious inhibitory controls (DNIC) attenuate temporal summation of second pain in normal males but not in normal females or fibromyalgia patients. *Pain* 2003; 101:167–174.

Tracey I, Ploghaus A, Gati JS, et al. Imaging attentional modulation of pain in the periaqueductal gray in humans. *J Neurosci* 2002; 22(7):2748–2752.

Villanueva L, Le Bars D. The activation of bulbo-spinal controls by peripheral nociceptive inputs: diffuse noxious inhibitory controls (DNIC). *Biol Res* 1995; 28:113–125.

Villanueva L, De Pommery J, Menétrey D, Le Bars D. Spinal afferent projections to subnucleus reticularis dorsalis in the rat. *Neurosci Lett* 1991; 134:98–102.

Villanueva L, Bernard JF, Le Bars D. Distribution of spinal cord projections from the medullary subnucleus reticularis dorsalis and the adjacent cuneate nucleus: a *Phaseolus vulgaris* leucoagglutinin (PHA-L) study in the rat. *J Comp Neurol* 1995; 352:11–32.

Villanueva L, Bouhassira D, Le Bars D. The medullary subnucleus reticularis dorsalis (SRD) as a key link in both the transmission and modulation of pain signals. *Pain* 1996; 67:231–240.

Villanueva L, Desbois C, Le Bars D, Bernard JF. Organization of diencephalic projections from the medullary subnucleus reticularis dorsalis and the adjacent cuneate nucleus: a retrograde and anterograde tracer study in the rat. *J Comp Neurol* 1998; 390:133–160.

Villemure C, Bushnell MC. Cognitive modulation of pain: how do attention and emotion influence pain processing? *Pain* 2002; 95(3):195–199.

Wall PD. Introduction. In: Wall PD, Melzack R (Eds). *Textbook of Pain,* 2nd ed. Edinburgh: Churchill Livingstone, 1989, pp 1–18.

Wall PD. Pain in context: the intellectual roots of pain research and therapy. In: Devor M, Wiesenfeld-Hallin Z, Rowbotham MC (Eds). *Proceedings of the 9th World Congress on Pain,* Progress in Pain Research and Management, Vol. 16. Seattle: IASP Press, 1999, pp 19–33.

Weiller C, May A, Limmroth V, et al. Brain stem activation in spontaneous human migraine attacks. *Nat Med* 1995; 1(7):658–660.

Woolf CJ, Mitchell D, Barrett GD. Antinociceptive effect of peripheral segmental electrical stimulation in the rat. *Pain* 1980; 8:237–252.

Yaksh TL. Direct evidence that spinal serotonin and noradrenaline terminals mediate the spinal antinociceptive effects of morphine in the periaqueductal grey. *Brain Res* 1979; 160:180–185.

Yezierski RP, Gerhart KD, Schrock BJ, Willis WD. A further examination of effects of cortical stimulation on primate spinothalamic tract cells. *J Neurophysiol* 1983; 49:424–441.

Yuan B, Morrow T, Casey KL. Corticofugal influences of S1 cortex on ventrobasal thalamic neurons in the awake rat. *J Neurosci* 1986; 6:3611–3617.

Zubieta JK, Smith YR, Bueller JA, et al. Regional mu opioid receptor regulation of sensory and affective dimensions of pain. *Science* 2001; 293:311–315.

Correspondence to: Luis Villanueva, DDS, PhD, INSERM E-216, Faculté de Chirurgie Dentaire, 11 Boulevard Charles de Gaulle, 63000 Clermont-Ferrand, France. Tel: 33-4-7317-7312; Fax: 33-4-7317-7306; email: luis.villanueva@u-clermont1.fr.

Part V

Novel Therapeutic Strategies: Preclinical and Clinical Approaches

*The Pain System in Normal and Pathological States:
A Primer for Clinicians,* Progress in Pain Research
and Management, Vol. 31, edited by Luis Villanueva,
Anthony Dickenson, and Hélène Ollat, IASP Press,
Seattle, © 2004.

14

Can the Evaluation of Drugs in Animal Pain Models Reliably Predict the Ability to Produce Clinical Analgesia?

Raymond G. Hill

*The Neuroscience Research Centre, Merck, Sharp and Dohme Research
Laboratories, Harlow, Essex, United Kingdom*

In the recent past, experimental work using traditional animal models, such as the carrageenan inflamed rat paw (Tjolsen and Hole 1997; Cowan 1999), has successfully predicted the analgesic properties of the cyclo-oxygenase 2 (COX-2) inhibitors (coxibs) and their utility in treating human pain conditions (see Boyce et al. 2001). Experimental work using such tests has been less successful, however, in predicting the clinical potential of other putative analgesics such as novel neuropeptide receptor antagonists (for review see Boyce et al. 2001; Boyce and Hill 2004). It is therefore relevant to ask, in a global sense, whether animal tests can always be assumed to be reliably predictive as we go forward and try to exploit potential novel pain targets emerging from knowledge of the human genome and those of other animal species. If the answer is negative, then it is necessary for those working in the field to cooperate in the discovery of new and better tests that will be more reliably predictive. The issue does not simply concern the availability of alternative tests, as many tests are already described in the literature (see Tjolsen and Hole 1997; Cowan 1999), but whether these tests have cross-species predictive value. In some cases, animal models that ought to be more reliable, by definition, will be based on the use of transgenic or gene knockout animals to validate a particular gene product as a target (see Akopian et al. 1999). In other cases, for example where there are observed interspecies differences in tissue distribution and in the pharmacology of neurotransmitters and their receptors, these factors are likely to make tests less predictive. This possibility is especially likely where there are differences between the critical binding sites of G-protein-coupled receptors across species such that agents optimized for binding to the human receptor may not be efficacious at the receptors found in those small animals commonly used in antinociceptive testing, and vice versa (see Boyce and Hill 2004 for discussion). Recent advances in the development of more disease-relevant models (see Monassi et al. 2003) and the use of imaging techniques that allow similar surrogate endpoints to be used in small animals and in human subjects (see Hill 2003) are encouraging steps in the right direction.

DEFINING THE PROBLEM

Until comparatively recently there was no issue to address because most drugs discovered and developed for use as analgesics in human subjects were variations on the common themes of opioids or nonsteroidal anti-inflammatory drugs (NSAIDs). Furthermore, the compounds of interest were evaluated in tests that had been optimized to show activity in these classes of drug by using calibration agents such as aspirin and morphine that had long been known to have analgesic properties in the clinical situation. For erudite reviews of the historical context, see Cowan (1999) and Tjolsen and Hole (1997). The increase in our knowledge of sensory neurotransmission processes in the last two decades of the 20th century had already started to generate targets that could not be validated in this time-honored way. This problem has now been compounded by the recent emergence of gene-based targets, where there is often no pre-existing base of pharmacological knowledge on which to design an experimental paradigm. It is arguable that the most important advances in drug-based treatment of pain have come from empirical observations on drugs that were introduced to therapeutics for an entirely different indication such as epilepsy or depression (see Dickinson et al. 2003). A posteriori experiments have sometimes been able to show antinociceptive properties when these drugs are subsequently tested in laboratory animals, but we now need to be able to predict such activity de novo in a reliable way or to accept that experimental medicine studies in human volunteers will have to take the place of unpredictive animal studies, in some cases at least.

WHAT ARE ANIMAL MODELS MODELING?

One complication that the experimental pharmacologist faces when scanning the literature for animal models that might be useful in the evaluation of putative analgesic drugs is that out of the plethora of reasons for setting up such models, drug evaluation is not the most common rationale. Much work on peripheral nerve lesions, for example, has had as its driver the desire to produce animals with a phenotype resembling the symptoms of patients experiencing neuropathic pain. The outcome of such studies has been remarkably successful, and it now possible to produce at will a group of rats that display regional hyperalgesia and allodynia (e.g., Dickenson et al. 2001). However, in terms of response to analgesic drugs, there is no a priori reason why the pharmacological phenotype of such an animal model should resemble its behavioral phenotype. Indeed, it has been postulated that for some purposes separate tests of pharmacological and physiological phenotype might be needed to adequately characterize the actions of a drug in a small laboratory animal (see Boyce and Hill 2004). It is also worth considering the hierarchy of quantitative measurements that might be made in order to record the effects of a drug on nociception. An objective measurement of, say, the firing of a single dorsal horn secondary sensory neuron may be a harder endpoint than a behavioral escape response, but it is a reductionist measurement that assumes that the spinal dorsal horn is the most important site of action for the drug in question. The behavioral measure, although less precise, is a more holistic endpoint that makes no assumptions other than the crucial one of a basic similarity between the physiology and pharmacology of the animal being studied as a model and that of the human. The only unequivocal animal model would be one derived from an understanding of the molecular mechanism of the particular human painful condition being modeled. This approach may not be generally feasible at the present time. A useful discussion of this dilemma in the context of neuropathic pain is found in Hansson et al. (2001). Cowan (1999) and Tjolsen and Hole (1997) describe the spectrum of currently available animal tests and their limitations.

DIFFERENCES AMONG SPECIES IN THE RESPONSE TO PUTATIVE ANALGESIC DRUGS

Perhaps the best recent example is the failure of the clinical evaluation of the substance P-receptor antagonists to confirm the analgesic potential of these agents suggested by a variety of animal pharmacology tests. This situation has been described in detail in a number of recent reviews (e.g., Boyce and Hill 2004) and so will only be given a brief treatment here.

Substance P has long been considered a prime candidate as a pain messenger because anatomical and immunochemical studies have shown its expression in small unmyelinated sensory fibers (Nagy et al. 1981) that transmit noxious information to the spinal cord. Substance P is released into the dorsal horn of the spinal cord following intense noxious stimulation (Duggan

et al. 1987). When applied onto the dorsal horn neurons, substance P produces prolonged excitation that resembles the activation observed following
noxious stimulation (Henry 1976). More recent work has shown that following peripheral noxious stimulation, neurokinin 1 (NK1) receptors become
internalized on dorsal horn neurons and that this effect can be blocked by
NK1-receptor antagonists (Mantyh et al. 1995). Based on this and other
evidence, the expectation was that centrally acting NK1-receptor antagonists
would be antinociceptive in animals and analgesic in humans and would
constitute a novel class of analgesic drugs.

One of the initial problems encountered with the evaluation of substance
P-receptor antagonists as potential analgesics was the marked species difference in NK1-receptor pharmacology. Compounds optimized for NK1 receptors expressed in humans typically have low affinity for these receptors in
rats or mice, the species most commonly used for antinociceptive studies
(Cowan 1999), and so the need for high doses in these species produced data
that were confounded by off-target activity (Rupniak et al. 1993). However,
good evidence from well-controlled studies in appropriate species (gerbils,
guinea pigs) with a substance P pharmacology similar to that in humans now
demonstrates unequivocally that substance P/NK1-receptor antagonists do
possess antinociceptive effects in animals. Persuasive preclinical data support an analgesic potential for substance P antagonists, particularly in pain
conditions associated with inflammation, nerve injury, and visceral pain
conditions. The analgesic profile of substance P antagonists in animals is
similar to that of the NSAIDs (Boyce and Hill 2004). However, the clinical
trial data available to date in dental postoperative pain, migraine, and a
variety of other pain conditions, obtained with compounds from a number of
different companies, indicate that substance P-receptor blockade does not
produce analgesia in human, even though coxibs and NSAIDs are effective
in at least some of the clinical paradigms used (Boyce and Hill 2004). In at
least two cases the negative data were obtained with substance P antagonist
drugs that were shown by PET studies to have been used at doses producing
full receptor occupancy in the brain.

Another example of species differences confounding analgesic drug research comes from studies on the role of drugs that block the cholecystokinin (CCK) receptor as adjuvants for opioid analgesics. In rats it is apparent
that block of the CCK_2 receptor potentiates the antinociceptive effects of
morphine, but in clinical studies, blocking the CCK_2 receptor with the antagonist L-365,260 failed to potentiate the effects of morphine in patients
with chronic neuropathic pain (McCleane 2003). This difference may be
explained by human subjects having CCK_1 receptors rather than CCK_2 receptors in the relevant anatomical locations in the spinal cord.

Where a novel target with no clinical precedent is selected, the predictive value of animal experiments is unknown. For example, impressive amelioration of the symptoms of experimental diabetic neuropathy has recently been demonstrated in rats following administration of sonic hedgehog protein (Calcutt et al. 2003). There is some uncertainty as to how well the administration of streptozotocin (the diabetes model used by Calcutt et al.) mimics the symptoms of human diabetic neuropathy. When this uncertainty is coupled to the differences in peripheral nerve regeneration capacity between rats and humans, the clinical outcome of studies with sonic hedgehog protein is not immediately predictable.

PREDICTIONS FROM HUMAN GENETICS AND NEW TARGETS FROM GENE CHIP EXPERIMENTS: HELP OR HINDRANCE?

It is tempting to suggest that there must be an important genetic component in many pain states. For example, not every patient who experiences a zoster infection suffers the distress of postherpetic neuralgia, and injury to peripheral nerves does not automatically lead to neuropathic pain. There are sex-related differences in the perception of pain in humans (e.g., see Cairns et al. 2001) and in the response to some opioid analgesic drugs (Gear et al. 1999; Zubieta et al. 2002). Recent evidence suggests that the *mc1r* gene is crucial in the response of female mice and humans to κ-opioids (Mogil et al. 2003). If we could understand at the genetic level why some patients are more likely to be victims of intractable pain, we might be able to produce better animal models. Human genetic disorders leading to changes in pain perception are uncommon, perhaps because of the essential survival value of the ability to feel pain. However, when such mutations can be studied, they provide the best evidence we can have for the involvement of a particular gene product in nociception. Perhaps the most extreme condition reported in humans is the congenital insensitivity to pain associated with defects in the nerve growth factor (NGF) signaling system, such as mutations in the gene coding the TrkA receptor at which the growth factor acts (see Bonkowsky et al. 2003). The phenotype of patients with this rare disorder indicates that blocking the effects of NGF would produce analgesia and also that this treatment would be associated with unacceptable side effects. A less extreme pain-related polymorphism has been reported by Zubieta et al. (2003), who showed that individuals homozygous for the met[158] allele of catechol-O-methyltransferase had a higher sensitivity to pain than did those who were homozygous for the val[158] allele.

The evaluation of the effects of peripheral nerve lesions or local inflammation on nociceptive behavior has recently developed into a detailed examination of the effects of these insults on the regulation of gene expression. In some cases it is unquestioned that such investigations help us validate drug targets or elucidate novel mechanisms of action, particularly when specific questions are asked about the regulation of a small number of mechanistically related genes. The increased availability of gene arrays has allowed investigations in which more global studies can be conducted on the effects on thousands of genes in parallel (see Wang et al. 2002). Such studies generate enormous data sets showing downregulation of some genes and upregulation of others, contributing to the overall message that chronic pain results from a complex, interconnected series of events. They do not, however, tell us how to use this information to provide a better animal model of the human pain experience.

The most abundant targets remain G-protein-coupled receptors; new members of this group continue to be discovered, although we are probably close to knowing the identity of all of the genes coding this family of proteins. For example, the Mrg or sensory-neuron-specific receptors (SNSRs) (Dong et al. 2001; Lembo et al. 2002) have recently been discovered specifically located on small (presumably nociceptive) sensory neurons. These receptors are substrates for a number of naturally occurring neuropeptides with the highest affinity to a family of opioid peptides known as bovine adrenal medullary peptides (BAMs), although their binding is not opioid-like as it is not sensitive to opioid receptor antagonists (Lembo et al. 2002). There are marked species differences in the number of these receptors and in the precise populations of dorsal root ganglion cells on which they are found. Unless the homologue of the most important human member of this family can be identified, there is little chance of making a knockout mouse that might help researchers to evaluate the utility of the target, and the evaluation of blocking drugs optimized for the human receptor(s) in small animals is likely to be very difficult.

THE UTILITY OF TRANSGENIC ANIMALS

It is interesting to note that the evidence obtained from studies with NK1-receptor knockout mice supporting the role of substance P and NK1 receptors in pain is less compelling than has been reported for nonpeptide antagonists, and it is relevant to ask whether the search for such compounds to evaluate as analgesics would have been so widely followed if the phenotype of the knockout mice had been known before the discovery of nonpeptide antagonists. It is not clear why there should be differences in the antinociceptive profile of NK1-receptor antagonists and in the phenotype of NK1 knockout mice. Nonspecific actions of NK1-receptor antagonists contributing to the antinociceptive effects can probably be ruled out because many of the studies with antagonist drugs were well-controlled, with enantioselective antagonism being demonstrated (Boyce and Hill 2004). It seems most likely that the differences may relate to compensatory changes in the knockout mice as a result of the lifelong absence of NK1 receptors, but it is intriguing to speculate that knockout mice may be a more discriminant model than the use of a blocking drug in a wild-type animal. The predictive value of the phenotype of knockout mice is not always certain, and the phenotype of the COX-1 and COX-2 knockouts (see Ballou et al. 2000) did not predict that the full spectrum of analgesia obtainable with an NSAID could be achieved with an agent that selectively blocks only COX-2 (see Boyce et al. 2001). The phenotype of the microsomal prostaglandin E (PGE)-synthase knockout mouse predicts that drugs which block this enzyme would have interesting potential as anti-inflammatory analgesics (Trebino et al. 2003), but in view of the COX-knockout data, it is questionable how reliable this prediction will turn out to be.

A gene deletion mutant mouse lacking functional DREAM (downstream regulatory element antagonistic modulator, which suppresses transcription from human prodynorphin) has now been engineered (Cheng et al. 2002); this mouse shows a striking reduction in its responses both to acute noxious stimuli and to inflammatory hyperalgesia but otherwise has a wild-type behavioral phenotype. The role of dynorphin in controlling nociceptive threshold is complex; it can be antinociceptive by acting as an agonist at κ-opioid receptors but can also be pronociceptive through a facilitatory action at NMDA receptors (see Vogt 2002). The decreased sensitivity to noxious stimuli in DREAM knockout mice seems to be due to increased activity of dynorphin at κ-opioid receptors because it was restored to the level seen in wild-type mice by administration of the selective κ-opioid receptor antagonist nor-binaltorphimine (Cheng et al. 2002). It is difficult at present to see how a DNA-binding protein such as DREAM could be addressed as a drug discovery target, and thus the knockout mice are currently of little value in facilitating analgesic drug discovery.

At the present time one can only conclude that transgenic mice, especially knockouts, are useful in the study of analgesic phenomena but that by themselves they do not fill the need for fully predictive models capable of identifying the best targets for analgesic drug discovery.

CAN WE BRIDGE THE GAP BETWEEN LABORATORY ANIMALS AND HUMANS?

It is important to realize that although animal models of pain states can produce a simple, reproducible, and consistent phenotype (see Dickenson et al. 2001), the typical human pain patient (see, e.g., Samanta et al. 2003) displays a complex, variable, and often progressive phenotype. Put simply, the condition we seek to model is not itself easily characterized. A clinical expert in the field concluded that a mechanism-based classification of pain is currently not feasible (Hansson 2003). It is therefore necessary for us to focus on what is achievable and to accept that although clinical pain may not be easily modeled, there may be certain common features between the clinical pain experience and what one can measure in experimental animal tests. These common features may allow successful predictive drug evaluations to be conducted. The most favorable situation would be produced by identifying a parameter that could be quantified in a small laboratory animal, then utilized in human experimental medicine studies in volunteers, and lastly used as a surrogate endpoint in patients. It is noteworthy that the measures that best illustrate the patient's pain experience (e.g., inability to sleep or to walk without assistance or discomfort) are not often the measures chosen by the pain scientist for study in experimental animals. It is pleasing to acknowledge that progress is being made; recent publications indicate that a number of groups are now trying to study their animal subjects in the same manner as patients using appropriate chronic endpoints. For example, Monassi et al. (2003) have been able to demonstrate that a subpopulation of a group of rats subjected to sciatic nerve injury displayed social interaction and sleep/waking changes typical of those reported in patients with chronic pain. Kerins et al. (2003) showed that inflammation of the temporomandibular joint in rats produced changes in meal pattern and duration that were normalized following administration of the NSAID analgesic, ibuprofen. Similarly, Nagakura et al. (2003) were able to dissect out the time course and progression of allodynia and hyperalgesia in rats with arthritis induced by complete Freund's adjuvant. There was surprisingly good correlation between the activity of analgesic drugs in these rats and their observed utility in arthritic patients; morphine, tramadol, indomethacin, and diclofenac all effectively relieved joint hyperalgesia. Villaneuva (2000) has pointed out that chronic pain in humans is not always associated with tissue damage or injury. This observation underlines the importance of using novel integrative approaches to bridge the gap between experimental and clinical pain.

One recent report (Butelman et al. 2003) described the study of capsaicin-induced hypersensitivity in unanesthetized primates. This test has also been used in conscious human volunteers (Petersen et al. 2003), but even this approach is not without its pitfalls. When the anticonvulsant lamotrigine was studied in human volunteers it failed to show analgesic efficacy in this paradigm, even though it has demonstrated utility in some neuropathic pain patients (Petersen et al. 2003). The authors concluded that the analgesic effects of this drug depend on some nerve-injury-induced abnormality that cannot be simulated in healthy volunteers.

It is becoming increasingly apparent that there is developmental learning in pain-related systems in animals and in humans (Waldenstrom et al. 2003) and that even humans can be sorted into graded nociceptive categories using an experimental medicine approach (Coghill et al. 2003).

THE FUTURE?

There is no doubt that broad-based holistic approaches are need to evaluate new analgesic drugs. However, some techniques, such as neuronal ensemble recordings, which are accessible for animal studies, are not easily used in human studies (see Villaneuva 2000). The advances in the use of imaging techniques, especially in functional magnetic resonance imaging (fMRI), provides our best chance of developing a truly bridging technology between animal and human experimental subjects and patient populations (Jones et al. 2003). Borsook et al. (2003) have recently been able to show somatotopic activation of the human trigeminal ganglion using fMRI following either innocuous or noxious stimuli applied to the peripheral receptive fields on the head, indicating that spatial resolution is no longer a limiting factor. Strigo et al. (2003) have been able to show differences in the pattern of brain activation following either visceral or somatic sensory stimulation and distinct fMRI activation patterns depending on whether the stimuli applied were noxious or innocuous. Studies with analgesic drug regimens are starting to appear, and the placebo response is being characterized (Benedetti et al. 2003). It is therefore appropriate to show a measure of optimism about the prospects for modeling pain states in animals and in humans and for the likelihood of being able to obtain information reliably predicting analgesic efficacy.

However, it is also important not to oversimplify the problem facing us. Jones et al. (2003) express it thus: "The brain does not share the construct for pain perception and treatment that the medical profession would like to impose upon it. It is premature to reclassify pain on a physiological basis." We still cannot answer the key questions of whether there is a behavioral or physiological event that can be unequivocally interpreted as signaling pain in nonhuman species and whether there is a single or multiple paradigm that can be used reliably to predict clinical analgesic efficacy. It is indisputable, however, that if we do succeed in unraveling these complexities, our success will owe much to the pioneering studies of Jean-Marie Besson and his colleagues on the physiological and functional anatomical basis of pain perception.

REFERENCES

Akopian AN, Souslova V, England S, et al. The tetrodotoxin-resistant sodium channel SNS has a specialized function in pain pathways. *Nat Neurosci* 1999; 2:541–548.

Ballou L, Botting R, Goorha S, et al. Nociception in cyclo-oxygenase isoenzyme-deficient mice. *Proc Natl Acad Sci USA* 2000; 97:10272–10276.

Benedetti F, Pollo A, Lopiano L, et al. Conscious expectation and unconscious conditioning in analgesic, motor and hormonal placebo/nocebo responses. *J Neurosci* 2003; 23:4315–4323.

Bonkowsky JL, Johnson J, Carey JC, et al. An infant with primary tooth loss and palmar hyperkeratosis: a novel mutation in the NTRK1 gene causing congenital insensitivity to pain with anhidrosis. *Pediatrics* 2003; 112:237–241.

Borsook D, DaSilva AFM, Ploghaus A, et al. Specific and somatotopic functional magnetic resonance imaging activation in the trigeminal ganglion by brush and noxious heat. *J Neurosci* 2003; 23:7897–7903.

Boyce S, Hill RG. Substance P (NK1) receptor antagonists—analgesics or not? In: Holzer P (Ed). *Tachykinins,* Handbook of Experimental Pharmacology, Vol. 164. Berlin: Springer-Verlag, 2004, pp 441–457.

Boyce S, Ali Z, Hill RG. New developments in analgesia. *Drug Discovery World* 2001:2:31–35.

Butelman ER, Ball JW, Harris TJ, et al. Topical capsaicin-induced allodynia in unanaesthetized primates: pharmacological modulation. *J Pharm Exp Ther* 2003; 306:1106–1114.

Cairns BE, Hu JW, Arendt-Nielsen L, et al. Sex-related differences in human pain and rat afferent discharge evoked by injection of glutamate into the masseter muscle. *J Neurophysiol* 2001; 86:782-791.

Calcutt NA, Allendoerfer KL, Mizisin AP, et al. Therapeutic efficacy of sonic hedgehog protein in experimental diabetic neuropathy. *J Clin Invest* 2003; 111:507–514.

Cheng H-YM, Pitcher GM, Laviolette SR, et al. DREAM is a critical transcriptional repressor for pain modulation. *Cell* 2002; 108:31–43.

Coghill RC, McHaffie JG, Yen Y-F. Neural correlates of interindividual differences in the subjective experience of pain. *Proc Natl Acad Sci USA* 2003; 100:8538–8542.

Cowan A. Animal models of pain. In: Sawynok J, Cowan A (Eds). *Novel Aspects of Pain Management.* New York: Wiley-Liss, 1999, pp 21–47.

Dickenson AH, Matthews EA, Suzuki R. Central nervous system mechanisms of pain in peripheral neuropathy. In: Hansson PT, Fields HL, Hill RG, Marchettini P (Eds). *Neuropathic Pain: Pathophysiology and Treatment,* Progress in Pain Research and Management, Vol. 21. Seattle: IASP Press, 2001, pp 85–106.

Dickinson T, Lee K, Spanswick D, Munro FE. Leading the charge–pioneering treatments in the fight against neuropathic pain. *Trends Pharmacol Sci* 2003; 24:555–557.

Dong X, Han S-K, Zylka MJ, Simon MI, Anderson DJ. A diverse family of GPCRs expressed in specific subsets of nociceptive sensory neurons. *Cell* 2001; 106:619–632.

Duggan AW, Morton CR, Zhao ZQ, et al. Noxious heating of the skin releases immunoreactive substance P in the substantia gelatinosa of the cat: a study with antibody microprobes. *Brain Res* 1987; 403:345–349.

Gear RW, Miaskowski C, Gordon NC, et al. The kappa opioid nalbuphine produces gender- and dose-dependent analgesia and antianalgesia in patients with postoperative pain. *Pain* 1999; 83:339–345.

Hansson P. Difficulties in stratifying neuropathic pain by mechanisms *Eur J Pain* 2003; 7:353–357.

Hansson P, Lacerenza M, Marchettini P. Aspects of clinical and experimental neuropathic pain: the clinical perspective. In: Hansson PT, Fields HL, Hill RG, Marchettini P (Eds). *Neuropathic Pain: Pathophysiology and Treatment,* Progress in Pain Research and Management, Vol. 21. Seattle: IASP Press, 2001, pp 1–18.

Henry JL. Effects of substance P on functionally identified units in cat spinal cord. *Brain Res* 1976; 114:439–451.

Hill RG. New targets for analgesic drugs. In: Dostrovsky JO, Carr DB, Koltzenburg M (Eds). *Proceedings of the 10th World Congress on Pain,* Progress in Pain Research and Management, Vol. 24. Seattle: IASP Press, 2003, pp 419–436.

Jones AKP, Kulkarni B, Derbyshire SWG. Pain mechanisms and their disorders. *Br Med Bull* 2003; 65:83–93.

Kerins CA, Carlson DS, McIntosh JE, et al. Meal pattern changes associated with temporomandibular joint inflammation/pain in rats: analgesic effects. *Pharmacol Biochem Behav* 2003; 75:181–189.

Lembo PMC, Grazzini E, Groblewski T, et al. Proenkephalin A gene products activate a new family of sensory neuron-specific GPCRs. *Nat Neurosci* 2002; 5:201–209.

Mantyh PW, DeMaster E, Malhotra A, et al. Receptor endocytosis and dendrite reshaping in spinal neurons after somatosensory stimulation. *Science* 1995; 268:1629–1632.

McCleane GJ. A randomised, double-blind, placebo-controlled crossover study of the cholecystokinin 2 antagonist L-365,260 as an adjunct to strong opioids in chronic human neuropathic pain. *Neurosci Lett* 2003; 338:151–154.

Mogil JS, Wilson SG, Chesler EJ, et al. The melanocortin-1 receptor gene mediates female specific mechanisms of analgesia in mice and humans. *Proc Natl Acad Sci USA* 2003; 100:4867–4872.

Monassi CR, Bandler R, Keay KA. A subpopulation of rats show social and sleep-waking changes typical of chronic neuropathic pain following peripheral nerve injury. *Eur J Neurosci* 2003; 17:1907–1920.

Nagakura Y, Okada M, Kohara A, et al. Allodynia and hyperalgesia in adjuvant-induced arthritic rats: time course of progression and efficacy of analgesics. *J Pharmacol Exp Ther* 2003; 306:490–497.

Nagy JI, Hunt SP, Iversen LL, et al. Biochemical and anatomical observations on the degeneration of peptide-containing primary afferent neurons after neonatal capsaicin. *Neuroscience* 1981; 6:1923–1934.

Petersen KL, Maloney A, Hoke F, et al. A randomized study of the effect of oral lamotrigine and hydromorphone on pain and hyperalgesias following heat/capsaicin sensitization. *J Pain* 2003; 4:400–406.

Rupniak NM, Boyce S, Williams AR, et al. Antinociceptive activity of NK1 receptor antagonists: non-specific effects of racemic RP67580. *Br J Pharmacol* 1993; 110:1607–1613.

Samanta J, Kendall J, Samanta A. Polyarthralgia. *BMJ* 2003; 326:859.

Strigo IA, Duncan GH, Bolvin M, et al. Differentiation of visceral and cutaneous pain in the human brain. *J Neurophysiol* 2003; 89:3294–3303.

Tjolsen A, Hole K. Animal models of analgesia. In: Dickenson A, Besson J-M (Eds). *The Pharmacology of Pain,* Handbook of Experimental Pharmacology, Vol. 130. Berlin: Springer-Verlag, 1997, pp 1–20.

Trebino CE, Stock JL, Gibbons CP, et al. Impaired inflammatory and pain responses in mice lacking an inducible prostaglandin E synthase. *Proc Natl Acad Sci USA* 2003; 100:9044–9049.

Villaneuva L. Is there a gap between preclinical and clinical studies of analgesia? *Trends Pharmacol Sci* 2000; 21:461–462.

Vogt BA. Knocking out the DREAM to study pain. *N Engl J Med* 2002; 347:362–364.

Wang H, Sun H, Della Penna K, et al. Chronic neuropathic pain is accompanied by global changes in gene expression and shares pathobiology with neurodegenerative diseases *Neuroscience* 2002; 114:529–546.

Waldenstrom A, Thelin J, Thimansson E, et al. Developmental learning in a pain-related system: evidence for a cross-modality mechanism. *J Neurosci* 2003; 23:7719–7725.

Zubieta J-K, Smith YR, Bueller JA, et al. μ-Opioid receptor-mediated antinociceptive responses differ in men and women. *J Neurosci* 2002; 22:5100–5107.

Zubieta J-K, Heitzeg MM, Smith YR, et al. COMT val[158] genotype affects μ-opioid neurotransmitter responses to a pain stressor. *Science* 2003; 299:1240–1243.

Correspondence to: Raymond G. Hill, PhD, Licensing and External Research, Europe, Merck, Sharp and Dohme Research Laboratories, Terlings Park, Harlow, Essex, CM20 2QR, United Kingdom. Email: hillr@merck.com.

The Pain System in Normal and Pathological States: A Primer for Clinicians, Progress in Pain Research and Management, Vol. 31, edited by Luis Villanueva, Anthony Dickenson, and Hélène Ollat, IASP Press, Seattle, © 2004.

15

Bone Cancer Pain: Mechanisms and Potential Therapies

Patrick W. Mantyh

Neurosystems Center and Departments of Preventive Sciences, Psychiatry, Neuroscience, and Cancer Center, University of Minnesota, and Veterans Affairs Medical Center, Minneapolis, Minnesota, USA

Although bone cancer pain can be severe and is relatively common, as it frequently arises from metastases from breast, prostate, and lung tumors, relatively little is known about the basic mechanisms that generate and maintain this type of chronic pain. To begin to define the mechanisms that give rise to bone cancer pain, we developed a mouse model using the intramedullary injection of osteolytic sarcoma cells into the mouse femur (Fig. 1) (Schwei et al. 1999). Critical to this model is ensuring that the tumor cells are confined within the marrow space of the injected femur and that they do not invade adjacent soft tissues, which would directly affect the joints and the muscles, making behavioral analysis problematic (Schwei et al. 1999; Honore et al. 2000a; Luger et al. 2001). Following injection the tumor cells proliferate, and ongoing, movement-evoked, and mechanically evoked pain-related behaviors develop that increase in severity with time (Table I). These pain behaviors correlate with the progressive tumor-induced bone destruction that ensues, which appears to mimic the condition in patients with primary or metastatic bone cancer. These models have allowed us to gain mechanistic insights into how cancer pain is generated and how the sensory information it initiates is processed as it moves from sense organ to the cerebral cortex under a constantly changing molecular architecture. As detailed below, these insights promise to fundamentally change the way cancer pain is controlled.

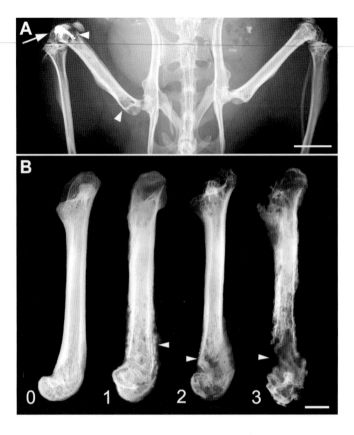

Fig. 1. Progressive destruction of mineralized bone in mice with bone cancer. (A) Low-power anterior-posterior radiograph of mouse pelvis and hindlimbs after a unilateral injection of sarcoma cells into the distal part of the femur and closure of the injection site with an amalgam plug (arrow), which prevents the tumor cells from growing outside the bone (Honore et al. 2000a). (B) Radiographs show the progressive loss of mineralized bone caused by tumor growth and represent the stages of bone destruction in the murine femur. At week 1 there is a minor loss of bone near the distal head (arrow); at week 2, substantial loss of mineralized bone at both the proximal and distal (arrow) heads; and at week 3, loss of mineralized bone throughout the entire femur and fracture of the distal head (arrow). Scale bar: 2 mm. Modified from Schwei et al. (1999).

PRIMARY AFFERENT SENSORY NEURONS

Primary afferent sensory neurons are the gateway by which sensory information from peripheral tissues is transmitted to the spinal cord and brain (Fig. 2), and these neurons innervate the skin and every internal organ of the body, including mineralized bone, marrow, and periosteum. The cell bodies of sensory fibers that innervate the head and body are housed in the trigeminal and dorsal root ganglia, respectively, and can be divided into two

Table I
Ongoing, movement-evoked, and mechanically evoked pain-related behaviors increase
in severity with time in the mouse femur model of bone cancer pain

Pain Behavior	Naive	Sham	Sarcoma		
			Day 6	Day 10	Day 14
I. Ongoing Pain (over 2-minute period)					
Guarding (sec)	0.4 ± 0.2	1.4 ± 0.5	2.1 ± 0.5	*4.3 ± 0.8*	*15.2 ± 3.3*
No. flinches	1.7 ± 0.7	3.1 ± 0.7	7.7 ± 1.6	*13.0 ± 2.0*	*24.5 ± 3.8*
II. Movement-Evoked Pain					
Ambulatory pain					
Forced†	4.7 ± 0.3	4.4 ± 0.3	3.8 ± 0.4	*2.5 ± 0.3*	*2.3 ± 0.3*
Normal‡	4.0 ± 0.0	3.9 ± 0.1	3.7 ± 0.4	*3.5 ± 0.3*	*2.7 ± 0.3*
Palpation-evoked pain (over 2-minute period)					
Guarding (sec)	0.4 ± 0.4	1.4 ± 0.5	1.9 ± 0.6	*7.1 ± 0.6*	*18.1 ± 4.0*
No. flinches	2.0 ± 1.2	3.1 ± 0.7	7.0 ± 2.1	*19.0 ± 1.1*	*30.5 ± 5.1*

Note: Italic type denotes significant difference from sham surgery ($P < 0.05$).
† Forced ambulation on rotarod. Score: 5 (normal) to 0 (impaired).
‡ Limb use during normal ambulation. Score: 4 (normal) to 0 (impaired).

major categories: myelinated A fibers and smaller-diameter unmyelinated C fibers. Nearly all large-diameter myelinated Aβ fibers normally conduct non-noxious stimuli applied to the skin, joints, and muscles, and thus these large sensory neurons usually do not conduct noxious stimuli (Djouhri et al. 1998). In contrast, most small-diameter sensory fibers—unmyelinated C fibers and finely myelinated A fibers—are specialized sensory neurons known as nociceptors, whose major function is to detect environmental stimuli that are perceived as harmful and convert them into electrochemical signals that are then transmitted to the central nervous system (CNS). Unlike primary sensory neurons involved in vision or olfaction, which are required to detect only one type of sensory stimulus (light or chemical odorants, respectively), individual primary sensory neurons of the pain pathway have the remarkable ability to detect a wide range of stimulus modalities, including those of a physical and chemical nature (Basbaum and Jessel 2000; Julius and Basbaum 2001). To accomplish this, nociceptors express an extremely diverse repertoire of transduction molecules that can sense forms of noxious stimulation (thermal, mechanical, and chemical), albeit with varying degrees of sensitivity.

The past few years have seen remarkable progress toward understanding the signaling mechanisms and specific molecules that nociceptors use to detect noxious stimuli. For example, the vanilloid receptor TRPV1 (formerly known as VR1), which is expressed by most nociceptors, detects heat

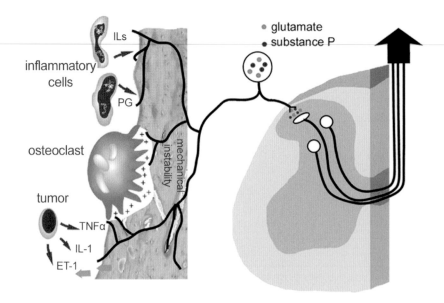

Fig. 2. Sensory neurons and detection of noxious stimuli due to tumor cells. Nociceptors use a diversity of signal-transduction mechanisms to detect noxious physiological stimuli, and many of these mechanisms may be involved in driving cancer pain. Thus, when nociceptors are exposed to products of tumor cells, tissue injury, or inflammation, their excitability is altered, and this nociceptive information is relayed to the spinal cord and then to higher centers of the brain. Some of the mechanisms that appear to be involved in generating and maintaining cancer pain include activation of nociceptors by factors such as extracellular protons (+), endothelin-1 (ET-1), interleukins (ILs), prostaglandins (PG), and tumor necrosis factor α (TNF-α).

(Kirschstein et al. 1999) and also appears to detect extracellular protons (Bevan and Geppetti 1994; Caterina et al. 2000; Welch et al. 2000) and lipid metabolites (Tominaga et al. 1998; Nagy and Rang 1999). In order to detect noxious mechanical stimuli, nociceptors express mechanically gated channels that initiate a signaling cascade upon excessive stretch (Price et al. 2001). The cells also express several purinergic receptors capable of sensing adenosine triphosphate (ATP), which may be released from cells upon excessive mechanical stimulation (Krishtal et al. 1988; Xu and Huang 2002).

To sense noxious chemical stimuli, nociceptors express a complex array of receptors capable of detecting inflammation-associated factors released from damaged tissue. These factors include protons (Bevan and Geppetti 1994; Caterina et al. 2000), endothelins (Nelson and Carducci 2000), prostaglandins (Alvarez and Fyffe 2000), bradykinin (Alvarez and Fyffe 2000), and nerve growth factor (McMahon 1996). Aside from providing promising targets for the development of more selective analgesics, identification of receptors expressed on the nociceptor surface has increased our understanding of how different tumors generate cancer pain in the peripheral tissues they invade and destroy.

In addition to expressing channels and receptors that detect tissue injury, sensory neurons are highly "plastic" in that they can change their phenotype in the face of a sustained peripheral injury. Following tissue injury, sensory neuron subpopulations alter patterns of signaling peptide and growth factor expression (Woolf and Salter 2000). This change in phenotype of the sensory neuron in part underlies peripheral sensitization, whereby the activation threshold of nociceptors is lowered so that a stimulus that would normally be mildly noxious is perceived as highly noxious (hyperalgesia). Damage to a peripheral tissue also activates previously "silent" or "sleeping" nociceptors, which then become highly responsive both to normally non-noxious stimuli (allodynia) and to noxious stimuli (hyperalgesia).

There are several examples of nociceptors that undergo peripheral sensitization in experimental cancer models (Schwei et al. 1999; Honore et al. 2000a; Luger et al. 2001). In normal mice, the neurotransmitter substance P is synthesized by nociceptors and released in the spinal cord in response to a noxious, but not to a non-noxious, palpation of the femur. In mice with bone cancer, normally nonpainful palpation of the affected femur induces the release of substance P from primary afferent fibers that terminate in the spinal cord. Substance P in turn binds to and activates the neurokinin-1 receptor that is expressed by a subset of spinal cord neurons (Mantyh et al. 1995a; Hunt and Mantyh 2001). Similarly, normally non-noxious palpation of tumor-bearing limbs of mice with bone cancer also induces the expression of c-fos protein in spinal cord neurons. In normal animals that do not have cancer, only noxious stimuli will induce the expression of c-fos in the spinal cord (Hunt et al. 1987). Thus, peripheral sensitization of nociceptors appears to be involved in the generation and maintenance of bone cancer pain.

PROPERTIES OF TUMORS THAT EXCITE NOCICEPTORS

Tumor cells and tumor-associated cells that include macrophages, neutrophils, and T-lymphocytes secrete a wide variety of factors that sensitize or directly excite primary afferent neurons (Fig. 2). These include prostaglandins (Nielsen et al. 1991; Galasko 1995), endothelins (Nelson and Carducci 2000; Davar 2001), interleukins 1 and 6 (Watkins et al. 1995; Leskovar et al. 2000; Opree and Kress 2000), epidermal growth factor (Stoscheck and King 1986), transforming growth factor (Poon et al. 2001; Roman et al. 2001), and platelet-derived growth factor (Daughaday and Deuel 1991; Radinsky 1991; Silver 1992). Receptors for many of these factors are expressed by primary afferent neurons. Each of these factors may play an important role in generating pain in particular forms of cancer, and therapies that block two of these factors, prostaglandins and endothelins, are currently approved for use in patients with other (noncancer) indications.

Prostaglandins are pro-inflammatory lipids that are formed from arachidonic acid by the action of cyclooxygenase (COX) and other downstream synthetases. There are two distinct forms of the COX enzyme, COX-1 and COX-2. Prostaglandins are involved in the sensitization or direct excitation of nociceptors by binding to several prostanoid receptors (Vasko 1995). Several tumor cells and tumor-associated macrophages express high levels of COX-2 and produce large amounts of prostaglandins (Dubois et al. 1996; Molina et al. 1999; Kundu et al. 2001; Ohno et al. 2001; Shappell et al. 2001).

The COX enzymes are a major target of current medications, and COX inhibitors are commonly administered for reducing both inflammation and pain. A major problem with using nonselective COX inhibitors such as aspirin or ibuprofen to block cancer pain is that these compounds inhibit both COX-1 and COX-2, and inhibition of the constitutively expressed COX-1 can cause bleeding and ulcers. In contrast, the new COX-2 inhibitors or coxibs preferentially inhibit COX-2 and avoid many of the side effects of COX-1 inhibition, which may allow their use in treating cancer pain. Other experiments have suggested that COX-2 is involved in angiogenesis and tumor growth (Masferrer et al. 2000; Moore and Simmons 2000), so in cancer patients, in addition to blocking cancer pain, COX-2 inhibitors may have the added advantage of reducing the growth and metastasis of the tumor. COX-2 antagonists show significant promise for alleviating at least some aspects of cancer pain, although clearly more research is required to fully define the actions of COX-2 in different types of cancer.

A second pharmacological target for treating cancer pain is the peptide endothelin-1 (Fig. 3). Several tumors, including prostate cancer, express high levels of endothelins (Shankar et al. 1998; Kurbel et al. 1999; Nelson and Carducci 2000), and clinical studies have reported a correlation between the severity of the pain in patients with prostate cancer and plasma levels of endothelins (Nelson et al. 1995). Endothelins could contribute to cancer pain by directly sensitizing or exciting nociceptors, given that a subset of small unmyelinated primary afferent neurons express receptors for endothelin (Pomonis et al. 2001). Direct application of endothelin to peripheral nerves activates primary afferent fibers and induces pain behaviors (Davar et al. 1998). Like prostaglandins, endothelins that are released from tumor cells are also thought be involved in regulating angiogenesis (Dawas et al. 1999) and tumor growth (Asham et al. 1998), suggesting again that endothelin antagonists may be useful not only in inhibiting cancer pain but in reducing the growth and metastasis of the tumor.

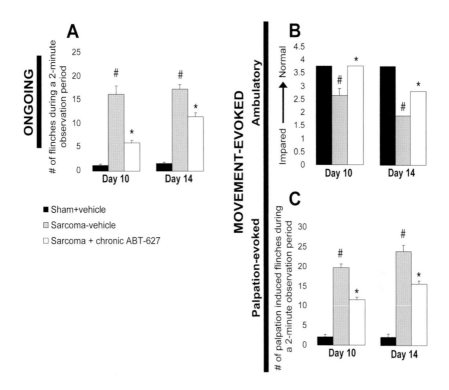

Fig. 3. Selective endothelin-A-receptor (ET$_A$R) inhibition attenuates ongoing and move-ment-evoked bone cancer pain behaviors. The number of spontaneous flinches of the cancerous limb over a 2-minute observation period was used as a measure of ongoing pain (A). Parameters of movement-evoked pain include assessment of the sarcoma-bearing limb during normal ambulation in an open field (B). Quantification of the number of flinches evoked by normally non-noxious palpation of the sarcoma-bearing limb over a 2-minute observation period following palpation was used as a measure of palpation-evoked pain (C). All pain behaviors were significantly reduced 10 and 14 days after sarcoma injection with chronic administration of ABT-627 beginning at 6 days after sarcoma injection: bars show means ± SEM. # $P < 0.05$ versus sham; * $P < 0.05$ versus sarcoma + vehicle group. Note that the ability of chronic ET-1-receptor inhibition to attenuate ongoing pain was significantly reduced from day 10 to day 14 after sarcoma injection. Modified from Peters et al. (2004).

TUMOR-INDUCED RELEASE OF PROTONS AND ACIDOSIS

Tumor cells become ischemic and undergo apoptosis as the tumor bur-den exceeds its vascular supply (Helmlinger et al. 2002). Local acidosis, the accumulation of acid metabolites, is a hallmark of tissue injury (Reeh and Steen 1996; Julius and Basbaum 2001). In the past few years the concept that sensory neurons can be directly excited by protons or acidosis has generated intense research and clinical interest. Studies have shown that subsets of sensory neurons express different acid-sensing ion channels (ASICs) (Olson et al. 1998; Julius and Basbaum 2001). The two major classes of ASICs expressed by nociceptors are TRPV1 (Caterina et al. 1997; Tominaga et al. 1998) and ASIC-3 (Bassilana et al. 1997; Olson et al. 1998; Sutherland et al. 2000). Both of these channels are sensitized and excited by a decrease in pH. More specifically, TRPV1 is activated when the pH falls below 6.0, while the pH that activates ASIC-3 appears to be highly dependent on the coexpression of other ASIC channels in the same nociceptor (Lingueglia et al. 1997).

There are several mechanisms by which a decrease in pH could be involved in generating and maintaining cancer pain. As tumors grow, tumor-associated inflammatory cells invade the neoplastic tissue and release protons that generate local acidosis (Helmlinger et al. 2002). A second mechanism by which acidosis may occur is apoptosis of the tumor cells. Release of intracellular ions may generate an acidic environment that activates signaling by ASICs expressed by nociceptors.

Tumor-induced release of protons and acidosis may be particularly important in the generation of bone cancer pain. Both osteolytic (bone-destroying) and osteoblastic (bone-forming) cancers involve a significant proliferation and hypertrophy of osteoclasts (Clohisy et al. 2000). Osteoclasts are terminally differentiated, multinucleated cells of the monocyte lineage that are uniquely designed to resorb bone by maintaining an extracellular microenvironment of acidic pH (4.0–5.0) at the interface between osteoclast and mineralized bone (Delaisse and Vaes 1992). Studies have shown significant expression of ASIC (Olson et al. 1998) and TRPV1 (Tominaga et al. 1998; Guo et al. 1999) in peptidergic afferent fibers, and we have localized peptidergic fibers in bone marrow and cortical bone (Mach et al. 2002). This evidence suggests that exposure of these sensory fibers to the osteoclast's acidic extracellular microenvironment could activate resident proton-sensitive ion channels, stimulating pain sensation. Recent experiments in a murine model of bone cancer pain reported that osteoclasts play an essential role in cancer-induced bone loss, and that osteoclasts contribute to the etiology of bone cancer pain (Honore et al. 2000a; Luger et al. 2001). Recent work has shown that osteoprotegerin (Honore et al. 2000) and a bisphosphonate (Fulfaro et al. 1998; Mannix et al. 2000; Clohisy et al. 2001), both of which are known to induce osteoclast apoptosis, are effective in decreasing osteoclast-induced bone cancer pain (Fig. 4). Similarly, TRPV1 or ASIC antagonists may be used to reduce pain in patients with soft tumors or bone cancer by blocking excitation of the ASICs on sensory neurons.

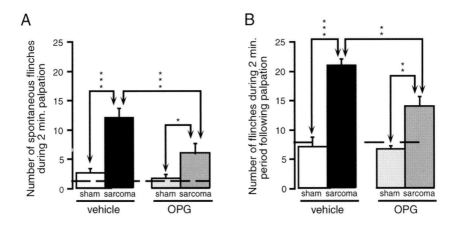

Fig. 4. Attenuation of bone cancer pain by osteoprotegerin (OPG). Histograms show that administration of OPG beginning 6 days after tumor implantation attenuated both (A) spontaneous and (B) palpation-evoked pain in mice at day 17 following tumor implantation (modified from Honore et al. 2000a). OPG is a naturally occurring protein that is a secreted decoy receptor that inhibits osteoclast differentiation, proliferation, and hypertrophy, resulting in reduced osteoclast activity and bone resorption.

RELEASE OF GROWTH FACTORS BY TUMOR CELLS

One of the most important discoveries in the past decade has been the demonstration that the biochemical and physiological status of sensory neurons is maintained and modified by factors derived from the innervated tissue. Changes in the periphery associated with inflammation, nerve injury, or tissue injury are mirrored by changes in the phenotype of sensory neurons (Honore et al. 2000b,c,d). After peripheral nerve injury, expression of a subset of neurotransmitters and receptors by damaged sensory neurons is altered in a highly predictable fashion. These changes are caused, in part, by a change in the tissue level of several growth factors released from the environment local to the injury site, including nerve growth factor (NGF) (Fu and Gordon 1997; Koltzenburg 1999; Fukuoka et al. 2001) and glial-derived neurotrophic factor (GDNF) (Boucher and McMahon 2001; Hoke et al. 2002). These neurochemical changes can be reversed in a receptor-specific fashion by intrathecal or peripheral application of NGF or GDNF (Bennett et al. 1996, 1998; Boucher et al. 2000; Ramer et al. 2000).

While the level of NGF expression reportedly correlates with the extent of pain in pancreatic cancer (Zhu et al. 1999; Schneider et al. 2001), relatively little is known about how other tumors affect the synthesis and release of growth factors. However, one certainty is that the repertoire of growth factors to which the sensory neuron is exposed will change as the developing tumor invades the peripheral tissue that the neuron innervates. Thus, in addition to a disruption of the growth factors normally released by the intact peripheral tissue, one can expect release of a variety of additional growth factors by tumor cells as well as by tumor-infiltrating leukocytes, which can comprise up to 80% of the total tumor mass (Zhang et al. 2002). Activated leukocytes synthesize and release high levels of several growth factors (Stoscheck and King 1986; Daughaday and Deuel 1991; Radinsky 1991; Silver 1992; Leon et al. 1994; Caroleo et al. 2001; Poon et al. 2001; Roman et al. 2001), and thus one would expect a significant change in the phenotype and response

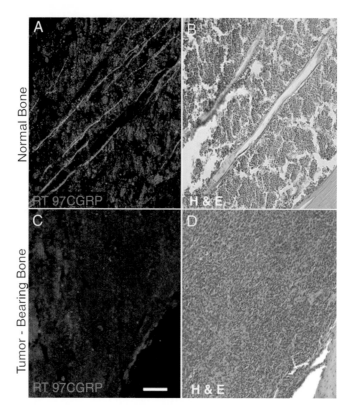

Fig. 5. Sensory nerve fibers in the marrow of the mouse femur are destroyed by invading sarcoma tumor cells. Confocal (A and C) images show calcitonin gene-related peptide (CGRP, green) and neurofilament-200 (RT-97, red) and serially adjacent sections (B and D) stained with hematoxylin and eosin (H and E, B and D) in the normal (A and B) and tumor-bearing (C and D) marrow. In the normal marrow, CGRP- and RT-97-expressing sensory fibers are generally associated with the vasculature (A and B), whereas 14 days following injection and confinement of the tumor cells to the marrow space (C and D), few, if any, CGRP- or RT-97-expressing sensory fibers can be detected. Scale bar = 150 μm.

characteristics of the sensory neurons following tumor invasion of a peripheral organ.

While tumor growth alters the invaded tissue, it is also clear that the affected tissue also influences the phenotype of the invading tumor cell (Mundy 2002). Because the local environment can influence the molecules that tumor cells express and release, it follows that the same tumor in the same individual may be painful at one site of metastasis but not at another. Clinical observations reveal that pain from cancer can be perplexing because the size, location, or type of cancer tumor does not necessarily predict

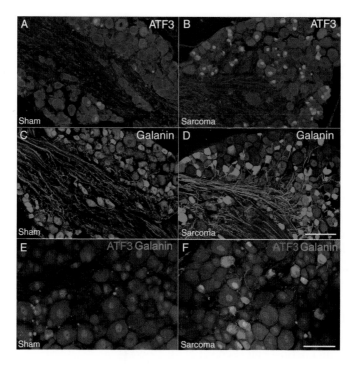

Fig. 6. Tumor-induced destruction of sensory nerve fibers in the tumor-bearing bone results in the upregulation of activated transcription factor-3 (ATF-3) and galanin in the cell body of sensory neurons that innervate the tumor-bearing femur. Neurons in the normal L2 dorsal root ganglia express low levels of both ATF-3 (A) and the neuropeptide galanin (C), whereas 14 days following injection and confinement of sarcoma cells to the marrow space, there is a marked upregulation of both ATF-3 and galanin in sensory neurons in the L2 dorsal root ganglia ipsilateral to the tumor-bearing bone. Many sensory neurons that show an upregulation of galanin in response to tumor-induced destruction of sensory fibers in the bone also show upregulation of ATF-3 in their nucleus (compare E vs. F). These data suggest that as tumor cells invade the bone, sensory nerve fibers that normally innervate the bone are destroyed, resulting in the generation of the neurochemical signature of neuropathy in sensory neurons that innervate the tumor-bearing bone. Scale bar = 100 μm. Modified from Ghilardi et al. (2003).

symptoms. Different patients with the same cancer may have vastly different symptoms. Kidney cancer may be painful in one person and asymptom-
atic in another. Metastases to bone in the same individual may cause pain at
the site of a rib lesion, but not at that of a humeral lesion. Small cancer
deposits in bone may be very painful, while large soft-tissue cancers may be
painless (Mantyh et al. 2002). Important areas for future research include
identification of tissue-specific mechanisms of cancer pain, comparing soft
tissue with bone, as well as site-specific mechanisms, comparing flat bones
(ribs) with tubular bones (femurs). It will also be of interest to determine
patient-specific factors that influence disease progression and its relationship to pain perception.

TUMOR-INDUCED DISTENSION AND DESTRUCTION
OF SENSORY FIBERS

In general, previous reports have suggested that tumors are not highly
innervated by sensory or sympathetic neurons (O'Connell et al. 1998; Seifert
and Spitznas 2001; Terada and Matsunaga 2001). However, in many cancers, rapid tumor growth frequently entraps and injures nerves, causing mechanical injury, compression, ischemia, or direct proteolysis (Mercadante
1997). Proteolytic enzymes produced by the tumor can also injure sensory
and sympathetic fibers, causing neuropathic pain.

The capacity of a tumor to injure and destroy peripheral nerve fibers has
been directly observed in an experimental model of bone cancer. Following
injection and containment of lytic murine sarcoma cells in the intramedullary space of the mouse femur, tumor cells grow in the marrow space and
disrupt innervating sensory fibers (Figs. 5 and 6). As the tumor cells grow
they first compress and then destroy both the hematopoietic cells of the
marrow and the sensory fibers that normally innervate the marrow, mineralized bone, and periosteum (Schwei et al. 1999).

While the mechanisms by which any neuropathic pain is generated and
maintained are still not well understood, several therapies that have proven
useful in the control of other types of neuropathic pain may also be useful in
treating tumor-induced neuropathic pain. For example, gabapentin, which
was originally developed as an anticonvulsant but whose mechanism of
action remains unknown, is effective in treating several forms of neuropathic pain and may also be useful in treating cancer-induced neuropathic
pain (Ripamonti and Dickerson 2001).

CENTRAL SENSITIZATION IN CANCER PAIN

A critical question is whether the spinal cord and forebrain also undergo significant neurochemical changes as a chronic cancer pain state develops. The murine cancer pain model revealed extensive neurochemical reorganization within spinal cord segments that receive input from primary afferent neurons innervating the cancerous bone (Honore et al. 2000a,c,d; Luger et al. 2001). These changes included astrocyte hypertrophy (Fig. 7) and

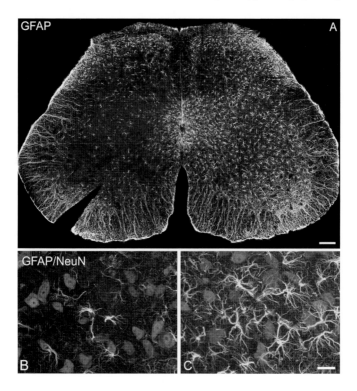

Fig. 7. Cancer-induced reorganization of the CNS. Chronic cancer pain not only sensitizes peripheral nociceptors, but also can induce significant neurochemical reorganization of the spinal cord. This reorganization may participate in the phenomenon of central sensitization, i.e., an increased responsiveness of spinal cord neurons involved in transmission of pain. (A) Confocal image of a coronal section of the mouse L4 spinal cord showing glial fibrillary acidic protein (GFAP)-positive astrocytes (white) that have undergone hypertrophy on the side ipsilateral to the tumor-bearing bone. Panels B and C show higher magnification of the ipsilateral and contralateral dorsal horn seen in panel A, with colocalization of the neuron-specific antibody NeuN. While the astrocytes (spindle-shaped cells) have undergone a massive hypertrophy, there does not appear to be any significant loss of NeuN-positive neurons. Scale bars: A, 200 μm; B and C, 30 μm. Modified from Schwei et al. (1999).

upregulation of the prohyperalgesic peptide dynorphin. Spinal cord neurons that normally would only be activated by noxious stimuli were activated by non-noxious stimuli. These spinal cord changes were attenuated by blocking the tumor-induced tissue destruction and pain (Honore et al. 2000a; Luger et al. 2001). Together, these neurochemical changes suggest that cancer pain induces and is at least partially maintained by a state of central sensitization, in which an increased transmission of nociceptive information allows normally non-noxious input to be amplified and perceived as noxious stimuli.

Once nociceptive information has been transmitted to the spinal cord by primary afferent neurons, it can travel via multiple ascending "pain" pathways that project from the spinal cord to higher centers of the brain. Classically, the main emphasis in examining the ascending conduction of pain has been placed on spinothalamic tract neurons. However, data from recent clinical studies have necessitated a reassessment of this position by showing significant attenuation of some forms of difficult-to-control visceral cancer pain following lesion of the axons of nonspinothalamic tract neurons (Willis et al. 1999; Nauta et al. 2000). Together these data suggest that one reason that cancer pain is frequently perceived as such an intense and disturbing pain is that it ascends to higher centers of the brain via multiple parallel neuronal pathways. Importantly for cancer patients, many of whom frequently experience anxiety or depression, it is clear that higher centers of the brain can modulate the ascending conduction of pain. Descending pathways that modulate the ascending conduction of cancer pain may play an important role in either enhancing or inhibiting the patient's perception of pain. The general mood and attention of the patient thus may be significant factors in determining the pain's intensity and degree of unpleasantness.

A CHANGING SET OF FACTORS MAY DRIVE CANCER PAIN WITH DISEASE PROGRESSION

Cancer pain frequently becomes more severe as the disease progresses, and adequate control of cancer pain becomes more difficult to achieve without encountering significant unwanted side effects (Payne 1998; Payne et al. 1998; Foley 1999; Portenoy and Lesage 1999; de Wit et al. 2001). While tolerance may contribute to the escalation of the dose of analgesics required to control cancer pain, a compatible possibility is that with the progression of the disease, different factors assume greater importance in driving cancer pain. For example, in the mouse model of bone cancer, as tumor cells first begin to proliferate, pain-related behaviors start to occur long before any significant bone destruction is evident. This pain may be due to prohyperalgesic factors such as prostaglandins and endothelin that are released by the growing tumor cells and subsequently activate nociceptors in the marrow. Pain at this stage might be attenuated by COX-2 inhibitors and endothelin antagonists. As the tumor continues to grow, sensory neurons innervating the marrow are compressed and destroyed, causing a neuropathic pain to develop that may best respond to treatment with drugs such as gabapentin that are known to attenuate noncancer-induced neuropathic pain. When the tumor begins to induce proliferation and hypertrophy of osteoclasts, the pain due to excessive osteoclast activity might be largely blocked by anti-osteoclastogenic drugs such as bisphosphonates or osteoprotegerin (Fig. 4). As the tumor cells completely fill the intramedullary space, tumor cells begin to die, generating an acidic environment; antagonists to TRPV1 or ASICs may attenuate the pain induced by this acidosis. Finally, as bone destruction compromises the mechanical strength of the bone, antagonists that block the mechanically gated channels and/or ATP receptors in the richly innervated periosteum may attenuate movement-evoked pain.

While the above pattern of tumor-induced tissue destruction and nociceptor activation may be unique to bone cancer, an evolving set of nociceptive events probably occurs in other cancers. This complex pattern may in part explain why cancer pain is frequently difficult to treat and why it is so heterogeneous in nature and severity. Changes in tumor-induced tissue injury, in nociceptor activation, and in the brain areas involved in transmitting these nociceptive signals as the disease progresses suggest that different therapies will be efficacious at particular stages of the disease. Understanding how tumor cells differentially excite nociceptors at different stages of the disease, and how the phenotype of nociceptors and CNS neurons involved in nociceptive transmission change as the disease progresses, should allow a mechanistic approach to designing more effective therapies to treat cancer pain.

FUTURE DIRECTIONS

For the first time, animal models of cancer pain are now available that mirror the clinical picture of patients with cancer pain. Information generated from these models should elucidate the mechanisms that generate and maintain different types of cancer pain. Many of these cancer models have been developed in mice and rats, but implantation of human tumors in immunocompromised rodent strains should allow examination of the pain that different human tumors generate. These animal models may also offer insight into one of the major conundrums of cancer pain: that the severity of cancer pain is so variable from patient to patient, from tumor to tumor, and even from site to site. Newer molecular techniques using microarrays and proteomics should reveal which specific features of different tumors are important in inducing cancer pain. Once we have determined the mechanisms by which the different types of cancer induce pain, we can identify molecular targets and develop mechanism-based therapies. Ultimately, the key will be to integrate information about tumor biology and the host's response to neoplasia with our understanding of how chronic pain is generated and maintained. These studies should improve the quality of life of all those who suffer from cancer pain.

ACKNOWLEDGMENTS

Supported by National Institutes of Health grants from the National Institute of Neurologic Disorders and Stroke (NS23970) and the National Institute for Drug Abuse (DA11986), National Institute of Dental and Craniofacial Research Dentist Scientist Award (DSA) DE00270 and training grant DE07288, and a Merit Review from the Veterans Administration.

REFERENCES

Alvarez FJ, Fyffe RE. Nociceptors for the 21st century. *Curr Rev Pain* 2000; 4(6):451–458.
Asham EH, Loizidou M, Taylor I. Endothelin-1 and tumour development. *Eur J Surg Oncol* 1998; 24(1):57–60.
Basbaum AI, Jessel TM. The perception of pain. In: Kandel ER, Schwartz JH, Jessell TM (Eds). *Principles of Neural Science.* New York: McGraw-Hill, 2000, pp 472–490.
Bassilana F, Champigny G, Waldmann R, et al. The acid-sensitive ionic channel subunit ASIC and the mammalian degenerin MDEG form a heteromultimeric H^+-gated Na^+ channel with novel properties. *J Biol Chem* 1997; 272(46):28819–28822.
Bennett DL, French J, Priestley JV, McMahon SB. NGF but not NT-3 or BDNF prevents the A fiber sprouting into lamina II of the spinal cord that occurs following axotomy. *Mol Cell Neurosci* 1996; 8(4):211–220.
Bennett DL, Michael GJ, Ramachandran N, et al. A distinct subgroup of small DRG cells express GDNF receptor components and GDNF is protective for these neurons after nerve injury. *J Neurosci* 1998; 18(8):3059–3072.
Bevan S, Geppetti P. Protons: small stimulants of capsaicin-sensitive sensory nerves. *Trends Neurosci* 1994; 17(12):509–512.
Boucher TJ, McMahon SB. Neurotrophic factors and neuropathic pain. *Curr Opin Pharmacol* 2001; 1(1):66–72.
Boucher TJ, Okuse K, Bennett DL, et al. Potent analgesic effects of GDNF in neuropathic pain states. *Science* 2000; 290(5489):124–127.
Caroleo MC, Costa N, Bracci-Laudiero L, Aloe L. Human monocyte/macrophages activate by exposure to LPS overexpress NGF and NGF receptors. *J Neuroimmunol* 2001; 113(2):193–201.

Caterina MJ, Schumacher MA, Tominaga M, et al. The capsaicin receptor: a heat-activated ion channel in the pain pathway. *Nature* 1997; 389(6653):816–824.

Caterina MJ, Leffler A, Malmberg AB, et al. Impaired nociception and pain sensation in mice lacking the capsaicin receptor. *Science* 2000; 288(5464):306–313.

Clohisy DR, Perkins SL, Ramnaraine ML. Review of cellular mechanisms of tumor osteolysis. *Clin Orthop Res* 2000a; (373):104–114.

Clohisy DR, Ramnaraine ML, Scully S, et al. Osteoprotegerin inhibits tumor-induced osteoclastogenesis and bone growth in osteopetrotic mice. *J Orthop Res* 2000b; 18(6):967–976.

Clohisy DR, O'Keefe PF, Ramnaraine ML. Pamidronate decreases tumor-induced osteoclastogenesis in mice. *J Orthop Res* 2001; 19(4):554–558.

Daughaday WH, Deuel TF. Tumor secretion of growth factors. *Endocrinol Metab Clin North Am* 1991; 20(3):539–563.

Davar G. Endothelin-1 and metastatic cancer pain. *Pain Med* 2001; 2(1):24–27.

Davar G, Hans G, Fareed MU, et al. Behavioral signs of acute pain produced by application of endothelin-1 to rat sciatic nerve. *Neuroreport* 1998; 9(10):2279–2283.

Dawas K, Laizidou M, Shankar A, et al. Angiogenesis in cancer: the role of endothelin-1. *Ann R Coll Surg Engl* 1999; 81:306–310.

Delaisse J-M, Vaes G. Mechanism of mineral solubilization and matrix degradation in osteoclastic bone resorption. In: Rifkin BR, Gay CV (Eds). *Biology and Physiology of the Osteoclast.* Ann Arbor: CRC, 1992, pp 289–314.

de Wit R, van Dam F, Loonstra S, et al. The Amsterdam Pain Management Index compared to eight frequently used outcome measures to evaluate the adequacy of pain treatment in cancer patients with chronic pain. *Pain* 2001; 91(3):339–349.

Djouhri L, Bleazard L, Lawson SN. Association of somatic action potential shape with sensory receptive properties in guinea-pig dorsal root ganglion neurones. *J Physiol* 1998; 513(Pt 3):857–872.

Dubois RN, Radhika A, Reddy BS, Entingh AJ. Increased cyclooxygenase-2 levels in carcinogen-induced rat colonic tumors. *Gastroenterology* 1996; 110(4):1259–1262.

Foley KM. Advances in cancer pain. *Arch Neurol* 1999; 56(4):413–417.

Fu SY, Gordon T. The cellular and molecular basis of peripheral nerve regeneration. *Mol Neurobiol* 1997; 14(1–2):67–116.

Fukuoka T, Kondo E, Dai Y, et al. Brain-derived neurotrophic factor increases in the uninjured dorsal root ganglion neurons in selective spinal nerve ligation model. *J Neurosci* 2001; 21(13):4891–4900.

Fulfaro F, Casuccio A, Ticozzi C, Ripamonti C. The role of bisphosphonates in the treatment of painful metastatic bone disease: a review of phase III trials. *Pain* 1998; 78(3):157–169.

Galasko CS. Diagnosis of skeletal metastases and assessment of response to treatment. *Clin Orthop* 1995; (312):64–75.

Ghilardi JR, Luger NM, Keyser CP, et al. A neuropathic component to bone cancer pain. *Soc Neurosci Abstr* 2003; 815.9.

Guo A, Vulchanova L, Wang J, et al. Immunocytochemical localization of the vanilloid receptor 1 (VR1): relationship to neuropeptides, the P2X3 purinoceptor and IB4 binding sites. *Eur J Neurosci* 1999; 11(3):946–958.

Helmlinger G, Sckell A, Dellian M, et al. Acid production in glycolysis-impaired tumors provides new insights into tumor metabolism. *Clin Cancer Res* 2002; 8(4):1284–1291.

Hoke A, Gordon T, Zochodne DW, Sulaiman OA. A decline in glial cell-line-derived neurotrophic factor expression is associated with impaired regeneration after long-term Schwann cell denervation. *Exp Neurol* 2002; 173(1):77–85.

Honore P, Luger NM, Sabino MA, et al. Osteoprotegerin blocks bone cancer-induced skeletal destruction, skeletal pain and pain-related neurochemical reorganization of the spinal cord. *Nat Med* 2000a; 6(5):521–528.

Honore P, Menning PM, Rogers SD, et al. Neurochemical plasticity in persistent inflammatory pain. *Prog Brain Res* 2000b; 129:357–363.

Honore P, Rogers SD, Schwei MJ, et al. Murine models of inflammatory, neuropathic and cancer pain each generates a unique set of neurochemical changes in the spinal cord and sensory neurons. *Neuroscience* 2000c; 98(3):585–598.

Honore P, Schwei J, Rogers SD, et al. Cellular and neurochemical remodeling of the spinal cord in bone cancer pain. *Prog Brain Res* 2000d; 129:389–397.

Hunt SP, Mantyh PW. The molecular dynamics of pain control. *Nat Rev Neurosci* 2001; 2(2):83–91.

Hunt SP, Pini A, Evan G. Induction of c-fos-like protein in spinal cord neurons following sensory stimulation. *Nature* 1987; 328(6131):632–634.

Julius D, Basbaum AI. Molecular mechanisms of nociception. *Nature* 2001; 413(6852):203–210.

Kirschstein T, Greffrath W, Busselberg D, Treede RD. Inhibition of rapid heat responses in nociceptive primary sensory of rats by vanilloid receptor antagonists. *J Neurophysiol* 1999; 82(6):2853–2860.

Koltzenburg M. The changing sensitivity in the life of the nociceptor. *Pain* 1999; (Suppl 6):S93–102.

Krishtal OA, Marchenko SM, Obukhov AG. Cationic channels activated by extracellular ATP in rat sensory neurons. *Neuroscience* 1988; 27(3):995–1000.

Kundu N, Yang QY, Dorsey R, Fulton AM. Increased cyclooxygenase-2 (COX-2) expression and activity in a murine model of metastatic breast cancer. *Int J Cancer* 2001; 93(5):681–686.

Kurbel S, Kurbel B, Kovacic D, et al. Endothelin-secreting tumors and the idea of the pseudoectopic hormone secretion in tumors. *Med Hypotheses* 1999; 52(4):329–333.

Leon A, Buriani A, Dal Toso R, et al. Mast cells synthesize, store, and release nerve growth factor. *Proc Natl Acad Sci USA* 1994; 91:3739–3743.

Leskovar A, Moriarty LJ, Turek JJ, et al. The macrophage in acute neural injury: changes in cell numbers over time and levels of cytokine production in mammalian central and peripheral nervous systems. *J Exp Biol* 2000; 203:1783–1795.

Lingueglia E, Weille JR, Bassilana F, et al. A modulatory subunit of acid sensing ion channels in brain and dorsal root ganglion cells. *J Biol Chem* 1997; 272:29778–29783.

Luger NM, Honore P, Sabino MAC, et al. Osteoprotegerin diminishes advanced bone cancer pain. *Cancer Res* 2001; 61(10):4038–4047.

Mach DB, Rogers SD, Sabino MC, et al. Origins of skeletal pain: sensory and sympathetic innervation of the mouse femur. *J Neurosci* 2002; 113(1):155–166.

Mannix K, Ahmedazai SH, Anderson H, et al. Using bisphosphonates to control the pain of bone metastases: evidence based guidelines for palliative care. *Palliat Med* 2000; 14:455–461.

Mantyh PW, DeMaster E, Malhotra A, et al. Receptor endocytosis and dendrite reshaping in spinal neurons after somatosensory stimulation. *Science* 1995a; 268(5217):1629–1632.

Mantyh PW, Allen CJ, Ghilardi JR, et al. Rapid endocytosis of a G protein-coupled receptor: substance P evoked internalization of its receptor in the rat striatum in vivo. *Proc Natl Acad Sci USA* 1995b; 92(7):2622–2626.

Mantyh PW, Clohisy DR, Koltzenburg M, Hunt SP. Molecular mechanisms of cancer pain. *Nat Rev Cancer* 2002; 2(3):201–209.

Masferrer JL, Leahy KM, Koki AT, et al. Antiangiogenic and antitumor activities of cyclooxygenase-2 inhibitors. *Cancer Res* 2000; 60(5):1306–1311.

McMahon SB. NGF as a mediator of inflammatory pain. *Philos Trans R Soc Lond B Biol Sci* 1996; 351(1338):431–440.

Mercadante S. Malignant bone pain: pathophysiology and treatment. *Pain* 1997; 69(1-2):1–18.

Molina MA, Sitja-Arnau M, Lemoine MG, et al. Increased cyclooxygenase-2 expression in human pancreatic carcinomas and cell lines: growth inhibition by nonsteroidal anti-inflammatory drugs. *Cancer Res* 1999; 59(17):4356–4362.

Moore BC, Simmons DL. COX-2 inhibition, apoptosis, and chemoprevention by nonsteroidal anti-inflammatory drugs. *Curr Med Chem* 2000; 7(11):1131–1144.

Mundy GR. Metastases to bone: causes, consequences, and therapeutic opportunities. *Nat Rev Cancer* 2002; 2:584–593.

Nagy I, Rang H. Noxious heat activates all capsaicin-sensitive and also a sub-population of capsaicin-insensitive dorsal root ganglion neurons. *Neuroscience* 1999; 88(4):995–997.

Nauta HJW, Soukup VM, Fabian RH, et al. Punctate midline myelotomy for the relief of visceral cancer pain. *J Neurosurg* 2000; 92(Suppl 2S):125–130.

Nelson JB, Carducci MA. The role of endothelin-1 and endothelin receptor antagonists in prostate cancer. *BJU Int* 2000; 85(Suppl 2):45–48.

Nelson JB, Hedican SP, George DJ, et al. Identification of endothelin-1 in the pathophysiology of metastatic adenocarcinoma of the prostate. *Nat Med* 1995; 1(9):944–999.

Nielsen OS, Munro AJ, Tannock IF. Bone metastases: pathophysiology and management policy. *J Clin Oncol* 1991; 9(3):509–524.

O'Connell JX, Nanthakumar SS, Nielsen GP, Rosenberg AE. Osteoid osteoma: the uniquely innervated bone tumor. *Modern Pathol* 1998; 11(2):175–180.

Ohno R, Yoshinaga K, Fujita T, et al. Depth of invasion parallels increased cyclooxygenase-2 levels in patients with gastric carcinoma. *Cancer* 2001; 91(10):1876–1881.

Olson TH, Riedl MS, Vulchanova L, et al. An acid sensing ion channel (ASIC) localizes to small primary afferent neurons in rats. *Neuroreport* 1998; 9(6):1109–1113.

Opree A, Kress M. Involvement of the proinflammatory cytokines tumor necrosis factor-alpha, IL-1 beta, and IL-6 but not IL-8 in the development of heat hyperalgesia: effects on heat-evoked calcitonin gene-related peptide release from rat skin. *J Neurosci* 2000; 20(16):6289–6293.

Payne R. Practice guidelines for cancer pain therapy: issues pertinent to the revision of national guidelines. *Oncology* 1998; 12(11A):169–175.

Payne R, Mathias SD, Pasta DJ, et al. Quality of life and cancer pain: satisfaction and side effects with transdermal fentanyl versus oral morphine. *J Clin Oncol* 1998; 16(4):1588–1593.

Peters CM, Lindsay TH, Pomonis JD. Endothelin and the tumorigenic component of bone cancer pain. *Neuroscience* 2004; 126:1043–1052.

Pomonis JD, Rogers SD, Peters CM, et al. Expression and localization of endothelin receptors: implication for the involvement of peripheral glia in nociception. *J Neurosci* 2001; 21(3):999–1006.

Poon RT, Fan ST, Wong J. Clinical implications of circulating angiogenic factors in cancer patients. *J Clin Oncol* 2001; 19(4):1207–1225.

Portenoy RK, Lesage P. Management of cancer pain. *Lancet* 1999; 353(9165):1695–1700.

Portenoy RKD, Payne D, Jacobsen P. Breakthrough pain: characteristics and impact in patients with cancer pain. *Pain* 1999; 81(1–2):129–134.

Price MP, McIlwrath SL, Xie JH, et al. The DRASIC cation channel contributes to the detection of cutaneous touch and acid stimuli in mice. *Neuron* 2001; 32(6):1071–1083.

Radinsky R. Growth factors and their receptors in metastasis. *Semin Cancer Biol* 1991; 2(3):169–177.

Ramer MS, Priestley JV, McMahon SB. Functional regeneration of sensory axons into the adult spinal cord. *Nature* 2000; 403(6767):312–316.

Reeh PW, Steen KH. Tissue acidosis in nociception and pain. *Prog Brain Res* 1996; 113:143–151.

Ripamonti C, Dickerson ED. Strategies for the treatment of cancer pain in the new millennium. *Drugs* 2001; 61(7):955–977.

Roman C, Saha D, Beauchamp R. TGF-beta and colorectal carcinogenesis. *Microsc Res Tech* 2001; 52(4):450–457.

Schneider MB, Standop J, Ulrich A, et al. Expression of nerve growth factors in pancreatic neural tissue and pancreatic cancer. *J Histochem Cytochem* 2001; 49(10):1205–1210.

Schwei MJ, Honore P, Rogers SD, et al. Neurochemical and cellular reorganization of the spinal cord in a murine model of bone cancer pain. *J Neurosci* 1999; 19(24):10886–10897.

Seifert P, Spitznas M. Tumours may be innervated. *Virchows Arch* 2001; 438(3):228–231.

Shankar A, Loizidou M, Aliev G, et al. Raised endothelin 1 levels in patients with colorectal liver metastases. *Br J Surg* 1998; 85(4):502–506.

Shappell SB, Manning S, Boeglin WE, et al. Alterations in lipoxygenase and cyclooxygenase-2 catalytic activity and mRNA expression in prostate carcinoma. *Neoplasia* 2001; 3(4):287–303.

Silver BJ. Platelet-derived growth factor in human malignancy. *Biofactors* 1992; 3(4):217–227.

Stoscheck CM, King LE Jr. Role of epidermal growth factor in carcinogenesis. *Cancer Res* 1986; 46(3):1030–1037.

Sutherland S, Cook S, Ew M. Chemical mediators of pain due to tissue damage and ischemia. *Prog Brain Res* 2000; 129:21–38.

Terada T, Matsunaga Y. S-100-positive nerve fibers in hepatocellular carcinoma and intrahepatic cholangiocarcinoma: an immunohistochemical study. *Pathol Int* 2001; 51(2):89–93.

Tominaga M, Caterina MJ, Malmberg AB, et al. The cloned capsaicin receptor integrates multiple pain-producing stimuli. *Neuron* 1998; 21(3):531–543.

Vasko MR. Prostaglandin-induced neuropeptide release from spinal cord. *Prog Brain Res* 1995; 104:367–380.

Watkins LR, Goehler LE, Relton J, et al. Mechanisms of tumor necrosis factor-alpha (TNF-alpha) hyperalgesia. *Brain Res* 1995; 692(1–2):244–250.

Welch JM, Simon SA, Reinhart PH. The activation mechanism of rat vanilloid receptor 1 by capsaicin involves the pore domain and differs from the activation by either or heat. *Proc Natl Acad Sci USA* 2000; 97(25):13889–13894.

Willis WD, Al-Chaer ED, Quast MJ, Westlund KN. A visceral pain pathway in the dorsal column of the spinal cord. *Proc Natl Acad Sci USA* 1999; 96(14):7675–7679.

Woolf CJ, Salter MW. Neuronal plasticity: increasing the gain in pain. *Science* 2000; 288(5472):1765–1769.

Xu GY, Huang LYM. Peripheral inflammation sensitizes P2X receptor-mediated responses in dorsal root ganglion neurons. *J Neurosci* 2002; 22(1):93–102.

Zhang F, Lu W, Dong Z. Tumor-infiltrating macrophages are involved in suppressing growth and metastasis of human prostate cancer cells by INF-beta gene therapy in nude mice. PG-2942-51. *Clin Cancer Res* 2002; 8(9).

Zhu ZW, Friess H, diMola FF, et al. Nerve growth factor expression correlates with perineural invasion and pain in human pancreatic cancer. *J Clin Oncol* 1999; 17(8):2419–2428.

Correspondence to: Patrick W. Mantyh, PhD, Neurosystems Center, University of Minnesota, 18-154 Moos Tower, 515 Delaware Street SE, Minneapolis, MN 55455, USA. Tel: 612-626-0180; Fax: 612-626-2565; email: manty001@umn.edu.

The Pain System in Normal and Pathological States: A Primer for Clinicians, Progress in Pain Research and Management, Vol. 31, edited by Luis Villanueva, Anthony Dickenson, and Hélène Ollat, IASP Press, Seattle, © 2004.

16

Neuropathic Pain: Sensory Loss, Hypersensitivity, and Spread of Pain

Troels S. Jensen and Nanna B. Finnerup

Department of Neurology and Danish Pain Research Center, Aarhus University, Aarhus, Denmark

Our understanding of nociceptive processing and plastic changes after persistent noxious input or nerve damage has increased considerably within the last two decades. Damage to the somatosensory nervous system carries a potential risk for development of neuropathic pain. Such pain is long-lasting, reduces quality of life, and also diminishes working capacity and increases the need for health care. It is now well known that injury to the peripheral (PNS) or the central nervous system (CNS) produces a cascade of neurobiological events in those parts of the brain receiving information from the injured area (for review see Besson 1999; Julius and Basbaum 2001; Mantyh et al. 2001; Watkins et al. 2001; Scholz and Woolf 2002). Damage to the nociceptive transmission system often manifests as increased sensitivity. We can explore the changes in the nervous system at various levels: molecular, cellular, and clinical.

At the molecular level, formation of new channels, upregulation of certain receptors, downregulation of others, expression of novel receptors, and induction of new genes are some of the biological features that, alone or in concert, may contribute to hyperexcitability.

These molecular changes translate into numerous cellular manifestations that include spontaneous discharges in nociceptors, reduced threshold to depolarization of cell bodies, an increased response to suprathreshold stimulation, recruitment of silent nociceptors, expansion of receptive fields, changes in cell phenotypes, and as a consequence, secondary changes in spinal cord and brain relay stations (Dubner 1991; Hunt and Mantyh 2001; Scholz and Woolf 2002). The clinical manifestations of this array of neuronal events are less clear, but probably include exaggerated and prolonged pain, different types of evoked pain, and an extraterritorial spread of pain to nondamaged tissue (Koltzenburg 1998; Hansson et al. 2001; Koltzenburg and Scadding 2001; Jensen and Baron 2003). It is now clear that a series of mechanisms are involved in generating neuropathic pain and that we lack a simple way to correlate each mechanism with particular signs and symptoms (Jensen and Baron 2003).

The possible translation of neuronal hyperexcitability into clinical symptoms deserves great attention because this area represents a window to understanding potential mechanisms underlying various neuropathic pain conditions and thereby a rational approach for how to target these conditions pharmacologically. However, at present the relationship between signs and symptoms and mechanisms is unclear because one mechanism may give rise to several symptoms and one specific symptom can be caused by different mechanisms (Woolf and Decosterd 1999; Hansson et al. 2001; Jensen et al. 2001; Jensen and Baron 2003).

An important clinical observation in neuropathic pain is the combination of sensory loss due to damage of transmitting pathways and the paradox of hypersensitivity phenomena in the painful area. The abnormal sensitivity is sometimes confined to the denervated territory and sometimes extends beyond the damaged territory (for review, see Hansson et al. 2001; Jensen et al. 2001). The mechanisms behind these sensory changes in the painful area after peripheral or central nerve lesions have caused some confusion.

This chapter summarizes clinical manifestations of neuropathic pain after peripheral nerve injury and after damage to the CNS, with particular emphasis on sensory abnormalities.

ETIOLOGY OF NEUROPATHIC PAIN

The essential pathological feature in neuropathic pain is a lesion of the afferent transmission system, either in the PNS or CNS, resulting in partial or complete loss of input to the nervous system with corresponding negative sensory phenomena such as partial or complete anesthesia in the damaged area. The reduction of afferent input caused by the nervous system lesion is also the starting point for regeneration and disinhibition with secondary development of hypersensitivity resulting in various positive symptoms.

The etiology behind neuropathic pain ranges from benign to malignant, from traumatic to metabolic, and from vascular to immunological. The listed causes (Table I) are incomplete. Woolf et al. (1998) have suggested a mechanism-based classification. They attempted to determine the mechanism involved in a particular pain patient, such as allodynia due to increased firing from sensitized nociceptors. It is beyond the scope of this chapter to present

Table I
Classification of neuropathic pain according
to disease and anatomical region

Peripheral	Spinal	Brain
Neuropathies	Multiple sclerosis	Stroke
Herpes zoster	Spinal cord injury	Multiple sclerosis
Nerve injuries	Arachnoiditis	Neoplasms
Amputations	Neoplasms	Syringomyelia
Plexopathies	Syringomyelia	Parkinson's disease?
Radiculopathies	Spinal stroke	Epilepsy?
Avulsions		
Neoplasms		
Trigeminal neuralgia		

a detailed description of current mechanisms, some of which are still hypo-thetical (for review, see Woolf and Mannion 1999; Woolf and Salter 2000; Hunt and Mantyh 2001; Julius and Basbaum 2001; Scholz and Woolf 2002). In brief, mechanisms of neuropathic pain include: (1) Pathological activity or sensitized nociceptors with recruitment of silent nociceptors and ectopic activity in spinal ganglion cells. The increased afferent neuronal barrage sensitizes dorsal horn neurons. (2) A severe loss of small-fiber input may give rise to central sensitization due to a spinal reorganization from sprout-ing of large myelinated fibers into superficial "nociceptive" laminae in the dorsal horn. (3) Inflammation of nerve trunks with corresponding ectopic nerve activity represents a source for central sensitization. (4) Sympathetic activity may sensitize nociceptors. (5) Altered spinal and brain processing due to plastic changes with recruitment of new brain areas usually not in-volved in pain. The complexity of neuropathic pain is underscored by the fact that certain mechanisms are not necessarily involved in all neuropathic pain conditions, in group of patients with the same pain condition, or even in the same patient. For example, a patient with postherpetic neuralgia may at one time point have electric jerks of pain and later in the course of the disease may have pain dominated by a touch-evoked allodynia.

SENSORY ABNORMALITIES IN NEUROPATHIC PAIN

SENSORY LOSS AND PAIN

An essential part of neuropathic pain is a loss (partial or complete) of sensory function in the painful area (Table II). In some patients the sensory deficit may be gross, in others subtle. Bedside testing using pinprick, strok-ing with a cotton –swab, or a thermal stimulus (e.g., thermorollers kept at

Table II
Assessment of negative sensory symptoms or signs in neuropathic pain

Negative Sensory Symptoms/Signs	Clinical Examination	Laboratory Test	Extending?*
Reduced detection threshold to touch	Touch skin with cotton wool	Graded von Frey hair	No
Reduced detection and pain threshold to pinprick	Prick skin with a pin (single stimuli)	von Frey hair specific (e.g., 100 g)	No
Reduced detection and pain threshold to cold/warm	Thermal response to 20°C and 45°C	Thermotest	No
Reduced detection threshold to vibration	Tuning fork on malleolus	Vibrometer	No

* Extending beyond the damaged innervation area.

20°C or 40°C) often suffice to demonstrate a sensory loss. In cases with minimal loss of sensory function, quantitative psychophysical measures (using thermographs, von Frey hairs, and algometers) may aid in demonstrating minor changes (Hanssson et al. 2001; Jensen and Gottrup 2003). Peripheral nerve injuries produce a wide range of sensory abnormalities, which may involve several sensory modalities. In patients with central lesions, neuropathic pain is linked to a partial or complete loss of spinothalamic functions. The corresponding sensory deficit may be dissociated with a decrease in thermal and pinprick sensations and a relative preservation of vibration and other lemniscal somatosensory functions. For example, in post-stroke pain, large-scale studies suggest that sensory deficit is a necessary, albeit not a sufficient condition, for the occurrence of pain (Vestergaard et al. 1995). In central pain due to spinal cord injury, recent studies indicate that sensory loss and areas with hypersensitivity are characteristic features (for review, see Finnerup and Jensen 2004). It remains to be seen whether similar patterns also occur in other central neuropathic pain states.

Recording the distribution of sensory loss on a drawing is an important initial step for pain assessment. The distribution of sensory loss can determine whether deficits are confined to one or several nerves, fascicles, nerve roots, dermatomes, or to the somatosensory map of damaged brain structures. Such drawings also help to distinguish between organic and nonorganic sensory disturbances and help determine whether sensory loss is part of a somatization disorder. In general. sensory loss is confined to the innervation territory corresponding to the damaged part of the nervous system, be it peripheral or central. In patients with somatization disorders, the apparent sensory loss does not correspond to the anatomical organization of the nervous system. The area of sensory loss can be measured to follow any changes in size. Such procedures are useful for recording the progression of a particular condition or a patient's recovery. Proposed automatic drawing systems may produce more accurate measurements.

SENSORY HYPERSENSITIVITY AND PAIN

Hyperalgesia (an increased response to noxious stimuli), and allodynia (pain evoked by non-noxious mechanical or thermal stimuli) are typical elements of neuropathic pain. Three types of mechanical hyperalgesia are generally distinguished: (1) static hyperalgesia evoked by gentle skin pressure, (2) punctate hyperalgesia evoked by punctate skin stimulation, and (3) touch (dynamic) allodynia produced by light brushing of the skin. Both cold and heat stimuli can evoke abnormal pain: (1) cold hyperalgesia produced by cold stimuli applied to skin, and (2) heat hyperalgesia evoked by heat stimuli to the skin.

Allodynia or hyperalgesia can be quantified by measuring intensity, threshold for elicitation, duration, and area of allodynia (Jensen and Gottrup 2003). The evocation of pain by a stimulus implies that a complete abolition of afferent information does not give rise to allodynia. Nevertheless, on occasions, despite a complete injury, abnormal sensations may subsequently develop, manifesting as anesthesia dolorosa in the deafferented body part. These phenomena can probably be ascribed to spontaneous firing in nerve sprouts, to alteration in peripheral innervation territory, to an expansion of receptive fields of sensitized central neurons that have lost their normal innervation, or to a combination of such mechanisms. Hyperalgesia can be provoked in normal persons following blockade of large-diameter afferent fibers. Pinprick or cold are now perceived as burning or squeezing pain, which suggests that afferent fibers under normal conditions inhibit dorsal horn neuronal activity. This inhibition may be disrupted in neuropathic pain.

Hyperpathia is a variant of hyperalgesia and allodynia and the prototypic disorder in neuropathic pain that involves loss of nerve fibers. In these cases a stimulus of an intensity that exceeds sensory threshold suddenly evokes an explosive pain response from cutaneous areas with increased sensory detection threshold. Hyperpathia reflects the peripheral or central deafferentation leading to both an elevation of threshold and central hyperexcitability due to lost or abnormal input from afferents.

DISTRIBUTION OF SENSORY HYPERSENSITIVITY

As for sensory loss, it is essential to map the distribution of sensory hypersensitivity to determine whether it corresponds to the innervation territory of a sensory nerve, a fascicle, a nerve root, a spinal cord segment, or a cerebral structure (Table III). We have only limited data on the sensory distribution of these phenomena. In general, the distribution of spontaneous or evoked positive sensory phenomena may correspond to the innervation territory of the damaged part of the nervous system, but it may also be a fraction of or extend beyond the innervation territories. The discrepancy between areas of negative and positive sensory phenomena has created some confusion in efforts to clarify mechanisms. For example, in some patients an extension of the distribution of positive sensory phenomena may be a consequence of central sensitization in a spinal cord segment due to peripheral nerve damage. Other patients can have positive sensory phenomena without detectable signs of nerve damage. It is possible that a general sensitization— merely as a consequence of pain—may explain the sensory hyperphenomena seen in these cases. Such phenomena have been described in ill-defined disorders such as irritable bowel disease after cervical distortions ("whiplash syndrome") and in diffuse musculoskeletal disorders such as fibromyalgia.

Table III
Assessment of positive sensory symptoms or signs in neuropathic pain

Positive Sensory Symptoms	Clinical Examination	Laboratory Test*	Extending?†
Spontaneous Pain			
Paresthesia	Pain intensity	Area, pain intensity	yes
Dysesthesia	Pain intensity	Area, pain intensity	yes
Paroxysms	Number, intensity	Threshold for evocation	?
Superficial burning pain	Pain intensity	Area, pain intensity	yes
Deep pain	Pain intensity	Area, pain intensity	?
Evoked Pain			
Touch-evoked hyperalgesia	Stroke skin with painter's brush	Evoked pain to touch	yes
Static hyperalgesia	Gentle mechanical pressure	Evoked pain to pressure	yes
Punctate hyperalgesia	Prick skin with pin	von Frey hair	yes
Punctate repetitive hyperalgesia (wind-up-like pain)	Prick skin with pin 2 times/second for 30 seconds	von Frey hair	yes
Aftersensation	Measure pain duration after stimulation	Measure pain duration after stimulation	yes
Cold hyperalgesia	Stimulate skin with cool metal roller	Evoked pain to cold stimuli	yes
Heat hyperalgesia	Stimulate skin with hot metal roller	Evoked pain to heat stimuli	yes

* Neuropathic area in cm^2 and pain intensity on a scale of 0–10.
† Extending beyond the damaged innervation area.

Although the mechanisms giving rise to pain may seem similar in cases with and without nerve damage, from a clinical and a treatment point of view it is essential to distinguish between these entirely different conditions.

STIMULUS-INDEPENDENT AND STIMULUS-DEPENDENT NEUROPATHIC PAIN

Clinically, neuropathic pains are characterized by spontaneous, ongoing types of pain termed *stimulus-independent,* and various types of evoked pain termed *stimulus-dependent,* which reflect the hyperexcitability in the nervous system (Dubner 1991; Coderre and Katz 1997; Woolf and Decosterd 1999; Koltzenburg and Scadding 2001).

STIMULUS-INDEPENDENT PAIN

These pains are spontaneous and may be continuous or paroxysmal. They can be shooting, shock-like, aching, cramping, crushing, smarting, or burning. Episodic, paroxysmal types of pain, lasting for seconds, are shooting, electric, shock-like, or stabbing. In its most typical form, paroxysmal pain occurs in tic douloureux, in entrapment neuropathies, after amputation, and in luetic diseases (Baron 2000; Jensen and Baron 2003). In tabes dorsalis (neurosyphilis), shooting pains are often described as transverse lightening pains in the legs provoked by emotional stress (Boivie 1999). Shooting pain can occur in cases with nerve compression (e.g., slipped disk, vertebral compression, neoplastic nerve compression, and entrapment syndromes).

The mechanism underlying these pains is assumed to reflect an increased discharge in sensitized C nociceptors. Alternatively, a sensation of burning or dysesthesia might be due to increased activity in sensitized receptors associated with large myelinated A fibers.

STIMULUS-DEPENDENT PAINS

The stimulus-evoked pains are classified according to the stimulus type that provokes them. Among several types of evoked pains, the most prominent are mechanical and thermal. Some patients may experience several of these phenomena; others may have only one type of hyperalgesia. For example, patients with nerve injury pain or amputation may have trigger points to mechanical stimuli, but with entirely normal thermal sensation. In patients with neuropathy, cold allodynia may be the only abnormality. A series of stimuli thus must be used to document or exclude abnormality. The evoked pains are usually brief, lasting only for the period of stimulation, but sometimes they can persist even after cessation of stimulation, causing aftersensations that can last for minutes, hours, or perhaps days (Gottrup et al. 2003). In such cases, distinguishing between evoked and spontaneous types of pain can be difficult. Although a certain cluster of signs and symptoms seems to be linked to neuropathic pain, to date it has not been possible in large sample studies to use signs and symptoms to distinguish pain patients with definite nerve damage from those unlikely to have nerve damage (Rasmussen et al. 2004).

PERIPHERAL NEUROPATHIC PAIN

In peripheral nerve injury the sensory loss on the body corresponds to the territory that has been denervated. Often surrounding this area is a territory with abnormal positive sensory phenomena including hyperalgesia and allodynia. In patients with amputation or plexus avulsion, the abnormal extraterritorial symptoms may include phantom sensations in anesthetic or lost body parts; these phantom sensations can either be painful or nonpainful. In addition, in some patients sensations are referred from body parts with a distribution that seems to correspond to spinal or brainstem segments adjacent to those that have lost their normal afferent input (T.S. Jensen et al., unpublished observations). The spinal neuronal hyperexcitability may in turn give rise to *secondary* cortical reorganization phenomena. In fact, several studies using various imaging techniques have confirmed that cortical reorganization occurs in upper-limb amputees with expansion of surrounding areas such as facial areas into the denervated hand area (for review, see Flor et al. 1995, 2001).

Fig. 1 shows an example of a patient with a previous plexus avulsion of the brachial plexus leaving that caused an anesthetic and paralytic arm. However, stimulation of non-anesthetic body parts on the skin near the affected region produced referred sensations into the anesthetic arm. These observations may be compatible with a primary neuronal hyperexcitability in spinal segments that have lost their normal patterned input. Rostral and caudal spread of neuronal hyperexcitability explains the evocation of hypersensitivity in neighboring dermatomes and referral into anesthetic body parts.

SENSITIZATION OF PRIMARY AFFERENT NOCICEPTORS

Pain is normally elicited by activating receptors of unmyelinated (C) and thinly myelinated (Aδ) primary afferents. Under normal conditions C nociceptors and Aδ nociceptors are silent and respond only to vigorous,

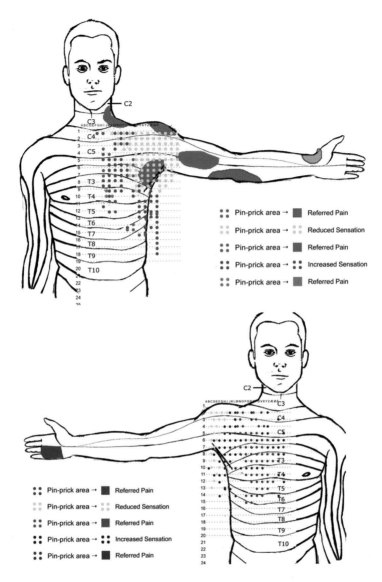

Fig. 1. Distribution of areas of sensory loss (yellow) and sites from which stimulation with a von Frey hair elicited referral into the anesthetic and deafferented hand in a 43-year-old man with a plexus avulsion of C4 to T1, a corresponding paralysis of the left arm, and a sensory loss in dermatomes C4 to T1.

potentially noxious stimuli. Models of peripheral nerve injury have shown abnormal nociceptor sensitization in the absence of acute tissue injury or inflammation or abnormal spontaneous afferent activity. After lesioning. peripheral nerve fibers exhibit spontaneous activity and an increased sensitivity to various chemical, thermal. and mechanical stimuli (Chabal et al. 1989, 1992; Wall and Gutnick 1974; Michaelis et al. 1997). Abnormal activity occurs not only at the peripheral terminal, but also along the peripheral nerve (ectopic activity) and in the dorsal root ganglion (DRG) cells. This pattern indicates that the CNS receives an abnormal input from at least three sources: sensitized nociceptors, ectopic foci along the nerve, and spontaneously active neurons within the DRG.

This ectopic activity following nerve injury is accompanied by increased expression of ion channels, in particular sodium channels (Novakovic et al. 1998) and receptors. The accumulation of sodium channels and receptors at sites of ectopic impulse generation may be one of the mechanisms responsible for lowering action potential threshold and for generating spontaneous activity in damaged primary afferents (Devor and Seltzer 1999; Julius and Basbaum 2001).

Microneurographic recordings from transected nerves in amputees with phantom limb pain (Nystrom and Hagbarth 1981) show spontaneous afferent activity; likewise, recordings from patients with mechanical or heat hyperalgesia exhibit sensitized C nociceptors innervating the painful region (Orstavik et al. 2003).

Indirect evidence for C-fiber sensitization is increased pain reported by patients with postherpetic neuralgia following topical application of the C-fiber excitant capsaicin (Petersen et al. 2000). Topical application of the local anesthetic lidocaine, which blocks ectopic impulse transmission in primary afferent nociceptors, relieves pain (Fields et al. 1998). Thus, sensitized nociceptors may not only be a source for spontaneous pain but also a site giving rise to different types of evoked pain.

Evoked pains are not confined to superficial tissue but can also occur as deep pain that is usually poorly localized. Patients with acute demyelinating polyradiculopathy report deep proximal aching pain in addition to paroxysmal pain. Deep aching pain is the most prevalent type in patients with polyneuropathy (Otto et al. 2003). It is uncertain whether this pain is due to an abnormal activity in small primary afferents from nervi nervorum or to a central sensitization, in which cutaneous afferent fibers terminate on second-order neurons also receiving convergent input from deep structures such as muscle.

CENTRAL SENSITIZATION: *INCREASED* PERIPHERAL INPUT

Central sensitization is a plastic change of cellular excitability in second- or higher-order transmission neurons. While usually described after tissue damage, such sensitization can also occur after nerve injury. The central sensitization elicited from the periphery may cause the dynamic mechanical allodynia produced by light tactile stimuli. Once central sensitization is established with an allodynia mediated by Aβ-fiber input, it can be maintained by input from C nociceptors (Gracely et al. 1992). Further stimulating these nociceptors, for example, by heating, increases not only ongoing pain but also touch-evoked pain. Selective block of Aβ fibers eliminates the touch-evoked pain but not the ongoing pain (Gracely et al. 1992). Furthermore, with central sensitization Aδ afferents also gain access to secondary pain-signaling neurons, which may cause punctate mechanical allodynia and perhaps also cold allodynia.

Studies by several groups have indicated that sensitization of nociceptors to thermal stimuli is associated with central sensitization, which then manifests as allodynia to mechanical and thermal stimuli (Rowbotham and Fields 1996; Gottrup et al. 1998, 2000). Thermal hyperalgesia has two forms: heat hyperalgesia and cold hyperalgesia. While the former is rare in neuropathic pain, cold hyperalgesia is common and seems to involve several mechanisms. In patients with peripheral neuropathic pain, the secondary hyperalgesia manifested by a touch-evoked pain can be reduced by the intrathecal administration of NMDA-receptor antagonists (Kristensen et al. 1992), indicating that this effect is spinally rather than supraspinally mediated.

CENTRAL SENSITIZATION: *DECREASED* PERIPHERAL INPUT

Clinical observations show that lost input also can be associated with neuropathic pain. Reduced C-fiber input as a consequence of degeneration or deafferentation reduces synaptic contacts in the outer laminae of the dorsal horn. Moreover, recent studies have suggested that cell death of segmental interneurons may be one reason for development of hyperexcitability (Baba et al. 2003). As a consequence, Aβ-mechanoreceptive afferents, which normally terminate in deeper laminae (III and IV), grow into lamina II and directly contact the deafferented cells (Woolf et al. 1992). While these findings would explain the touch-evoked allodynia in patients with reduced or lost C-fiber input, more recent experimental findings have questioned this explanation. The experimental evidence for a deafferentation hyperexcitability is unclear, although clinical observations confirm such hyperexcitability (Watson et al. 1991; Nurmikko 2001). Pathological studies have demonstrated loss of nerve fibers or cell bodies in the peripheral nerve, the DRG, and the spinal cord in several painful sensory neuropathies including HIV-associated, diabetic, and idiopathic neuropathy. Skin biopsies and the anti-PGP 9.5 antibody, a pan-axonal marker, were used in patients with postherpetic neuralgia (PHN) and in herpes zoster patients without pain

(Rowbotham et al. 1996). In PHN a severe dendritic loss could be demonstrated on the affected side. C-fiber axon reflex reactions allow objective assessment of cutaneous C-fiber function in human skin (Fields et al. 1998). Histamine iontophoresis, which stimulates cutaneous C fibers, has been used in combination with laser-Doppler flowmetry to quantify the vascular response (Baron and Saguer 1993). In some patients with PHN the histamine-evoked axon reflex vasodilatation was impaired or abolished and the area of flare was decreased in skin regions with intense dynamic allodynia. Quantitative thermal sensory testing to assess C- and Aδ-fiber function revealed that some patients with acute herpes zoster and some chronic PHN patients have pathologically high thermal thresholds in areas with marked dynamic allodynia (Nurmikko et al. 1990). Similar findings have been seen in patients with neuropathic pain due to mastectomy (Gottrup et al. 2000).

It is clear that a subgroup of neuropathic pain patients has loss of cutaneous C nociceptors and coexisting allodynia. In such patients degeneration of central terminals of unmyelinated primary afferents induces a synaptic reorganization within the dorsal horn that leads to aberrant direct connections between Aβ-mechanoreceptive fibers and dorsal horn neurons that have lost their normal nociceptor input.

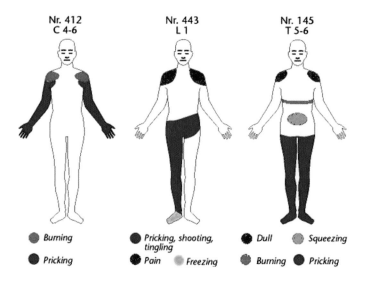

Fig. 2. Terms used to describe nociceptive and neuropathic at-level and below-level pain in patients with a cervical, lumbar, or thoracic spinal cord injury.

CENTRAL NEUROPATHIC PAIN

A characteristic neuropathic phenomenon after spinal cord injury is neuropathic pain at the injury level and at sites below that level. At the level of injury, pain manifests as a strip of sensory abnormality, while below that level it may occur as phantom pain in the anesthetic body part. The pain below injury level may be driven by populations of hyperexcitable neurons immediately rostral to the injury level that have intact central connections to the brain. In central post-stroke pain, the pain always occurs in a portion of the body part that has lost its afferent input. A hyperexcitability in neurons that have lost a normal afferent drive may underlie the pain in these cases.

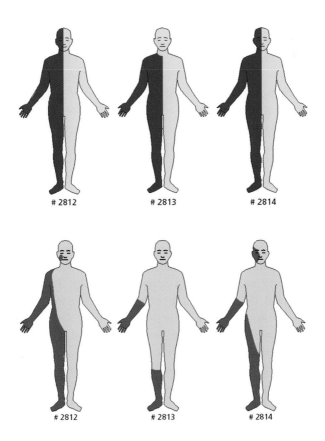

Fig. 3. Distribution of sensory abnormality (upper panel) and of pain (lower panel) in patients with pain due to a stroke in brain hemispheres contralateral to the sensory abnormalities and pain.

SPINAL CORD INJURY PAIN

Spinal cord injury (SCI) pain may occur in patients with spinal cord damage due to trauma or diseases such as multiple sclerosis, neoplasms, or spinal stroke (Table I). Studies report pain in an average of 70% of SCI patients, of whom one-third have severe pain. SCI leads to a wide range of sensory disturbances with both negative and positive symptoms. Patients may complain of ongoing stimulus-independent pain or dysesthesia at or below the level of injury; pain may be burning, freezing, squeezing, shooting, aching, pricking, or tingling (Fig. 2). Paresthesias may accompany these unpleasant sensations. Stimulus-dependent pain may occur at the level of injury or in a portion of the body below the injury level in cases of incomplete injuries.

The separation of SCI pain into "at-level" and "below-level" pain (Siddall et al. 2000) may indicate different mechanisms for these two types of pain. Below-level pain is considered to be a central pain caused by the spinal cord trauma, while at-level pain may have both peripheral (nerve root) and central (spinal cord) components. Accordingly, at-level pain tends to have an early onset, while below-level pain develops months or years after the spinal injury; despite treatment attempts, remission rates for both types are low (Siddall et al. 2003).

Neuropathic pain in SCI is distributed in an area of sensory loss. The dominating sensory deficit is abnormal spinothalamic function with altered sensitivity to temperature and pinprick (Bowsher 1996). Spinothalamic lesion, however, is not a sufficient condition because patients with such lesions may be pain free (Eide et al. 1996; Defrin et al. 2001; Finnerup et al. 2003a). Clinical examination and quantitative sensory testing indicate that thermal and tactile sensations may be equally severely affected in patients with and without pain, but evoked pains such as allodynia are more prevalent in pain patients and in areas of spontaneous pain. These findings have led to the proposal that neuronal hyperexcitability may be an additional factor required for development of neuropathic pain. One study separating SCI patients with at-level and below-level pain found a higher intensity of brush-evoked dysesthesia and pinprick hyperalgesia at the lesion level in patients with pain as opposed to those who were pain free (Finnerup et al. 2003a). These findings suggest that neuronal hyperexcitability expressed as hypersensitivity at the segmental lesion level is an important mechanism underlying pain below injury level. Additionally, magnetic resonance imaging revealed that pain patients had significantly more damage to the spinal gray matter at the rostral end of the spinal lesion compared to those without pain (Finnerup et al. 2003b). In animals with experimental lesions of the dorsal central gray matter, there are signs of sensory hypersensitivity and a corresponding neuronal hyperexcitability in the dorsal horn at or near the level of injury (Yezierski et al. 1998). Deafferentation from interruption of spinothalamic projections in combination with neuronal hyperexcitability at the segmental level of the injury may be important for the development of pain below injury level (Vierck et al. 2002; Finnerup et al. 2003b).

Sensory perception may also be altered in areas not directly affected by the spinal lesion. At trunk sites adjacent to the spinal injury site, sensory detection thresholds are lower in SCI patients with pain than in those without pain (Song et al. 1993; Cohen et al. 1996), while higher detection thresholds have been recorded in pain patients in areas innervated by the trigeminal nerve remote from the spinal injury (Finnerup et al. 2003c). This increase in detection thresholds remote from the spinal injury suggests that the central pain in SCI is not due to a generalized central sensitization leading to a general lowering of thresholds. Rather, the decreases in thresholds observed only near the injury level suggest a restricted hyperexcitability in segments close to the injury. It is not known whether the remote increases in threshold are due to recruitment of endogenous pain suppression systems, attentional deficits, or secondary changes in supraspinal structures.

POST-STROKE PAIN

Post-stroke pain, formerly known as thalamic pain. is a classic example of a central pain condition (Bowsher 1996). The condition is characterized by pain and sensory abnormalities in body parts damaged by a vascular lesion in the brain. Initially, the contralateral part of the thalamus was the presumed site, but subsequent studies have shown that the lesion can occur in any part of the brain where disruption of normal ascending somatosensory traffic would affect the sensory body functions. It is now believed that disruption of the spinothalamic tract plays an essential role in development of central pain. Accordingly, post-stroke pain has been described following lateral medullary infarctions, thalamic strokes, and various cortical lesions. While central pain was previously considered a rare condition, more recent studies indicate that it may occur in up to 8% of patients afflicted by a stroke. Patients generally complain of a burning, tightening, or squeezing sensation in body parts corresponding to the area that has been deafferented by the vascular lesion. Clinical examination indicates sensory abnormality with both hypo- and hypersensitivity. The hyposensitivity reflects the deafferentation caused by the lesion, while the islands of hypersensitivity reflect neuronal hyperexcitability, possibly due to the deafferentation (Jensen and Lenz 1995; Vestergaard et al. 1995; Boivie 1999). The pain is characteristically distributed within the territory with sensory abnormality and generally occupies only a fraction of that area (Fig. 3). These observations have led to the proposal that post-stroke pain may be due not only to a loss of spinothalamic input into certain parts of the brain, but also reflects a central neuronal hyperexcitability in neuronal populations that have lost their normal patterned (inhibitory?) input. Seen as such, post-stroke pain can be due to a disinhibition from cells that are normally under control from surrounding structures. Consistent with this observation, it has been possible to reduce central pain by substances that inhibit central neurons (Attal et al. 2000; Vestergaard et al. 2001).

HYPERALGESIA WITHOUT NERVE DAMAGE

Positive sensory symptoms sometimes occur in patients without nerve damage. This response is well described in patients with chronic musculoskeletal types of pain such as tension type headache, whiplash injuries, and fibromyalgia. In cases with hyperalgesia of undetermined origin, a careful neurological examination is crucial to document or refute damage to the nervous system. Electrophysiological imaging or other laboratory techniques may be helpful in documenting nerve damage. While the distribution of negative sensory phenomena provides the most reliable documentation of nerve damage, the extent of hyperalgesic phenomena is of less value due to the dynamic nature of the nervous system with the spread of neuronal hypersensitivity to non-damaged areas.

ACKNOWLEDGMENTS

The studies on which this chapter is based have in part been supported by grants from the Danish Pain Research Center, Danish Medical Research Council, Institute for Experimental Clinical Research University of Aarhus, Karen Elise Jensens Foundation, Ludvig og Sara Elsass' Foundation, and the Danish Society of Polio and Accident Victims.

REFERENCES

Attal N, Gaude V, Brasseur L, et al. Intravenous lidocaine in central pain: a double-blind, placebo-controlled, psychophysical study. *Neurology* 2000; 54:564–574.
Baba H, Ji RR, Kohno T, et al. Removal GABAergic inhibition facilitate A fiber-mediated excitatory transmission to the superficial spinal dorsal horn. *Mol Cell Neurosci* 2003; 24:818–830.

Baron R. Peripheral neuropathic pain: from mechanisms to symptoms. *Clin J Pain* 2000;16:s12–s20.

Baron R, Saguer M. Postherpetic neuralgia: are C-nociceptors involved in signalling and maintenance of tactile allodynia? *Brain* 1993; 116:1477–1496.

Besson J-M. The neurobiology of pain. *Lancet* 1999; 353:1610–1615.

Boivie J. Central pain. In: Wall PD, Melzack R (Eds). *Textbook of Pain,* 4th ed. Edinburgh: Churchill Livingstone, 1999, pp 879–914.

Bowsher D. Central pain: clinical and physiological characteristics. *J Neurol Neurosurg Psychiatry* 1996; 61:62–69.

Chabal C, Jacobson L, Russell LC, Burchiel KJ. Pain responses to perineuromal injection of normal saline, gallamine and lidocaine in humans. *Pain* 1989; 36:321

Chabal C, Jacobson L, Russell LC, Burchiel KJ. Pain responses to perineuromal injection of normal saline, epinephrine and lidocaine in humans. *Pain* 1992; 49:9–12.

Coderre TJ, Katz J. Peripheral and central hyperexcitability: differential signs and symptoms in persistent pain. *Behav Brain Sci* 1997; 20:404–419.

Cohen MJ, Song ZK, Schandler SL, Ho WH, Vulpe M. Sensory detection and pain thresholds in spinal cord injury patients with and without dysesthetic pain, and in chronic low back pain patients. *Somatosens Mot Res* 1996; 13:29–37.

Defrin R, Ohry A, Blumen N, Urca G. Characterization of chronic pain and somatosensory function in spinal cord injury subjects. *Pain* 2001; 89:253–263.

Devor M, Seltzer Z. Pathophysiology of damaged nerves in relation to chronic pain. In: Wall PD, Melzack R (Eds). *Textbook of Pain.* Edinburgh: Churchill Livingstone, 1999, pp 128–164.

Dubner R. Neuronal plasticity in the spinal and medullary dorsal horns: a possible role in central pain mechanisms. In: Casey KL (Eds). *Pain and Central Nervous Disease: The Central Pain Syndromes.* New York: Raven Press, 1991, pp 143–155.

Eide PK, Jorum E, Stenehjem AE. Somatosensory findings in patients with spinal cord injury and central dysaesthesia pain. *J Neurol Neurosurg Psychiatry* 1996; 60:411–415.

Fields HL, Rowbotham M, Baron R. Postherpetic neuralgia: irritable nociceptors and deafferentation. *Neurobiol Dis* 1998; 5:209–227.

Finnerup NB, Jensen TS. Spinal cord injury pain—mechanisms and treatment. *Eur J Neurol* 2004; 11:73–82.

Finnerup NB, Johannesen IL, Fuglsang-Frederiksen A, Bach FW, Jensen TS. Sensory function in spinal cord injury patients with and without central pain. *Brain* 2003a; 126:57–70.

Finnerup NB, Gyldensted C, Nielsen E, et al. MRI in chronic spinal cord injury patients with and without central pain. *Neurology* 2003b; 61:1569–1575.

Finnerup NB, Johannesen IL, Bach FW, Jensen TS. Sensory function above lesion level in spinal cord injury patients with and without pain. *Somatosens Mot Res* 2003c; 20:71–76.

Flor H, Elbert T, Knecht S, et al. Phantom limb pain as a perceptual correlate of cortical reorganization following arm amputation. *Nature* 1995; 375:482–484.

Flor H, Denke C, Schaefer M, Grüsser S. Sensory discrimination training alters both cortical reorganization and phantom limb pain. *Lancet* 2001; 357:1763–1764.

Gottrup H, Nielsen J, Arendt-Nielsen L, Jensen TS. The relationship between sensory thresholds and mechanical hyperalgesia in nerve injury. *Pain* 1998; 75:321–329.

Gottrup H, Andersen J, Arendt-Nielsen L, Jensen TS. Psychophysical examination in patients with postmastectomy pain. *Pain* 2000; 87:275–284.

Gottrup H, Kristensen AD, Bach FW, Jensen TS. Aftersensations in experimental and clinical hyperalgesia. *Pain* 2003; 103:157–164.

Gracely RH, Lynch SA, Bennett GJ. Painful neuropathy: altered central processing, maintained dynamically by peripheral input. *Pain* 1992; 51:175–194.

Hansson P, Lacerenza M, Marchettini P. Aspects of clinical and experimental neuropathic pain: the clinical perspective. In: Hansson PT, Fields HL, Hill RG, Marchettini P (Eds). *Neuropathic Pain: Pathophysiology and Treatment,* Progress in Pain Research and Management, Vol. 21. Seattle: IASP Press, 2001, pp 1–18.

Hunt SP, Mantyh PW. The molecular dynamics of pain control. *Nat Rev Neurosci* 2001; 2:83–91.

Jensen TS, Baron R. Translation of symptoms and signs into mechanisms in neuropathic pain. *Pain* 2003; 102:1–8

Jensen TS, Gottrup H. Assessment of neuropathic pain. In: Jensen TS, Wilson PR, Rice ASC (Eds). *Clinical Pain Management: Chronic Pain*. London: Arnold, 2003, pp 113–124.

Jensen TS, Lenz FA. Central post-stroke pain: a challenge for the scientist and the clinician. *Pain* 1995; 61:161–164.

Jensen TS, Gottrup H, Sindrup SH, Bach FW. The clinical picture of neuropathic pain. *Eur J Pharmacol* 2001; 429:1–11.

Julius D, Basbaum AI. Molecular mechanisms of nociception. *Nature* 2001; 413:203–210.

Koltzenburg M. Painful neuropathies. *Curr Opin Neurol* 1998; 11:515–521.

Koltzenburg M, Scadding J. Neuropathic pain. *Curr Opin Neurol* 2001; 14:641–647.

Kristensen JD, Svensson B, Gordh T Jr. The NMDA receptor antagonist CPP abolishes neurogenic "wind-up pain" after intrathecal administration in humans. *Pain* 1992; 51:249–253.

Mantyh PW, Cloihisy DR, Koltzenburg M, Hunt SP. Molecular mechanisms of cancer pain. *Nature Rev Cancer* 2001; 2:201–209.

Michaelis M, Vogel C, Blenk KH, Janig W. Algesics excite axotomised afferent nerve fibres within the first hours following nerve transection in rats. *Pain* 1997; 72:347–354.

Novakovic SD, Tzoumaka E, McGivern JG, et al. Distribution of the tetrodotoxin-resistant sodium channel PN3 in rat sensory neurons in normal and neuropathic conditions. *J Neurosci* 1998; 18:2174–2187.

Nurmikko TJ. Postherpetic neuralgia—a model for neuropathic pain. In: Hansson PT, Fields HL, Hill RG, Marchettini P (Eds). *Neuropathic Pain: Pathophysiology and Treatment, Progress in Pain Research and Management*, Vol. 21. Seattle: IASP Press, 2001, pp 151–167.

Nurmikko TJ, Rasanen A, Hakkinen V. Clinical and neurophysiological observations on acute herpes zoster. *Clin J Pain* 1990; 6:284–290.

Nystrom B, Hagbarth KE. Microelectrode recordings from transected nerves in amputees with phantom limb pain. *Neurosci Lett* 1981; 27:211–216.

Ochoa JL, Yarnitsky D. Mechanical hyperalgesias in neuropathic pain patients: dynamic and static subtypes. *Ann Neurol* 1993; 33:465–472.

Orstavik K, Weidner C, Schmidt R, et al. Pathological c-fibres in patients with a chronic painful condition. *Brain* 2003; 126:567–578.

Otto M, Bak S, Bach FW, Jensen TS, Sindrup SH. Pain phenomena and possible mechanisms in patients with painful polyneuropathy. *Pain* 2003; 101:187–192.

Petersen KL, Fields HL, Brennum J, Sandroni P, Rowbotham MC. Capsaicin evoked pain and allodynia in post-herpetic neuralgia. *Pain* 2000; 88:125–133.

Rasmussen PV, Sindrup SH, Jensen TS, Bach FW. Symptoms and signs in patients with suspected neuropathic pain. *Pain* 2004; in press.

Rowbotham MC, Fields HL. The relationship of pain, allodynia and thermal sensation in post-herpetic neuralgia. *Brain* 1996; 119(Pt 2):347–354.

Rowbotham MC, Yosipovitch G, Connolly MK, et al. Cutaneous innervation density in the allodynic form of postherpetic neuralgia. *Neurobiol Dis* 1996; 3:205–214.

Scholz J, Woolf CJ. Can we conquer pain? *Nat Neurosci* 2002; 5:1062–1067.

Siddall PJ, Yezierski RP, Loeser JD. Pain following spinal cord injury: clinical features, prevalence, and taxonomy. *IASP Newsletter* 2000; 3. Available at http://www.iasp-pain.org/ TC00-3.html.

Siddall PJ, McClelland JM, Rutkowski SB, Cousins MJ. A longitudinal study of the prevalence and characteristics of pain in the first 5 years following spinal cord injury. *Pain* 2003; 103:249–257.

Song ZK, Cohen MJ, Ament PA, et al. Two-point discrimination thresholds in spinal cord injured patients with dysesthetic pain. *Paraplegia* 1993; 31:425–493.

Vestergaard K, Nielsen J, Andersen G, et al. Sensory abnormalities in consecutive, unselected patients with central post-stroke pain. *Pain* 1995; 61:177–186.

Vestergaard K, Andersen G, Gottrup H, Kristensen BT, Jensen TS. Lamotrigine for central poststroke pain: a randomized controlled trial. *Neurology* 2001; 56:184–190.

Vierck CJ, Cannon RL, Stevens KA, Acosta-Rua AJ, Wirth ED. Mechanisms of increased pain sensitivity within dermatomes remote from an injured segment of the spinal cord. In: Yezierski RP, Burchiel KJ (Eds). *Spinal Cord Injury Pain: Assessment, Mechanisms, Management,* Progress in Pain Research and Management, Vol. 23. Seattle: IASP Press, 2002, pp 155–173.

Wall PD, Gutnick M. Ongoing activity in peripheral nerves: the physiology and pharmacology of impulses originating from a neuroma. *Exp Neurol* 1974; 43:580–593.

Watkins LR, Milligan ED, Maier SF. Glial activation: a driving force for pathological pain. *Trends Neurosci* 2001; 24:450–455.

Watson CPN, Deck JH, Morshead C, Van der Kooy D, Evans RJ. Postherpetic neuralgia: further post-mortem studies of cases with and without pain. *Pain* 1991; 44:105–117.

Woolf CJ, Decosterd I. Implications of recent advances in the understanding of pain pathophysiology for the assessment of pain in patients. *Pain* 1999; (Suppl 6):S141–S147.

Woolf CJ, Mannion RJ. Neuropathic pain: aetiology, symptoms, mechanisms, and management. *Lancet* 1999; 353:1959–1964.

Woolf CJ, Salter MW. Neuronal plasticity: increasing the gain in pain. *Science* 2000; 288:1765–1769.

Woolf CJ, Shortland P, Coggeshall RE. Peripheral nerve injury triggers central sprouting of myelinated afferents. *Nature* 1992; 355:75–78.

Woolf CJ, Bennett GJ, Doherty M, et al. Towards a mechanism-based classification of pain? *Pain* 1998; 77:227–229.

Yezierski RP, Liu S, Ruenes GL, Kajander KJ, Brewer KL. Excitotoxic spinal cord injury: behavioral and morphological characteristics of a central pain model. *Pain* 1998; 75:141–155.

Correspondence to: Prof. Troels S. Jensen, MD, PhD, Department of Neurology and Danish Pain Research Center, Aarhus University Hospital, DK-8000 Aarhus C, Denmark. Tel: 45-8949-3283; Fax: 45-8949-3300; email: tsj@akhphd.au.dk.

The Pain System in Normal and Pathological States:
A Primer for Clinicians, Progress in Pain Research
and Management, Vol. 31, edited by Luis Villanueva,
Anthony Dickenson, and Hélène Ollat, IASP Press,
Seattle, © 2004.

17

Novel Strategies for Neuropathic Pain

Didier Bouhassira and Nadine Attal

Center for the Evaluation and Treatment of Pain, INSERM E-332, Ambroise
Paré Hospital, Boulogne-Billancourt, France; and University of Versailles-
Saint-Quentin, France

According to the definition of the International Association for the Study
of Pain (IASP), the term *neuropathic pain* refers to all pains initiated or
caused by a primary lesion or dysfunction of the nervous system. This broad
category includes highly heterogeneous and difficult-to-treat clinical conditions associated with a large variety of lesions in the peripheral or central
nervous system (Woolf and Mannion 1999; Jensen et al. 2001). Thus, only
approximately one-third of patients achieve satisfactory relief with antidepressants and antiepileptics, which are considered the mainstay of treatment
(Sindrup and Jensen 1999, 2000). The heterogeneity of neuropathic pain
syndromes is apparent from the clinical examination of patients with various
painful symptoms including spontaneous pain, either continuous or paroxysmal, and evoked pain. The latter, which can be even more distressing than
spontaneous pain, is termed *allodynia* when pain is triggered by normally
non-noxious stimuli, and *hyperalgesia* when pain is an exaggerated response
to a normally noxious stimulus. Due to poor understanding of their pathophysiological mechanisms, the different neuropathic pain syndromes were
grouped together and treated in a uniform fashion. This empirical approach
might represent a major cause of therapeutic failures in these patients.

Over the last few years, several authors have proposed a new approach
to neuropathic and other types of pain based on the current understanding of
pain mechanisms and with the aim to target treatments specifically at those
mechanisms (Woolf et al. 1998; Woolf and Decosterd 1999; Woolf and
Mannion 1999; Woolf and Max 2001). Such a rational approach is attractive
but does not yet seem attainable, mainly due to the difficulties of translating
the pathophysiological mechanisms identified in animal studies to the clinical treatment of patients (Max 2000; Hansson 2003; Jensen and Baron 2003;

Fig. 1). More clinically oriented approaches seem to be more realistic and rapidly applicable. Several major questions must be readdressed in the clinical setting to help to determine: (1) whether pain associated with a nerve injury has specific features as compared with pain associated with other types of somatic lesions and (2) whether the clinical presentation or therapeutic response of neuropathic pains differs according to the anatomical location (e.g., peripheral versus central) or the cause of the lesion (e.g., postherpetic neuralgia, diabetes, or trauma). Such clinical studies should allow establishment of diagnostic criteria of neuropathic pain and identification of any distinct clinical subtypes (or syndromes) pertaining to the broad neuropathic pain category. This information is essential for proposing a consensual and operational definition of neuropathic pain, and more importantly, it could also lead to substantial improvement of therapeutic strategies. This chapter, presents recent data that tend to support the relevance of this clinical approach to neuropathic pain.

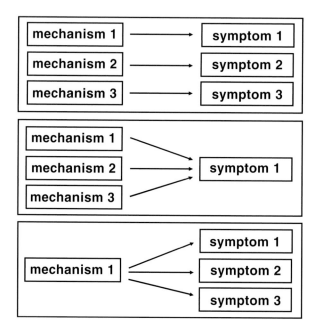

Fig. 1. Possible relationship between neuropathic pain symptoms and pathophysiological mechanisms. On the basis of the available experimental and clinical data, it is not yet possible to determine whether each symptom is sustained by a specific mechanism, whether a single symptom can be sustained by several mechanisms, or whether a single mechanism can explain several symptoms.

CLINICAL FEATURES AND DIAGNOSIS
OF NEUROPATHIC PAIN

The definition of neuropathic pain has long been a subject of controversy (e.g., Backonja 2003; Bennett 2003; Dworkin et al. 2003; Hansson 2003). Much discussion has revolved around the term "dysfunction," which many authors consider too vague. Indeed, according to the current definition, many conditions not associated with a clearly identified lesion, such as fibromyalgia, irritable bowel syndrome, stomatodynia, and migraine are sometimes included in this category because they could involve some dysfunctions of the nervous system. This issue is of major theoretical interest, but in our opinion, relevant pathophysiological and clinical data to validate any definition of neuropathic pain are still lacking.

Neuropathic pains are generally characterized by the association of unspecified positive and negative symptoms, but these pains still lack validated diagnostic criteria. Surprisingly few studies have directly compared the symptoms and signs associated with a nerve lesion to those of other somatic lesions (Boureau et al. 1990; Bennett et al. 2001; Krause and Backonja 2003). Furthermore, these studies had methodological limitations because they included patients without identified nerve lesions (e.g., complex regional pain syndrome [CRPS] type I), patients with pains presumably of mixed origin (e.g., lumboradicular or cervicobrachial neuralgia; Boureau et al. 1990; Bennett et al. 2001), or did not mention the causes of pain (Krause and Backonja 2003). It is thus difficult to determine the specific characteristics of pain that might be associated with a definite injury of the nervous system. We recently performed a prospective, multicenter study with a panel of French experts to compare directly patients with "pure" neuropathic pain due to a peripheral or central neurological lesion and patients with pain due to other somatic tissue injuries (Bouhassira et al. 2004a). This comparison was based on responses to a 17-item hetero-assessed questionnaire including pain descriptors and items related to clinical examination, both rated as present or absent. The most frequent causes of neuropathic pain were traumatic nerve injury, postherpetic neuralgia, and post-stroke pain. Osteoarthritis and common low back pain were the most frequent causes in the non-neuropathic pain group.

As shown in Table I, several pain descriptors such as "burning" and "shooting" and symptoms such as "tingling," "pins and needles," or "numbness" were highly prevalent and significantly more frequent in patients with a nerve injury, although none were specific. Not surprisingly, the clinical examination revealed hypoesthesia in most patients with a neurological lesion

Table I
Comparison of the pain descriptors in patients presenting with
neuropathic (n = 89) or non-neuropathic pains (n = 71)

Pain Descriptor	Neuropathic Pain (%)	Non-neuropathic Pain (%)	$P*$
Burning	68.3	30.4	<0.001
Squeezing	48.8	37.7	n.s.
Cold pain	25.6	10.1	0.01
Shooting	64.6	17.4	<0.001
Lancinating	75.6	65.2	n.s.
Tingling	59.8	15.9	<0.001
Pins and needles	65.9	17.4	<0.001
Itching	29.3	5.8	<0.001
Numbness	65.9	30.4	<0.001

Source: Data from Bouhassira et al. (2004a).
* χ^2 test.

(Table II). Evoked pains were also more frequent in these patients, with the exception of hypersensitivity to pressure. Thus, these results indicate that a relatively small number of descriptors can allow investigators to discriminate between pains associated with an injury to the nervous system and those related to other somatic lesions, which may well reflect differences in their underlying pathophysiological mechanisms. We could now use the same approach to determine, whether the features of pain due to a putative nervous system dysfunction (e.g., fibromyalgia or CRPS type I) are similar to or different from those of pain associated with a frank injury to the nervous system. Apart from clarifying the definition of neuropathic pain, such an approach might be helpful for proposing positive clinical diagnostic criteria. Such criteria would be of major interest in both daily practice and in the clinical research setting, especially for standardizing the selection of patients to be included in future therapeutical trials.

EVALUATION AND CLASSIFICATION
OF NEUROPATHIC PAIN

According to the data succinctly described above, a lesion of the nervous system tends to confer particular qualities to the painful symptoms. However, this category is highly heterogenous because it includes many different causes and types of lesions, and patients may report multiple combinations of symptoms including spontaneous and evoked pains. This situation raises two major clinical questions: (1) Is there one or are there several subtypes of neuropathic pains? and (2) What are the appropriate criteria for defining such subtypes? The cause or the anatomical location of the lesion and the symptoms could constitute relevant criteria for classification.

To address these questions, we need adequate methods for evaluating the different components of neuropathic pain. Current pain questionnaires, such as the McGill Pain Questionnaire (MPQ; Melzack 1975) or Brief Pain Inventory (BPI; Cleeland and Ryan 1994) are not specific enough for this purpose. Quantitative sensory testing (QST) appears to be particularly suitable for measuring evoked pain (Fruhstorfer et al. 1976; Hansson and Lindblom 1992). However, the limitations of QST are the length of time required for testing, the variability of the test-retest reliability, and the need for trained investigators to conduct the tests (Yarnitzky 1997). They are still difficult to use in multicenter studies with large patient cohorts. To address these questions, we developed and validated a 10-item self-questionnaire, the Neuropathic Pain Symptom Inventory (NPSI), specifically designed to assess the different components of neuropathic pain. We wanted to collect evidence on four components: spontaneous ongoing pain, paroxysmal pain, evoked pain, and paresthesia/dysesthesia. We conducted a complete validation study of this questionnaire in 176 patients with "pure" neuropathic pain due to a peripheral or central lesion (Bouhassira et al. 2004b). A factor analysis clearly identified five distinct dimensions of neuropathic pain. In particular, we identified two dimensions corresponding to superficial and deep spontaneous ongoing pain. The other factors corresponded to paroxysmal pain, evoked pain, and paresthesia. This analysis thus clearly demonstrated that neuropathic pain is a multidimensional entity.

Table II
Comparison of the clinical examination in patients presenting
with neuropathic ($n = 89$) or non-neuropathic pains ($n = 71$)

Clinical Finding	Neuropathic Pain (%)	Non-neuropathic Pain (%)	P*
Touch hypoesthesia	64.6	5.8	<0.001
Pressure hypoesthesia	69.5	10.1	<0.001
Heat hypoesthesia	70.7	5.8	<0.001
Cold hypoesthesia	67.1	4.3	<0.001
Brush allodynia	41.5	4.3	<0.001
Pressure allodynia	46.3	44.9	n.s.
Cold allodynia	28.0	4.3	<0.001
Heat allodynia	20.7	4.3	0.003

Source: Data from Bouhassira et al. (2004a).
* χ^2 test.

We used the NPSI to compare the frequency of descriptors in the different populations of neuropathic pain patients. First, we compared peripheral and central pain. As shown in Fig. 2, we found few differences,; only two items were slightly but significantly different between both groups. Pressure-evoked pain was more frequent in peripheral neuropathic pain, while cold-evoked pain was more frequent in central pain. However, further comparisons of the frequencies of descriptors between the various peripheral and central etiologies included in this study were less consistent. In fact, the six main etiological groups included in this study (i.e., postherpetic neuralgia, painful polyneuropathies, traumatic nerve injury, post-stroke pain, spinal cord trauma, and syringomyelia) appeared to be similar in terms of the frequency of the items. This finding was further confirmed by a multiple correspondence analysis, which did not show any association between the painful symptoms (or paresthesia/dysesthesia) and the cause or location of the lesion.

As a whole, these data suggest that the prevalence and frequency of neuropathic pain symptoms are "trans-etiological" and consequently that the cause and location of the lesion do not constitute relevant criteria for a subclassification of neuropathic pains. Thus, the current way of selecting patients based on the disease or topography of the lesion is not justified and probably not appropriate. Pharmacological trials also illustrate this point, showing that most systemic treatments of neuropathic pain have similar efficacy in various disease entities, such as postherpetic neuralgia, painful

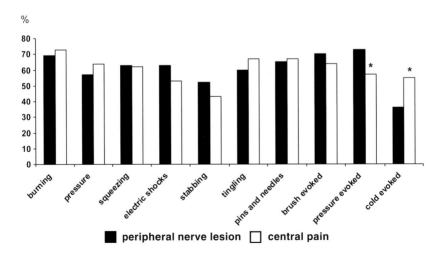

Fig. 2. Comparison (χ^2 test) of the percentage of neuropathic symptoms in patients with peripheral nerve lesions ($n = 120$) and central lesions ($n = 56$). * $P < 0.05$. Data from Bouhassira et al. (2004a).

polyneuropathies, and central pain, with a number needed to treat (NNT) ranging from 2.5 to 4 (Sindrup and Jensen 1999, 2000). This finding concerns antidepressants (McQuay et al. 1996; Sindrup and Jensen 2000), gabapentin (Backonja et al. 1998; Rowbotham et al. 1998; Rice and Maton 2001; Pandey et al. 2002), lamotrigine (Eisenberg et al. 2000; Vestergaard et al. 2001), and opioids and tramadol (Harati et al. 1998; Watson and Babul 1998; Sindrup et al. 1999; Boureau et al. 2003; Watson et al. 2003). Furthermore, in trials that included patients with various peripheral or central neuropathic pains, the level of the injury or its cause did not influence patients' analgesic response to opioids (Dellemijn et al. 1997; Rowbotham et al. 2003).

In contrast, our data tend to emphasize the advantage of a symptom-based approach to neuropathic pain. The relevance of such an approach has also been suggested by a series of pharmacological studies, particularly those using QST, which showed the differential or preferential effects of various agents on neuropathic pain symptoms. Thus, better effects on spontaneous pain compared to mechanical allodynia have been reported with lamotrigine and desipramine (Max et al. 1991; Vestergaard et al. 2001), while the reverse has been demonstrated with N-methyl-D-aspartic acid (NMDA) antagonists and opioids (Eide et al. 1994, 1995a,b; Leung et al. 2001; Attal et al. 2002; Wallace et al. 2002). Other studies have reported modality-specific effects on the various subtypes of allodynia (Eide et al. 1994, 1995a,b; Attal et al. 2000, 2002; Wallace et al. 2000; Leung et al. 2001). This finding is illustrated in particular by our studies of the sodium channel blocker intravenous (i.v.) lidocaine (Attal et al. 2000, 2004). In these studies, a similar pattern of effects was seen in patients with peripheral or central pain due to several causes. In both groups of patients, i.v. lidocaine preferentially reduced ongoing pain and mechanical allodynia, which suggests that these symptoms share some common mechanisms, whatever their cause. In contrast, cold allodynia/hyperalgesia was not significantly modified after lidocaine administration, suggesting that it is subserved by distinct mechanisms.

However, individual symptoms alone may not be sufficient to classify neuropathic pain syndromes, which show a constellation of various painful and nonpainful symptoms and signs of sensory deficits. A classification based on a combination of symptoms and signs might be more relevant (Jensen and Baron 2003). Such a classification should remain trans-etiological, given that one combination may be common to several etiologies. For instance, burning pain and brush-induced allodynia frequently coexist in both postherpetic neuralgia and central pain (Boivie et al. 1989; Nurmikko and Bowsher 1990; Bowsher 1996; Fields et al. 1998; Bouhassira et al.

2000; Pappagallo et al. 2000). Conversely, several different combinations may be observed in a given disease, such as postherpetic neuralgia, nerve trauma, or pain due to spinal cord injury (Fields et al. 1998; Bouhassira et al. 2000; Baumgartner et al. 2002). The mechanisms involved in individual pain symptoms might well depend on whether they pertain to one or another distinct combination. For instance, in a study of patients with HIV-related polyneuropathies, we observed a significant correlation between spontaneous pain intensity and the magnitude of mechanical static (punctate) hyperalgesia, which suggests common peripheral mechanisms for these two symptoms (Bouhassira et al. 1999). In contrast, the same symptom, such as burning pain due to various causes (postherpetic neuralgia, traumatic nerve lesions, or spinal cord injury) could involve distinct mechanisms depending on whether it is associated with mechanical allodynia and severe thermal deficits (Fields et al. 1998; Bouhassira et al. 2000; Baumgartner et al. 2002). Such a classification could have therapeutic implications. In patients with traumatic nerve injuries and postherpetic neuralgia, we recently demonstrated that i.v. lidocaine was more effective in patients with spontaneous (generally burning) pain combined with mechanical allodynia than in those with spontaneous pain only (Attal et al. 2004). Similar dissociated effects have been reported by studies using lamotrigine in patients with spinal cord injury pain (Finnerup et al. 2002). To confirm the clinical validity of such an approach, we need clinical and pharmacological studies in larger cohorts of patients with a detailed assessment of their various neuropathic pain symptoms and signs.

CONCLUSION

Pain associated with a nerve lesion represents a particular group of conditions that should be diagnosed based validated criteria, at least in the clinical research setting. Several lines of evidence indicate that neuropathic pains constitute a multidimensional category. Thus, the development of novel treatment strategies may well depend on the identification of relevant criteria that allow diagnosis and classification of patients in several subgroups who might respond differentially to the treatments. Numerous data tend to favor an approach based on symptoms, or combinations of symptoms, of neuropathic pain, but this approach should be confirmed in further studies. Whether it is legitimate (or useful) to incorporate other painful syndromes unrelated to a clearly identified lesion (e.g., fibromyalgia, stomatodynia, and irritable bowel syndrome) in this category still requires determination.

REFERENCES

Attal N, Gaudé V, Brasseur L, et al. Intravenous lidocaine in central pain: a double blind placebo controlled psychophysical study. *Neurology* 2000; 54:564–574.

Attal N, Guirimand F, Brasseur L, et al. Effects of IV morphine in central pain: a randomized placebo-controlled study. *Neurology* 2002; 58:554–563.

Attal N, Rouaud J, Brasseur L, Chauvin M, Bouhassira D. Systemic lidocaine in pain due to peripheral nerve injury and predictors of response. *Neurology* 2004; 62(2):218–225.

Backonja MM. Defining neuropathic pain. *Anesth Analg* 2003; 97:785–790.

Backonja M, Beydoyn A, Edwards KR, et al. for the Gabapentin Diabetic Neuropathy Study Group. Gabapentin for the symptomatic treatment of painful neuropathy in patients with diabetes mellitus. *JAMA* 1998; 280:1831–1836.

Baron R. Peripheral neuropathic pain: from mechanisms to symptoms. *Clin J Pain* 2000; 16(Suppl):S12–20.

Baumgartner U, Magerl W, Klein T, et al. Neurogenic hyperalgesia versus painful hypoalgesia: two distinct mechanisms of neuropathic pain. *Pain* 2002; 96:141–151.

Bennett GJ. Neuropathic pain: a crisis of definition? *Anesth Analg* 2003; 97:619–620.

Bennett M. The LANSS Pain Scale: the Leeds assessment of neuropathic symptoms and signs. *Pain* 2001; 92:147–157.

Boivie J, Leijon G, Johansson I. Central post-stroke pain—a study of the mechanisms through analyses of the sensory abnormalities. *Pain* 1989; 37:173–185.

Bouhassira D, Attal N, Willer JC, Brasseur L. Quantitative sensory testing in patients with painful or painless peripheral neuropathy due to HIV infection. *Pain* 1999; 80:265–272.

Bouhassira D, Attal N, Parker F, Brasseur L. Quantitative sensory testing in patients with painful or painless syringomyelia. In: Devor M, Rowbotham MC, Wiesenfeld-Hallin (Eds). *Proceedings of the 9th World Congress on Pain,* Progress in Pain Research and Management, Vol. 16. Seattle: IASP Press, 2000, pp 401–411.

Bouhassira D, Attal N, Boureau F, et al. Development and validation of a questionnaire for the diagnosis of neuropathic pain. *J Pain* 2004; 5(Suppl 1):115.

Bouhassira D, Attal N, Fermanian J, et al. Development and validation of the Neuropathic Pain Symptom Inventory. *Pain* 2004b; 108(3):248–257.

Boureau F, Doubrere JF, Luu M. Study of verbal description in neuropathic pain. *Pain* 1990; 42:145–152.

Boureau F, Legallicier P, Kabir-Ahmadi M. Tramadol in post-herpetic neuralgia: a randomized, double-blind, placebo-controlled trial. *Pain* 2003; 104:323–331.

Bowsher D. Central pain: clinical and physiological characteristics. *J Neurol Neurosurg Psychiatry* 1996; 61:62–69.

Cleeland CS, Ryan KM. Pain assessment: global use of the Brief Pain Inventory. *Ann Acad Med Singapore* 1994; 23:129–138.

Dellemijn PL, Vanneste JA. Randomised double-blind active-placebo controlled crossover trial of intravenous fentanyl in neuropathic pain. *Lancet* 1997; 349:753–758.

Dworkin RH, Backonja M, Rowbotham MC, et al. Advances in neuropathic pain: diagnosis, mechanisms, and treatment recommendations. *Arch Neurol* 2003; 60:1524–1534.

Eide PK, Jorum E, Stubhaub A, Bremmes J, Breivik H. Relief of post-herpetic neuralgia with the *N*-methyl-D-aspartic acid receptor antagonist ketamine: a double-blind, cross-over comparison with morphine and placebo. *Pain* 1994; 58:347–354.

Eide PK, Strubhaug A, Oye I, Breivik H. Continuous subcutaneous administration of the *N*-methyl-D-aspartic acid (NMDA) receptor antagonist ketamine in the treatment of post-herpetic neuralgia. *Pain* 1995a; 61:221–228.

Eide PK, Stubhaug A, Stenehjem AE. Central dysesthesia pain after traumatic spinal cord injury is dependent on *N*-methyl-D-aspartate receptor activation. *Neurosurgery* 1995b; 37:1080–1087.

Eisenberg E, Lurie Y, Braker C, Daoud D, Ishay A. Lamotrigine reduces painful diabetic neuropathy: a randomized, controlled study. *Neurology* 2001; 57:505–509.

Fields H, Rowbotham M, Baron R. Postherpetic neuralgia: irritable nociceptors and deafferentation. *Neurobiol Dis* 1998; 209–227.

Finnerup N, Sindrup SH, Bach FW, Johannesen IL, Jensen TS. Lamotrigine in spinal cord injury pain: a randomized controlled trial. *Pain* 2002; 96(3):375–383.

Fruhstorfer H, Lindblom U, Schmidt WC. Method for quantitative estimation of thermal thresholds in patients. *J Neurol Neurosurg Psychiatry* 1976; 39:1071–1075.

Hansson P. Difficulties in stratifying neuropathic pain by mechanisms. *Eur J Pain* 2003; 7:353–357.

Hansson P, Lindblom U. Hyperalgesia assessed with quantitative sensory testing in patients with neurogenic pain. In: Willis WD (Ed). *Hyperalgesia and Allodynia*. New York: Raven Press, 1992, pp 335–343.

Harati Y, Glooch C, Edelmann S, et al. Double blind randomized trial of tramadol for the treatment of the pain of diabetic neuropathy. *Neurology* 1998; 50:1842–1846.

Jensen TS, Baron R. Translation of symptoms and signs into mechanisms in neuropathic pain. *Pain* 2003; 102:1–8.

Jensen TS, Gottrup H, Sindrup SH, Bach FW. The clinical picture of neuropathic pain. *Eur J Pharmacol* 2001; 429:1–11.

Krause SJ, Backonja M. Development of a neuropathic pain questionnaire. *Clin J Pain* 2003; 19:306–314.

Leung A, Wallace MS, Ridgeway B, Yaksh T. Concentration-effect relationship of intravenous alfentanil and ketamine on peripheral neurosensory thresholds, allodynia and hyperalgesia of neuropathic pain. *Pain* 2001; 91:177–187.

Max MB. Is mechanism-based pain treatment attainable? Clinical trials issues. *J Pain* 2000; 1(Suppl 1):2–9.

Max MB, Kishore-Kumar R, Schafer SC, Meister B. Efficacy of desipramine in painful diabetic neuropathy: a placebo-controlled trial. *Pain* 1991; 45:3–9.

McQuay HJ, Tramer M, Nye BA, et al. A systematic review of antidepressants in neuropathic pain. *Pain* 1996; 68:217–227.

Melzack R. The McGill Pain Questionnaire: major properties and scoring methods. *Pain* 1975; 1:275–299.

Nurmikko T, Bowsher D. Somatosensory findings in postherpetic neuralgia. *J Neurol Neurosurg Psychiatry* 1990; 53:135–141.

Pandey CK, Bose N, Garg G, et al. Gabapentin for the treatment of pain in Guillain-Barre syndrome: a double-blinded, placebo-controlled, crossover study. *Anesth Analg* 2002; 95:1719–1723.

Pappagallo M, Oaklander AL, Quatrano-Piacentini AL. Clark Heterogenous patterns of sensory dysfunction in postherpetic neuralgia suggest multiple pathophysiologic mechanisms. *Anesthesiology* 2000; 92:691–698.

Rice AS, Maton S. Gabapentin in postherpetic neuralgia: a randomised, double blind, placebo controlled study. *Pain* 2001; 94:215–224.

Rowbotham M, Harden N, Stacey B, Bernstein P, Magnus-Miller L. For the Gabapentin Postherpetic Neuralgia Study Group. Gabapentin in the treatment of postherpetic neuralgia. *JAMA* 1998; 280:1837–1842.

Rowbotham MC, Twilling L, Davies PS, et al. Oral opioid therapy for chronic peripheral and central neuropathic pain. *N Engl J Med* 2003; 348:1223–1232.

Sindrup SH, Jensen TS. Efficacy of pharmacological treatment of neuropathic pain: an update and effect related to mechanism of drug action. *Pain* 1999; 81:389–400.

Sindrup SH, Jensen TS. Pharmacologic treatment of pain in polyneuropathy. *Neurology* 2000; 55:915–920.

Sindrup SH, Andersen G, Madsen C, et al. Tramadol relieves pain and allodynia in polyneuropathy: a randomised double blind controlled trial. *Pain* 1999; 83:85–90.

Sindrup SH, Bach FW, Madsen C, Gram LF, Jensen TS. Venlafaxine versus imipramine in painful polyneuropathy: a randomized, controlled trial. *Neurology* 2003; 60:1284–1289.

Vestergaard K, Andersen G, Gottrup H, Kristensen BT, Jensen TS. Lamotrigine for central poststroke pain: a randomized controlled trial. *Neurology* 2001; 56:184–190.

Wallace MS, Ridgeway BM, Leung AY, Gerayli A, Yaksh TL. Concentration-effect relationship of intravenous lidocaine on the allodynia of complex regional pain syndrome types I and II. *Anesthesiology* 2000, 92:75–83.

Wallace MS, Rowbotham MC, Katz NP, et al. A randomized, double-blind, placebo-controlled trial of a glycine antagonist in neuropathic pain. *Neurology* 2002; 59:1694–1700.

Watson CP, Babul N. Efficacy of oxycodone in neuropathic pain: a randomized trial in postherpetic neuralgia. *Neurology* 1998; 50:1837–1841.

Watson CP, Moulin D, Watt-Watson J, Gordon A, Eisenhoffer J. Controlled-release oxycodone relieves neuropathic pain: a randomized controlled trial in painful diabetic neuropathy. *Pain* 2003; 105:71–78.

Woolf CJ, Decosterd I. Implications of recent advances in the understanding of pain pathophysiology for the assessment of pain in patients. *Pain* 1999; (Suppl 6):141–147.

Woolf CJ, Mannion RJ. Neuropathic pain aetiology, symptoms, mechanisms and management. *Lancet* 1999, 353:1959–1964.

Woolf CJ, Max MB. Mechanism-based pain diagnosis: issues for analgesic drug development. *Anesthesiology* 2001; 95:241–249.

Woolf CJ, Bennett GJ, Doherty M, et al. Towards a mechanism-based classification of pain? *Pain* 1998; 77:227–229.

Yarnitsky D. Quantitative sensory testing. *Muscle Nerve* 1997; 20:198–204.

Correspondence to: Didier Bouhassira, MD, PhD, INSERM E-332, Hôpital Ambroise Paré, 9 Avenue Charles de Gaulle, 92 100 Boulogne-Billancourt, France. Tel: 33-1-4909-4556; Fax: 33-1-4909-4435; email: didier.bouhassira@apr.ap-hop-paris.fr.

The Pain System in Normal and Pathological States:
A Primer for Clinicians, Progress in Pain Research
and Management, Vol. 31, edited by Luis Villanueva,
Anthony Dickenson, and Hélène Ollat, IASP Press,
Seattle, © 2004.

18

Novel Strategies for Modern Neurosurgery

Jean Paul Nguyen, Jean Pascal Lefaucheur,
Karim Moubarak, Pierre Cesaro, Stéphane Palfi,
and Yves Keravel

Department of Neurosciences, INSERM U-421, Créteil, France

Many instances of chronic pain are now believed to have a neurological component, and most of the novel strategies for modern neurosurgery are oriented toward the treatment of neuropathic pain. Neurosurgical methods to treat neuropathic pain date back to lesional strategies used in the early 1900s, followed by neurostimulation methods used in the early 1960s. At the present time, spinal cord stimulation should be regarded as a routine therapy in selected neuropathic pain conditions (Linderoth and Meyerson 2001). Neuropathic pain secondary to a central nervous system lesion (central pain) or to a trigeminal nerve lesion (neuropathic facial pain) is generally difficult to treat. Drug treatments are usually not very effective, and spinal cord stimulation is unsuitable or ineffective. Stimulation of the ventralis caudalis nucleus of the thalamus, designed to improve neuropathic facial pain, has been disappointing. Pain secondary to a thalamic lesion (thalamic pain) is also generally refractory to thalamic stimulation. Because insufficient data were available to support the efficacy and safety of these procedures (including midbrain periaqueductal and periventricular gray stimulation), deep brain stimulation for pain was largely abandoned.

For these various reasons, the cortex stimulation technique, proposed by Tsubokawa and colleagues (1991), constituted a very promising alternative. Tsubokawa observed that central lesions in animals could induce the development of abnormal neuronal hyperactivity in the thalamus, and that this hyperactivity could be reduced by chronic stimulation of the sensorimotor cortex. The results of an initial series of patients with thalamic pain confirmed the efficacy of chronic cortex stimulation on this type of pain

(Tsubokawa et al. 1993). In this series, 67% of patients obtained marked and lasting improvement, a much higher success rate than that obtained with thalamic stimulation. Surprisingly, stimulation of the motor cortex was found to be more effective than stimulation of the sensory cortex, which sometimes even exacerbated pain. In 1993, Meyerson and colleagues confirmed that motor cortex stimulation (MCS) was effective against deafferentation pain. Meyerson's series mainly comprised patients with neuropathic facial pain. All of these patients improved, but MCS was not effective in two patients with central pain, in contrast with the results reported by Tsubokawa. This discordance can probably be explained by the fact that the surgical technique, at that time, was relatively imprecise and poorly reproducible, because the motor cortex was identified preoperatively by the position of the coronal suture and by scalp recording of somatosensory evoked potentials. The electrode placement technique could also increase the imprecision of the procedure, as it consisted of introducing a four-plate electrode into the epidural space via a standard burr hole (Nguyen et al. 1997). The accuracy of electrode positioning therefore essentially depended on the position of the burr hole. Because the position of the electrode often had to be changed during the operation, this technique was associated with a risk of epidural hematoma. With time, the technique has become more precise, with a lower risk of complications. In parallel with improvement of the technique, the results of other teams have shown that the indications for MCS could be extended to other types of pain (Nguyen et al. 1999; Franzini et al. 2000; Saitoh et al. 2000; Katayama et al. 2001; Roux et al. 2001b). This chapter will describe the various steps leading to improvement of the surgical procedure, the current main indications, and the various hypotheses concerning the mechanism of the analgesic action of chronic MCS.

TECHNIQUE FOR MOTOR CORTEX STIMULATION

PREOPERATIVE MAPPING OF THE MOTOR CORTEX

Clinicopathological and electrophysiological studies have long established that the primary motor cortex (Brodmann's area 4) is situated in the anterior part of the central sulcus and is the part of the cortex situated immediately anteriorly to this sulcus. Penfield's studies also demonstrated the somatotopic representation of the lower limbs, upper limbs, and face that are represented on the superior, middle, and inferior parts of the precentral gyrus, respectively (Penfield et al. 1950). The motor cortex can therefore be mapped indirectly by determining the anatomical position of the central sulcus (Fig. 1). This sulcus is visible on a computed tomography (CT) scan

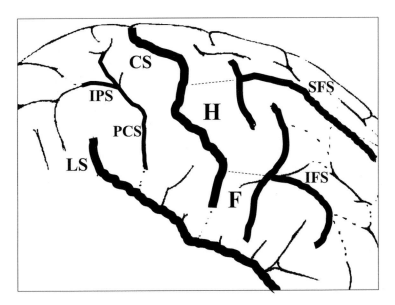

Fig. 1. Detail of the central region showing the position of the central sulcus (CS) and lateral sulcus (LS); the superior frontal sulcus (SFS), which is connected to the superior precentral sulcus; the inferior frontal sulcus (IFS), which is connected to the inferior precentral sulcus; and the postcentral sulcus (PCS), which is connected to the intraparietal sulcus (IPS).

and can be even more clearly visualized by magnetic resonance imaging (MRI). However, classical axial, frontal, and sagittal views are unsuitable for identifying the various zones (superior, middle, and inferior) of the central and precentral region. Progress in the field of digital image processing now allows identification of these various zones. These structures can be easily identified on images obtained after curved reconstruction following the curvature of the cortical surface (Lee et al. 1998). The ideal site of stimulation, based on our knowledge of the somatotopic representation of this region, can be easily determined on these images (Fig. 2).

Theoretically, to treat neuropathic facial pain, MCS should be applied to the lower part of the precentral gyrus corresponding to the representation of the face on the motor homunculus. According to the studies by Penfield et al. (1950), Woolsey et al. (1979), and MacCarthy et al. (1993), this zone is limited inferiorly by the frontoparietal operculum and lateral sulcus and superiorly by a horizontal line corresponding to a posterior continuation of the inferior frontal sulcus. The zone of stimulation for treatment of deafferentation pain affecting the upper limb is situated between the levels of the inferior and superior frontal sulci. The motor cortex situated between the levels of the superior frontal sulcus and longitudinal cerebral fissure corresponds to the

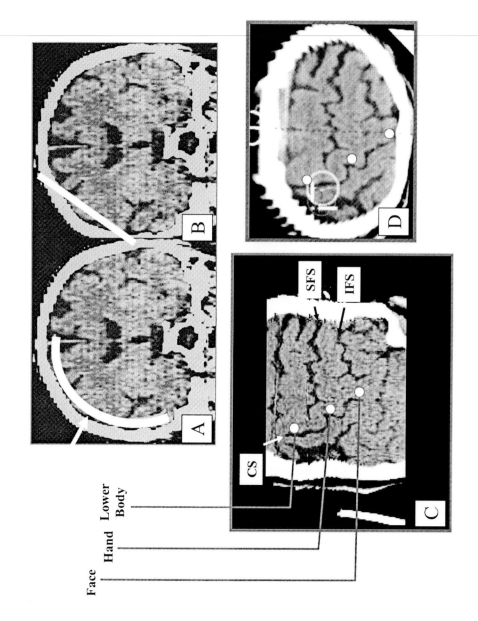

representation of the trunk and proximal part of the lower limbs. The distal part of the lower limbs is classically represented essentially in the internal surface of the hemisphere. However, Woolsey et al. (1979) showed that, in some cases, this representation could extend to the superior part of the hemisphere, even as far as the superior frontal sulcus.

These various functional zones are easily identified by neuronavigation systems, but at the present time, these systems are unable to perform curved reconstructions. However, oblique reconstructions, relatively parallel to the cortical surface, can easily be obtained. The various structures visualized by curved reconstructions (performed preoperatively) can be identified on these oblique reconstructions (Fig. 2), which can be used to define the same target. The neuronavigation system allows the center of the craniotomy to be placed very precisely over the target (Fig. 3).

Other examinations can also be helpful for preoperative target planning: functional MRI (fMRI) and especially transcranial magnetic stimulation (TMS). Functional MRI provides good visualization of the sensorimotor cortex, and its spatial resolution is sufficient to establish somatotopic maps (Rao et al. 1995). The results of fMRI are well correlated with the results of direct cortical stimulation and intraoperative somatosensory evoked potentials (Roux et al. 2001b). Some teams regularly use fMRI for preoperative motor cortex target planning (Sol 2001). TMS can also be used to identify the motor cortex (Migita et al. 1995) and can be combined with a neuronavigation system to precisely determine the cortical zone to be stimulated.

CRANIOTOMY

Several authors have demonstrated the advantages of craniotomy over a burr hole (Peyron et al. 1995; Ebel et al. 1996; Nguyen et al. 1999). By allowing suspension of the dura mater, a true craniotomy limits the risk of postoperative epidural hematoma. A craniotomy of 4–5 cm in diameter allows sufficient exploration of the central region to identify the appropriate area of the motor cortex to be stimulated. This larger access also allows a multi-plate electrode to be placed on the dura mater to optimize intraoperative electrophysiological testing. We use a 16-plate diagnostic electrode array

◄— **Fig. 2.** Superficial curved and oblique reconstructions. (A) Superficial curved reconstruction represented on panel C, visualizing the central sulcus (CS), superior frontal sulcus (SFS) and inferior frontal sulcus (IFS). White circles in panel C correspond to functional zones of the face, hand, and lower part of the body. (B) Superficial oblique reconstruction represented on panel D. This type of reconstruction can be used with all neuronavigation systems (so-called "surgeon's eye" or "tool view" function indicated by the arrow on panel A). The potential location of functional areas of the motor cortex is represented in panel D by white circles.

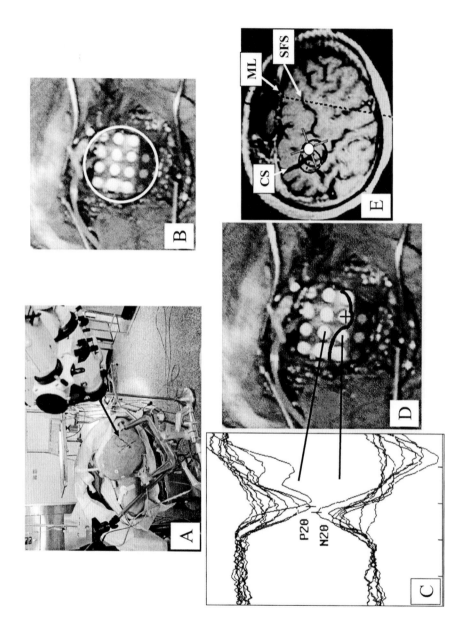

allowing recording of somatosensory evoked potentials (SEPs) as well as intraoperative MCS (Fig. 3).

INTRAOPERATIVE ELECTROPHYSIOLOGICAL TESTING

The first step of electrophysiological testing consists of confirming the position of the central sulcus detected by the neuronavigation system by recording SEPs. Theoretically, the polarity of the potentials recorded 20 ms after stimulation of the median nerve at the wrist is reversed across the central sulcus (N20/P20 phase shift). The zone of N20 potential recording is situated anteriorly to this sulcus and globally corresponds to the part of the motor cortex corresponding to representation of the hand. Potentials recorded after stimulation of the posterior tibial nerve or labial commissure are difficult to interpret and are consequently rarely used to identify the central sulcus. Fig. 3 shows the N20 and P20 waves recorded by the 16-plate diagnostic electrode applied to the dura mater. The good correlation between radiological and electrophysiological data can be easily verified in real time by using the pointer system or laser guidance beam of the neuronavigation system. In our experience, an excellent correlation has always been obtained between SEP data and the anatomical position of the central sulcus indicated by the neuronavigation system. In the case of severe deafferentation, SEPs may be difficult or even impossible to record. The absence of preoperative SEPs does not necessarily mean that they will be absent intraoperatively, because SEP recording from electrodes placed on the dura mater is more sensitive than scalp recording.

The second step consists of confirming the position of the motor cortex by stimulation. The objective of this step is to stimulate the contacts of the grid placed over the motor cortex to trigger muscle jerks in the zone corresponding to the pain. In the case of upper limb pain, those contacts providing the highest N20 potentials will be stimulated. For pain of the face and lower half of the body, contacts situated below or above this zone will be

---

← **Fig. 3.** Craniotomy and recording of somatosensory evoked potentials (SEPs). (A) The neuronavigation system ensures that the craniotomy (white circle on image B) is correctly centered over the target selected by imaging (black arrow). (B) A 16-plate electrode is placed on the dura mater. (C) SEPs are recorded by the 16-plate electrode after stimulation of the median nerve at the wrist. (D) The position of the electrodes at which the P20 (precentral) and N20 (postcentral) waves are recorded corresponds to the theoretical position of the central sulcus (black line). The good correspondence with the anatomical targeting (white circle on panel E) can be immediately verified during imaging (in this case MRI) by pointing (laser beam or cursor of neuronavigation system) to one of the plates (black cross) situated just anteriorly to the central sulcus (CS on panel E). ML: midline, SFS: superior frontal sulcus.

stimulated. The following stimulation parameters are generally used: pulse width: 1 ms, frequency: 16–20 Hz, intensity: 5–10 mA. The stimulation amplitude mainly varies according to the depth of general anesthesia and the distance between the dura mater and the cerebral cortex.

The site of the four-plate electrode for chronic stimulation depends on the results of the electrophysiological tests (SEPs and stimulation). The electrode is positioned perpendicularly in the direction of the central sulcus to ensure that at least one of the contacts is situated over the motor cortex, whose width varies considerably from one part of the central region to another. This positioning also allows verification of the potential analgesic efficacy of stimulation of the sensory cortex or premotor cortex. This electrode is sutured to the dura mater by two sutures. The electrode is connected to a lead wire that is tunneled out onto the skin to test the efficacy of stimulation for several days. In cases of patients presenting with pain in large areas of the body, two electrodes or a new type of electrode with eight contacts can be used. When the efficacy of stimulation has been confirmed, this temporary lead wire is replaced by a completely internalized lead wire connected to a pulse generator implanted subcutaneously, generally in the supraclavicular region.

STIMULATION PARAMETERS

Mean stimulation parameters based on our experience are as follows: frequency: 40 Hz (range: 25–55 Hz), pulse width: 82.4 µs (range: 60–180 µs), amplitude: 2.1 V (range: 1.3–4 V). Bipolar stimulation is used in most cases, with the negative pole overlying the motor cortex and the positive pole over the sensory cortex. Some teams (Tsubokawa et al. 1991; Meyerson et al. 1993; Mogilner and Rezai 2001) have obtained good results by using higher stimulation voltages, corresponding to about 70-80% of motor threshold values.

INDICATIONS AND OUTCOME

A review of the literature reveals two main indications for MCS: central pain and trigeminal neuropathic pain (Tsubokawa et al. 1991; Hosobuchi 1993; Meyerson et al. 1993; Canavero 1995, 1999; Herregodts et al. 1995; Migita et al. 1995; Peyron et al. 1995; Ebel et al. 1996; Nguyen et al. 1997; Rainov et al. 1997; Yamamoto et al. 1997; Garcia-Larrea et al. 1999; Mertens et al. 1999; Carroll et al. 2000; Franzini et al. 2000; Saitoh et al. 2000; Katayama et al. 2001; Mogilner and Rezai 2001; Pirotte et al. 2001; Roux et al. 2001a).

CENTRAL PAIN

Central pain, especially pain related to a thalamic lesion, theoretically constitutes the best indication for MCS. Moreover, Tsubokawa et al. (1991) developed this treatment modality specifically in order to treat this type of pain. In most cases published in the literature, pain is secondary to hemor-rhagic or ischemic stroke: 11 cases for Tsubokawa et al. (1993), 11 cases for Nguyen et al. (1999), 7 cases for Katayama et al. (1998), including 3 cases of Wallenberg syndrome, and 2 cases for Migita et al. (1995). Central pain can also be secondary to other causes: sequelae of head injury or thalamic abscess (Nguyen et al. 1999). The review of the literature indicates that 159 cases of central pain secondary to stroke have been published. It is difficult to analyze the results of these cases because the assessment criteria differ. When only very good results are considered (>50% reduction in pain intensity on the visual analogue scale [VAS]), the success rate is 52% (82/159 patients).

However, these results need to be modulated, as they do not take into account those patients who obtained a satisfactory improvement, without achieving a 50% improvement on the VAS. For example, in our series of 18 cases of central pain (Nguyen 2002), 7 (38.9%) obtained very marked im-provement (>60% improvement on the VAS), 8 (44.5%) obtained satisfac-tory improvement (40–60% improvement on the VAS), and 3 (16.6%) did not improve. The mean clinical follow-up was 46 months. More than 80% of patients declared that they were satisfied with the operation.

TRIGEMINAL NEUROPATHIC PAIN

Trigeminal neuropathic pain represents the second main indication. In most cases, pain is secondary to thermocoagulation of the trigeminal gan-glion (54.5%). In 36.3% of cases, pain is secondary to surgery to the maxil-lary sinus, posterior fossa or cavernous sinus (Nguyen et al. 1999).

Forty-five cases of trigeminal neuropathic pain have been reported in the literature. A very good improvement (>50% improvement on the VAS) was obtained in 33 patients (73%). These results also need to be modulated. In our series of 22 patients, 13 (59%) obtained very marked improvement, 5 (22.8%) obtained satisfactory improvement, and 4 did not improve (Nguyen 2002).

OUTCOME

Regardless of the method of evaluation used, the results obtained in the treatment of neuropathic facial pain are clearly better than those obtained in central pain. Katayama et al. (2001) showed that patients with central pain and a marked motor deficit have a significantly less favorable response to

MCS than other patients. In his series, Katayama observed that pain relief was satisfactory in 73% of patients who had mild or absent motor weakness. When there was moderate to severe motor weakness, MCS was of benefit in only 15% of the 13 patients ($P < 0.01$). When motor contractions could not be induced, only 9% of patients achieved pain relief. In our series, the mean (± SD) improvement on the VAS was 38.1% ± 8% in patients with motor weakness and 46.5% ± 9% in patients with no evidence of motor weakness. While similar to that reported by Katayama, the difference between the two groups was not significant in our series ($P = 0.53$).

Similarly, severe sensory deafferentation can also be considered to be a factor of poor prognosis. Drouot et al. (2002) measured non-nociceptive and nociceptive sensory thresholds in the painful area with the stimulator in the "off" and in the "on" position. All 13 patients who exhibited normal non-nociceptive thermal thresholds within the painful area benefited from MCS. Of the remaining 18 patients with altered thermal sensory thresholds, 8 patients nevertheless experienced good pain control with MCS. In these 8 "good responders," sensory thresholds were improved by switching MCS on. In contrast, the last 10 patients showed abnormal thermal thresholds that were not modified by switching MCS on, and they did not respond clinically to MCS. Therefore, "good responders" to MCS could be identified by the absence of alteration of non-nociceptive sensory modalities within the painful area, or by abnormal sensory thresholds that could be improved by MCS.

Repetitive transcranial magnetic stimulation (rTMS) of the motor cortex is a very useful tool for predicting the effect of stimulation by implanted electrodes (Lefaucheur et al. 2001a). We studied the effect of preoperative rTMS in seven patients with central pain (J.-P. Nguyen, unpublished data): three patients obtained a major analgesic effect, while the stimulation had no effect in the other four patients. All patients subsequently received MCS: the three patients benefited from rTMS were all improved by subsequent MCS (mean improvement on the VAS: 72% ± 14%) and the four patients who did not benefit from rTMS did not improve postoperatively (mean improvement on the VAS: 32.2% ± 11%). Although the difference was not significant ($P = 0.07$), these results confirm those reported in the literature (Lefaucheur et al. 2001b; Drouot et al. 2002).

OTHER INDICATIONS

Other indications for MCS are deafferentation pain of the upper limbs, lower limbs, or trunk. This type of pain can theoretically be improved by cervical or thoracic spinal cord stimulation, and MCS is generally only considered when these techniques have failed.

Several authors have demonstrated the efficacy of MCS in the treatment of *phantom limb pain*. However, discordant results have been reported. Overall (19 cases published in the literature), very good results were obtained in about 53% of patients. The results were less favorable in Katayama's series (Katayama et al. 2001), as only 20% patients were improved. According to this author, thalamic stimulation (nucleus ventralis caudalis) was more effective, accounting for 60% of the good results. Somatotopic modifications could account for these disappointing results of MCS. Functional MRI would theoretically be able to identify these changes and may explain the much better results obtained by Sol (2001).

Pain related to *brachial plexus injury* can also be treated by MCS. Results of the 18 cases published are relatively disappointing, as only 44% of patients improved. As in phantom limb pain, fMRI could be useful to detect somatotopic modifications, which may be considerable in the case of complete sensorimotor deficit. In this case, the absence of SEPs and the motor effect of cortical stimulation make target mapping considerably more difficult.

Similar problems are encountered in patients with pain related to complete *paraplegia or quadriplegia*. Curiously, the published results appear to be much better (seven out of eight patients improved). In all of these cases, treatment was designed to relieve pain below the lesion. Unilateral MCS has been shown to be effective even in the case of bilateral pain (Nguyen et al. 1999).

Only five cases have been published in which pain related to a *peripheral nerve lesion* was treated with MCS. Four of these five patients markedly improved. Some of these patients presented with nerve root or nerve trunk pain related to multi-operated neurofibromas in the context of von Recklinghausen disease (Nguyen et al. 1999; Smith et al. 2001). One case of intercostal postherpetic neuralgia responded favorably to MCS (Nguyen et al. 1999).

ADVERSE EFFECTS

Globally, 11.4% of published cases experienced an adverse effect. The most serious cases represent 3.6% of all cases: epidural or subdural hematoma (2.2%), epileptic seizures (0.7%) and speech disorders (0.7%). The low incidence of epileptic seizures during chronic stimulation shows that stimulation of the cortex through the dura with reasonable intensity is safe (Bezard et al. 1999). Skin ulceration and infection were reported in 0.7 and 2.2% of published cases, respectively.

MECHANISM OF ACTION OF MOTOR CORTEX STIMULATION

The mechanism of action of MCS has not been fully elucidated. In his first publications, Tsubokawa proposed the hypothesis that MCS antidromically activated neurons of the sensory cortex (Tsubokawa et al. 1993), allowing descending impulses to activate structures inhibiting the abnormal thalamic hyperactivity secondary to the deafferentation phenomenon. However, several results tend to refute this hypothesis, including clinical improvement after MCS of some patients with infarction of the postcentral region and the absence of modification of cerebral blood flow in the postcentral region on positron emission tomography (PET) scan during MCS (Garcia-Larrea et al. 1999).

In contrast, these studies showed that the most marked changes in regional blood flow in response to MCS mainly concerned the nucleus ventralis lateralis and the nucleus ventralis anterior of the thalamus. These structures are directly connected to the motor cortex, and direct activation of these nuclei can explain the effects of MCS on motor disorders, including improvement of spasticity (Garcia-Larrea et al. 1999) or tremor (Nguyen et al. 1998). The role of these structures in the analgesic effect is more difficult to explain. MCS also induces changes in blood flow in other structures more directly involved in pain mechanisms, especially the midline thalamic nuclei, anterior cingulate gyrus, insula, and the upper part of the brainstem (Garcia-Larrea et al. 1999). The role of the anterior cingulate gyrus and insula in pain mechanisms and their relations with the midline thalamic nuclei have been clearly established. Connections between these cortical regions and anterior thalamic nuclei have also been demonstrated (Garcia-Larrea et al. 1999).

It is now fairly well established that the analgesic effect of MCS depends on the zone of motor cortex stimulated. It is therefore essential to take the somatotopic organization of the cortex into account, because our studies (Nguyen et al. 1999) have demonstrated that the sites of stimulation effective against pain correspond to the sites at which intraoperative stimulation triggers motor responses (Fig. 4). MCS clearly stimulates the motor cortex as a whole, including the primary motor area (area 4) but also the premotor area (area 6). The results of MCS on phantom limb pain showed that somatotopic modifications must also be taken into account; such modifications can be demonstrated by fMRI and/or rTMS. Activation of inhibitory descending structures (especially anterior thalamic nuclei) may only be effective when the somatotopic organization of the motor cortex is taken into account. The direct action of the pyramidal tract on the posterior horn of the spinal cord certainly plays a major role in the analgesic effects of MCS (Coulter et al. 1974).

The specific structures activated by MCS also need to be defined: which layer of the cortex is involved, are cell bodies or axons activated, and are the pathways tangential or perpendicular to the cortical surface? Answers to these questions would probably allow more precise definition of stimulation parameters, which are currently only empirical. The difficulty of adjusting stimulation parameters is mainly due to the latency of the analgesic effect, as the effect of an adjustment can often only be determined on the following day or even several days after the procedure. In rare cases, the analgesic effect has been obtained within minutes following the start of stimulation. In these patients, the best effect was obtained with a relatively low stimulation amplitude, about 2 mA (2 V for an impedance of 1000 Ω) at a frequency of about 40 Hz, with a pulse width of 60 μs.

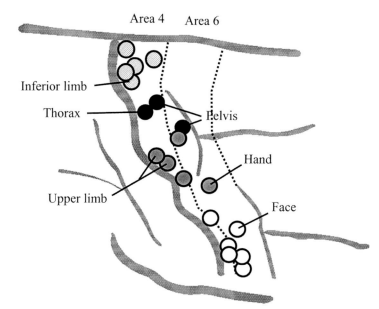

Fig. 4. Correlations between anatomical targeting and analgesic effects (19 patients obtaining an excellent or good analgesic result). White circles: region of the face. Gray circles: region of the upper limb. Black circles: pelvic region. Hatched circles: region of the lower limb. Vertical dotted lines indicate the theoretical position of the motor and premotor cortex. An analgesic effect on intercostal deafferentation pain was obtained by chronic stimulation of a zone situated between the level of the superior frontal sulcus and the midline. Several effective stimulation sites are situated in the premotor region. Improvement of pain in the inferior limb (including the foot) was obtained by stimulating contacts situated at the upper part of the cerebral convexity.

CONCLUSIONS

Motor cortex stimulation, recommended by Tsubokawa, is a promising treatment modality for deafferentation pain. It is essentially indicated for the treatment of pain that cannot be controlled by spinal cord stimulation: central pain and neuropathic facial pain. Optimal selection of the best indications must be based on a technique that precisely identifies the zone to be stimulated. A relatively large craniotomy and the use of a neuronavigation system appear to be essential. Other indications need to be confirmed, especially paraplegic pain, phantom limb pain, and plexus injury pain. In the field of phantom limb pain, the results show that thalamic stimulation should be also considered as a therapeutic option. The more systematic use of fMRI and transcranial magnetic stimulation will probably contribute to a broader range of indications for MCS. We also need to improve our understanding of the mechanisms of action of MCS.

REFERENCES

Bezard E, Boraud T, Nguyen JP, et al. Cortical stimulation and epileptic seizure: a study of the potential risk in primates. *Neurosurgery* 1999; 45:346–350.

Canavero S. Cortical stimulation for central pain. *J Neurosurg* 1995; 83:1117.

Canavero S, Bonicalzi V, Castellano G, Perozzo P, Massa-Micon B. Painful supernumerary phantom arm following motor cortex stimulation for central poststroke pain. *J Neurosurg* 1999; 91:121–123.

Carroll D, Joint C, Maartens N, et al. Motor cortex stimulation for chronic neuropathic pain: a preliminary study of 10 cases. *Pain* 2000; 84:431–437.

Coulter JD, Maunz RA, Willis WD. Effects of stimulation of sensorimotor cortex on primate spinothalamic neurons. *Brain Res* 1974; 64:351–356.

Drouot X, Nguyen JP, Peschanski M, Lefaucheur JP. The antalgic efficacy of chronic motor cortex stimulation is related to sensory changes in the painful zone. *Brain* 2002; 125:1660–1664.

Ebel H, Rust D, Tronnier V, Böker D, Kunze S. Chronic precentral stimulation in trigeminal neuropathic pain. *Acta Neurochir* 1996; 138:1300–1306.

Franzini A, Ferroli P, Servello D, Broggi G. Reversal of thalamic hand syndrome by long-term motor cortex stimulation. *J Neurosurg* 2000; 93:873–875.

Garcia-Larrea L, Peyron R, Mertens P, et al. Electrical stimulation of motor cortex for pain control: a combined PET-scan and electrophysiological study. *Pain* 1999; 83:259–273.

Herregodts P, Stadnik T, De Ridder F, D'Haens J. Cortical stimulation for central neuropathic pain: 3-D surface MRI for easy determination of the motor cortex. *Acta Neurochir Suppl* 1995; 64:132–135.

Hosobuchi Y. Motor cortical stimulation for control of central deafferentation pain. In: Devinsky O, Beric A, Dogari M (Eds). *Electrical and Magnetic Stimulation of the Brain and Spinal Cord*. New York: Raven Press, 1993, pp 215–217.

Katayama Y, Fukaya C, Yamamoto T. Poststroke pain control by chronic motor cortex stimulation: neurological characteristics predicting a favorable response. *J Neurosurg* 1998; 89:585–591.

Katayama Y, Yamamoto T, Kobayashi K, et al. Motor cortex stimulation for phantom limb pain: a comprehensive therapy with spinal cord and thalamic stimulation. *Stereotact Funct Neurosurg* 2001; 77:159–161.

Lee U, Bastos AC, Alonso-Vanegas MA, Morris R, Olivier A. Topographic analysis of the gyral patterns of the central area. *Stereotact Funct Neurosurg* 1998; 70:38–51.

Lefaucheur JP, Drouot X, Keravel Y, Nguyen JP. Pain relief induced by repetitive transcranial magnetic stimulation of precentral cortex. *Neuroreport* 2001a; 12:1–3.

Lefaucheur JP, Drouot X, Nguyen JP. Interventional neurophysiology for pain control: duration of pain relief following repetitive transcranial magnetic stimulation of the motor cortex. *Neurophysiol Clin* 2001b; 31:247–252.

Linderoth B, Meyerson BA. Central nervous system stimulation for neuropathic pain. In: Hansson PT, Fields HL, Hill RG, Marchettini P (Eds). *Neuropathic Pain: Pathophysiology and Treatment,* Progress in Pain Research and Management, Vol. 21. Seattle: IASP Press, 2001, pp 223–249.

McCarthy G, Allison T, Spencer DD. Localization of the face area of human sensorimotor cortex by intracranial recording of somatosensory evoked potentials. *J Neurosurg* 1993; 79:874–884.

Mertens P, Nuti C, Sindou M, et al. Precentral cortex stimulation for the treatment of central neuropathic pain. *Stereotact Funct Neurosurg* 1999; 73:122–125.

Meyerson BA, Lindblom U, Lind G, Herregodts P. Motor cortex stimulation as treatment of trigeminal neuropathic pain. *Acta Neurochir Suppl* 1993; 58:150–153.

Migita K, Tohru U, Kazunori A, Shuji M. Transcranial magnetic coil stimulation in patients with central pain: technique and application. *Neurosurgery* 1995; 36:1037–1040.

Mogilner AY, Rezai AR. Epidural motor cortex stimulation with functional imaging guidance. *Neurosurg Focus* 2001; 11:Article 4.

Nguyen JP. Motor cortex stimulation. *Abstracts: 10th World Congress on Pain.* Seattle: IASP Press, 2002, p 119.

Nguyen JP, Keravel Y, Feve A, et al. Treatment of deafferentation pain by chronic stimulation of the motor cortex: report of a series of 20 cases. *Acta Neurochir Suppl* 1997; 68:54–60.

Nguyen JP, Pollin B, Fève A, Geny C, Cesaro P. Improvement of action tremor by chronic cortical stimulation. *Mov Disord* 1998; 13:84–88.

Nguyen JP, Lefaucheur JP, Decq P, et al. Chronic motor cortex stimulation in the treatment of central and neuropathic pain: correlations between clinical, electrophysiological and anatomical data. *Pain* 1999; 82:245–251.

Penfield W, Rasmussen T. *The Cerebral Cortex of Man: A Clinical Study of Localization of Function.* New York: MacMillan, 1950.

Peyron R, Garcia-Larrea L, Deiber MP, et al. Electrical stimulation of precentral cortical area in the treatment of central pain: electrophysiological and PET study. *Pain* 1995; 62:275–286.

Pirotte B, Voordecker P, Joffroy F, et al. The Zeiss-MKM system for frameless image-guides approach in epidural motor cortex stimulation for central neuropathic pain. *Neurosurg Focus* 2001; 11:Article 3.

Rainov NG, Fels C, Heidecke V, Burkert W. Epidural electrical stimulation of the motor cortex in patients with facial neuralgia. *Clin Neurol Neurosurg* 1997; 99:205–209.

Rao SM, Binder JR, Hammeke TA, et al. Somatotopic mapping of the human primary motor cortex with functional magnetic resonance imaging. *Neurology* 1995; 45:919–924.

Roux FE, Ibarrola D, Lazorthes Y, Berry I. Chronic motor cortex stimulation for phantom limb pain: a functional magnetic resonance imaging study: technical case report. *Neurosurgery* 2001a; 48:681–688.

Roux FE, Ibarrola D, Tremoulet M, et al. Methodological and technical issues for integrating functional magnetic resonance imaging data in a neuronavigation system. *Neurosurgery* 2001b; 49:1145–1157.

Saitoh Y, Shibata M, Hirano SI, et al. Motor cortex stimulation for central and peripheral deafferentation pain. *J Neurosurg* 2000; 92:150–155.

Saitoh Y, Hirano SI, Kato A, et al. Motor cortex stimulation for deafferentation pain. *Neurosurg Focus* 2001; 11:Article 1.

Smith H, Joint C, Schlugman D, et al. Motor cortex stimulation for neuropathic pain. *Neurosurg Focus* 2001; 11:Article 2.

Sol JC, Casaux J, Roux FE, et al. Chronic motor cortex stimulation for phantom limb pain: correlations between pain relief and functional imaging studies. *Stereotact Funct Neurosurg* 2001; 77:172–176.

Tsubokawa T, Katayama Y, Yamamoto T, Hirayama T, Koyama S. Chronic motor cortex stimulation for the treatment of central pain. *Acta Neurochir* 1991; (Suppl 52):137–139.

Tsubokawa T, Katayama Y, Yamamoto T, Hirayama T, Koyama S. Chronic motor cortex stimulation in patients with thalamic pain. *J Neurosurg* 1993; 78:393–401.

Woolsey CN, Erickson TC, Gilson WE. Localization in somatic sensory and motor areas of human cerebral cortex as determined by direct recording of evoked potentials and electrical stimulation. *J Neurosurg* 1979; 51:476–506.

Yamamoto T, Katayama Y, Hirayama T, Tsubokawa T. Pharmacological classification of central post-stroke pain: comparison with the results of chronic motor cortex stimulation therapy. *Pain* 1997; 72:5–12.

Correspondence to: Jean Paul Nguyen, MD, Department of Neurosciences, INSERM U-421, CHU Henri Mondor, Créteil 94000, France.

The Pain System in Normal and Pathological States:
A Primer for Clinicians, Progress in Pain Research
and Management, Vol. 31, edited by Luis Villanueva,
Anthony Dickenson, and Hélène Ollat, IASP Press,
Seattle, © 2004.

19

Pain Matters: A Clinical Viewpoint

Henry J. McQuay

Pain Relief Unit, Churchill Hospital,
University of Oxford, Oxford, United Kingdom

MECHANISMS AND CONDITIONS

The mechanistic approach to pain is fashionable because it offers a useful theoretical basis and a cogent rationale for laboratory work. From the clinical standpoint there are shortcomings to an exclusively mechanistic approach, however. The column headings of the timing and mechanism matrix in Table I use nociceptive, neuropathic (peripheral and central), visceral, and combined as the mechanistic divisions. Even these broad distinctions present a pragmatic problem. The same drugs provide pain relief in nociceptive and visceral pain, with little hard evidence of any distinction in efficacy. The same drugs provide pain relief in peripheral and central neuropathic pain, again with little hard evidence of any distinction in efficacy. Thus, beyond the use of different drugs in neuropathic and nociceptive pain, we have little clinical evidence to support pharmacologically distinguishable mechanisms.

The row headings of the matrix are about the timing of the pain, about its duration and its frequency. The striking distinction for the clinician is the disparity between the duration of laboratory pain studies and the clinical setting. In fact, the clinician's acute pain is the scientists' chronic pain. This difference emphasizes the chronological difficulty in extrapolating from bench studies to the clinic, which adds to the other difficulties for the clinician in interpreting inflammatory and neuropathic models in the laboratory. This problem is reflected in the general dissatisfaction with bench models of pain states: "inflammatory" to the clinician describes the process involved in joint disease, but in the laboratory, where studies of long duration are problematic from an ethical standpoint, it sometimes seems to be a synonym for what clinicians might call acute pain.

Table I
Pain conditions by time and by mechanism

Time Frame	Nociceptive	Neuropathic		Visceral	Combined
		Peripheral	Central		
Acute	Postoperative pain, burns, sprains, strains			"Stone" pain, ulcer	
Inter-mittent or inciden-tal	Headache, migraine, osteoarthritis	Trigeminal neuralgia		Dysmenor-rhea, endo-metriosis, pelvic pain, irritable bowel syndrome, dyspepsia	Cancer
Chronic	Low back pain, rheuma-toid arthritis, osteoarthritis, fibromyalgia, myofascial pain	Post-herpetic neuralgia, diabetic neuropathy, nerve trauma	Spinal cord injury pain, poststroke pain, multiple sclerosis, Parkinson's	Pelvic pain	Cancer, low back pain with radiculo-pathy, whiplash

INCIDENCE AND PREVALENCE

Sometimes it appears that we focus on rare complaints rather than common ones, and at a time of diminishing research resources this can mean that we study only rare complaints and ignore the common. Fig. 1 shows the estimated prevalence for some common and some rarer pain complaints. This is not an argument for studying the common to the exclusion of the rare, but it is a plea not to exclude the common when studying the rare. Chronic pain, pain lasting 6 months or more, is reported by one in five people, rising to one in three for those over 67 years of age (Elliott et al. 1999; Eriksen et al. 2003). Most of those with chronic pain have suffered with it for more than 2 years. Musculoskeletal problems were the most prevalent chronic pain conditions in both the Danish and the Grampian surveys, and in the Grampian survey (Elliot et al. 1999) the two most common reasons for chronic pain were back pain, which varied little with age; and arthritis, which rose dramatically with age to affect a quarter of people who were over 60 years old. People treat their pain with prescription medicine, over-the-counter medicine, and alternative remedies. In Denmark, 2% of those questioned were taking weak opioids, defined as codeine or tramadol, and 1% were taking strong opioids, defined as opioids other than codeine or

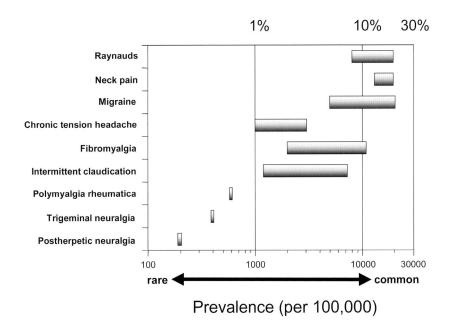

Fig. 1. Prevalence of some pain conditions. Data from McQuay et al. (in press).

tramadol (Eriksen et al. 2003). Of the 1,800 people reporting chronic pain, 9% were taking weak opioids and 3% strong opioids.

DISEASE BURDEN AND THE AGING POPULATION

In clinical pain studies we are ever more aware of looking at function as well as at pain intensity. Effective analgesia may enable the patient to be more active but may titrate to the same level of pain. If we do not measure the function then we miss the fact that the intervention is indeed making a difference. Analgesia will not reverse disability, but it may decrease the burden of the disease. Our estimates of this burden remain crude, but Elliott et al. (1999) showed that about a third of people reporting chronic pain were moderately or severely limited by their pain.

Sprangers et al. (2000) investigated this burden in a different way, by looking at scores on the Medical Outcomes Study Short Form 36 (SF-36) for people with a variety of different diseases. Surprising to me was that musculoskeletal disease was rated the most burdensome, worse than perhaps more obvious candidates such as cardiovascular or respiratory disease. The importance of this finding for pain clinicians is that with aging populations, musculoskeletal disease will become more prevalent. Treating their pain will be challenging, because older people have other diseases for which they take multiple medications. Effective and tolerable treatments in younger populations may be contraindicated or intolerable in older patients.

CHRONICITY

The importance of surgical procedures as a cause of chronic pain received further substantiation from Perkins and Kehlet (2000). They showed (Fig. 2) that patients having common procedures have a substantial chance of having chronic pain one year later.

One obvious question is why only some patients have chronic pain after surgery and not all, because the same nerves will be subject to damage. With this order of incidence, surgery is clearly one of the most common causes of nerve damage pain, but it is underinvestigated.

TREATMENT CHOICE AND EVIDENCE

As with the pain epidemiology evidence above, we now have methods and more evidence than we did 10 years ago to compare treatment efficacy and adverse effects.

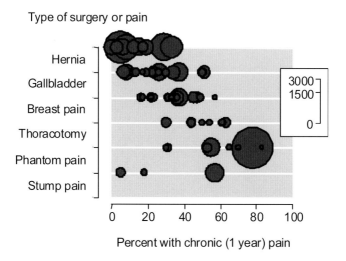

Fig. 2. Chronic pain after surgery. Data from Perkins and Kehlet (2000).

NON-OPIOID ANALGESICS

Using the information from single-dose randomized studies in postoperative pain, we can compare the efficacy of different analgesics in terms of the number needed to treat (NNT) for the outcome of at least 50% pain relief at 6 hours (Fig. 3). The lower the NNT, the more effective the drug.

This league table demonstrates the efficacy of nonsteroidal anti-inflammatory drugs (NSAIDs) as analgesics; single-dose oral opioids consistently perform relatively less well in these comparisons. The ranking is helpful for making decisions, and the methodology has revealed the benefits of combining opioid and non-opioid analgesics. This latter is important because individual small trials often fail to reveal the advantage of the combination over the component drugs, but the advantage is shown by meta-analysis. An additive effect of opioids and non-opioids is sufficient to justify clinical use when NSAIDs are contraindicated, but further work on the possibility of synergy would be helpful.

ANTIDEPRESSANTS AND ANTICONVULSANTS

The same meta-analytic techniques applied for anticonvulsants and antidepressants used to treat various forms of neuropathic pain show that effective drugs can produce NNTs of about 3 for 50% pain relief at 8 weeks

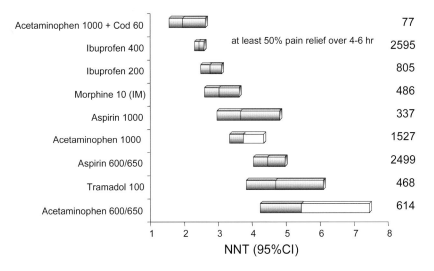

Fig. 3. Relative efficacy of selected analgesics for acute pain. Doses are in milligrams and are oral except for intramuscular morphine; numbers at right are numbers of patients given treatment. NNT = number needed to treat for the outcome of at least 50% pain relief at 6 hours. Data from Moore et al. (2003).

(Moore et al. 2003). A problem with some of the newer trials is that they used an enriched enrollment type of study design, excluding patients who had not responded previously to the drug under test. This problem means that the NNTs reported in the trial, while valid for that trial, overestimate the efficacy of the treatment for the neuropathic pain population at large.

Perhaps the biggest obstacle to progress here is the poor reporting of adverse effects in the studies. Patients will not persist with effective treatments that have substantial adverse effects. If trials report only the frequency of the adverse effects and not their severity then we struggle to define what constitutes "substantial." With antidepressants and anticonvulsants at least one patient in 30 will have to stop the drug because of adverse effects, and one patient in three will report "minor" adverse effects. The trials do not report severity, so that although frequency of minor adverse effects with antidepressants and anticonvulsants is about one in three, we have no idea whether these are more less severe for the two drug classes.

MIGRAINE MEDICATIONS

For migraine the league table of relative efficacy (Fig. 4) shows the greater efficacy of the triptans over older drugs, the dose-response relationships for particular triptans, and the effects of route (Moore et al. 2003). Subcutaneous sumatriptan 6 mg has an NNT of about 3, compared with oral doses of 100 mg with an NNT in excess of 5.

WHERE TRIAL DESIGNS FAIL US

The meta-analytic approaches above are only possible when there are good clinical trials. Many interventions used in the pain world have not been, or cannot be, subjected to clinical trial. Invasive interventions (injections and surgery) are one category in which we lack good trials. While it is often difficult to devise and use control interventions for these treatments, it is not impossible. When we do have high-quality trials, for instance injections for facet joint or epidural steroid injections for the management of back pain, they tend to be negative (Carette et al. 1991, 1997).

For many of the alternative or complementary treatments where we do have evidence, that evidence is profoundly negative, meaning that the treatments do not have analgesic efficacy. They may still make patients feel better, which is laudable in itself, but they do not significantly change pain outcomes compared with controls. For other treatments the problem is a lack of evidence rather than evidence of lack of effect. The reasons why these unproven therapies often seem (to the uncritical) to work include the fact

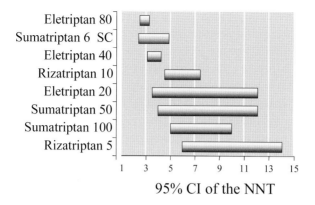

95% CI of the NNT

Fig. 4. Relative efficacy of triptans in migraine (sustained response over 24 hours). Data from Moore et al. (2003).

that many diseases are self-limiting or cyclical, the original diagnosis may be wrong, there may be mood improvement and a placebo effect, and the patients may have substantial psychological investment in the therapy.

Unfortunately, we still lack study designs that can help us to investigate packages of care, so it is difficult to untangle which are the beneficial components in a package of therapies. Cognitive-behavioral programs have proven benefit, but precisely which parts of the programs are the most important can be difficult to fathom. This is not to diminish the importance of psychology in pain management. Far from it, because much of what we do may facetiously be called psychiatry with needles. Thus is why study designs must be meticulous, to control for patients whose pain is really anxiety about the cause of their pain, or bitterness that they are the victim, people who are just happy being miserable or catastrophizing, or those whose expectations are hopelessly unrealistic. These "reality gaps" may be as simple as failing to acknowledge that even if the pain is relieved the disability will not improve and hence there may be no lessening of distress.

CARE PATHWAYS

A potentially fruitful way of looking at how and why we make decisions to change therapies in the management of particular pain conditions, the decision points in so-called care pathways, requires a new type of study architecture. Imagine that we had an algorithm to manage painful osteoarthritis. According to various guidelines, first-line treatment would be acetaminophen (paracetamol), followed, if analgesia were inadequate, by an

NSAID or coxib. We have little idea of the proportion of patients with painful osteoarthritis who would need to change from acetaminophen to an NSAID or coxib, and little idea of the proportion who would need to stop taking the NSAID or coxib because of adverse effects. The next treatment choice for patients with "acetaminophen-inadequate-analgesia" or who are "NSAID or coxib intolerant" may involve combination analgesics or even opioids.

Studying by treatment option within condition, as in the example above, is important, in acute as well as chronic pain, and the example shows how information on adverse effects, as well as on relative efficacy, is needed for clinical decision making. We have the raw rankings for relative efficacy of drug interventions across conditions, but we now need rankings of efficacy and tolerability within a condition, because that is the relevant clinical framework. In acute pain we need comparisons of the various pain treatments for pain after joint replacement, or, in neuropathic chronic pain, head-to-head comparisons of antidepressants and anticonvulsants.

It is perhaps from this type of comparison that we would gain information that is most directly applicable to the clinical context. An example would be the management of a 79-year-old woman suffering from rheumatoid arthritis and with widespread pains. She cannot take NSAIDs or coxibs because of gastrointestinal problems, she finds acetaminophen insufficient, even when combined with an opioid, and she is anticoagulated because of atrial fibrillation, precluding injections. Options are then severely limited, and by default optimal management may require strong opioids, a decision that remains controversial in noncancer pain.

Effective treatments cause adverse effects, and I have already stressed the problem of poor reporting of adverse effects in trials, even though that information was often gathered. The within-condition treatment comparisons proposed above will require strict attention to adverse effect reporting if they are to be useful.

DISCONNECTION BETWEEN BENCH AND CLINIC

Over the past decade clinicians have been dismayed by the failure of a number of promising ideas from basic research to produce clinical benefit. This is not an argument against basic research, but a signal perhaps that divorcing clinical and basic research can lead us down blind alleys. An example is preemptive analgesia, where a huge amount of clinical trial time and effort has failed to reveal any worthwhile benefit from giving the treatment before the pain as opposed to after pain onset. Again, this is not an argument that analgesia should be "withheld," or not given before the onset of pain, but rather that the timing confers no measurable advantage.

The fact that pain science is complicated, and is becoming more so, underlines the importance of basic and clinical interaction. Interdisciplinary collaboration is necessary to resolve the current debate about the mechanistic approach, where pragmatic clinicians know that the same drugs work, for instance antidepressants and anticonvulsants in neuropathic pain, independent of the underlying mechanism. Clinical trials that would show differential efficacy in conditions with different underlying mechanisms could illuminate this area. The danger is that the clinicians cannot keep up with the "peptide du jour" phenomenon and cannot see how that peptide fits into the overall picture. The clinician and the scientist then drift ever further apart.

Clinical pain research needs to be able to study packages of care, as well as to be able to study the efficacy of single interventions. Just as basic researchers need fresh thought about how to study neuropathic pain, clinicians need a methodology that will allow us to compare different packages of care, each with a raft of different interventions. Exciting times.

ACKNOWLEDGMENTS

This volume honors the contribution of Jean-Marie Besson to the study of pain. He has championed an open approach in which basic scientists and clinicians go forward together, the antithesis of a divided culture. Let us hope that we can follow in the footsteps of his huge achievement.

REFERENCES

Carette S, Marcoux S, Truchon R, et al. A controlled trial of corticosteroid injections into facet joints for chronic low back pain. *N Engl J Med* 1991; 325:1002–1007.

Carette S, Leclaire R, Marcoux S, et al. Epidural corticosteroid injections for sciatica due to herniated nucleus pulposus. *N Engl J Med* 1997; 336:1634–1640.

Elliott AM, Smith BH, Penny KI, Smith WC, Chambers WA. The epidemiology of chronic pain in the community. *Lancet* 1999; 354:1248–1252.

Eriksen J, Jensen MK, Sjogren P, Ekholm O, Rasmussen NK. Epidemiology of chronic non-malignant pain in Denmark. *Pain* 2003; 106:221–228.

McQuay HJ, Smith LA, Moore RA. Chronic non-malignant pain. In: Stevens A (Ed). *Health Care Needs,* in press.

Moore A, Edwards J, Barden J, McQuay H. *Bandolier's Little Book of Pain.* Oxford: Oxford University Press, 2003.

Perkins FM, Kehlet H. Chronic pain as an outcome of surgery. *Anesthesiology* 2000; 93:1123–1133.

Sprangers MAG, de Regt EB, Andries F, et al. Which chronic conditions are associated with better or poorer quality of life? *J Clin Epidemiol* 2000; 53:895–907.

Correspondence to: Henry J. McQuay, DM, Pain Relief Unit, Churchill Hospital, Headington, Oxford OX3 7LJ, United Kingdom. Email: henry.mcquay@balliol.ox.ac.uk.

Index

Progress in Pain Research and Management Series